Immediate Molar Implants

Dedication

Writing this book during a pandemic was a major challenge for us and our contributors, but we persisted. And what allowed us to remain optimistic was having the opportunity to interact with the very bright and talented graduate periodontic residents in both of our departments. It continues to be a humbling experience to interact with these outstanding young men and women, and it is to them that we dedicate this book.

Douglas Deporter & Mohammad Ketabi

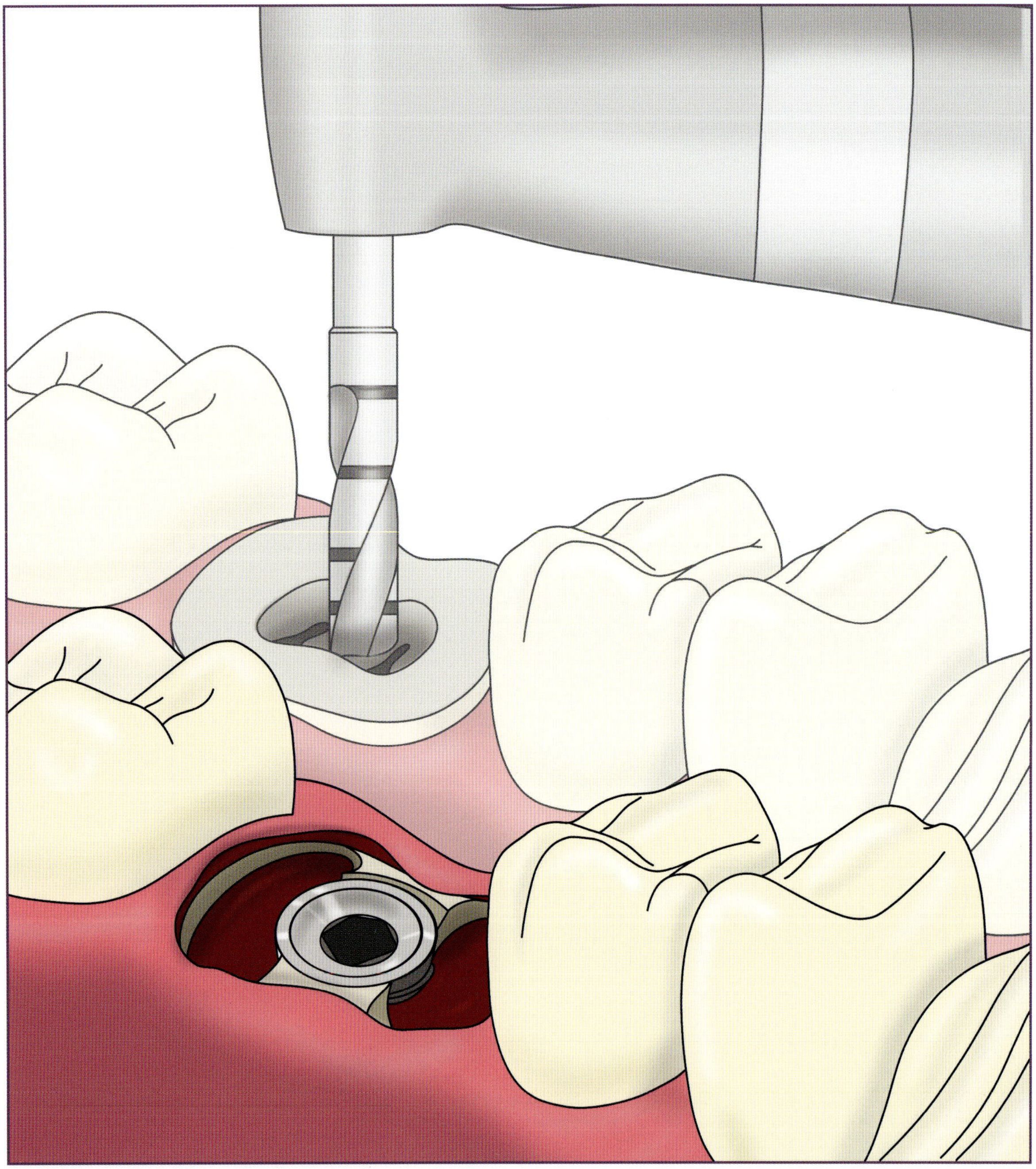

IMMEDIATE MOLAR IMPLANTS

Edited by

Douglas Deporter, DDS, Dipl Perio, PhD

Professor
Discipline of Periodontology and Oral Reconstruction Center
Faculty of Dentistry
University of Toronto
Toronto, Canada

Mohammad Ketabi, BDS, DDS, MDS

Professor
Department of Periodontology and Implant Dentistry
Faculty of Dentistry
Islamic Azad University, Isfahan Branch
Isfahan, Iran

Adjunct Professor
Faculty of Dentistry
University of Toronto
Toronto, Canada

QUINTESSENCE PUBLISHING

Berlin | Chicago | Tokyo
Barcelona | London | Milan | Mexico City | Paris | Prague | Seoul | Warsaw
Beijing | Istanbul | Sao Paulo | Zagreb

Library of Congress Cataloging-in-Publication Data

Names: Deporter, Douglas, editor. | Ketabi, Mohammad, editor.
Title: Immediate molar implants / edited by Douglas Deporter, Mohammad Ketabi.
Description: Batavia, IL : Quintessence Publishing Co, Inc, [2022] | Includes bibliographical references and index. | Summary: "This book systematically describes the current best practices for immediate implant placement in molar sites, including careful case selection, implant types, placement protocols, and adjunctive procedures to ensure implant success"-- Provided by publisher.
Identifiers: LCCN 2022017464 (print) | LCCN 2022017465 (ebook) | ISBN 9780867159547 (hardcover) | ISBN 9780867159813 (ebook)
Subjects: MESH: Immediate Dental Implant Loading | Molar | Dental Implants
Classification: LCC RK667.I45 (print) | LCC RK667.I45 (ebook) | NLM WU 640 | DDC 617.6/93--dc23/eng/20220801
LC record available at https://lccn.loc.gov/2022017464
LC ebook record available at https://lccn.loc.gov/2022017465

A CIP record for this book is available from the British Library.
ISBN: 978-0-86715-954-7

QUINTESSENCE PUBLISHING
USA

Quintessence Publishing Co, Inc
411 N Raddant Rd
Batavia, IL 60510
www.quintpub.com

5 4 3 2 1

Publishing Director: Bryn Grisham
Editor: Marieke Swerski
Design: Sue Zubek
Production: Sue Robinson

Printed in Croatia

CONTENTS

PREFACE

It is not that people lose their dreams because they've grown old—rather, they've grown old because they have lost their dreams.

My coeditor for this book, Mohammad Ketabi, reached out to me over a decade ago asking if he could visit with me on sabbatical for 6 months, and when he did come, we immediately felt simpatico working together. So comfortable in fact that he has spent similar academic visits every few years since then. On his last visit, he suggested that we undertake a systematic review on immediate molar implant (IMI) treatment, which we did and published in 2016.[1] A second paper outlining suggested guidelines for successful outcomes with IMIs followed in 2017.[2] Both of these publications generated enormous interest from others worldwide, so much so that we decided to undertake the current book project. Mohammad already had considerable experience using and teaching IMI methodology in Iran and elsewhere.

Make no mistake: Treating patients with IMIs is no romp in the park. Like the late luminary P-I Brånemark who conceived osseointegration as a medical breakthrough, those who pioneered the use of IMIs clearly knew the importance of dreaming and encouraged the rest of us to do so too. One by one, small modifications in technique have led to big gains for patients in less than a generation. However, the procedures using IMIs require careful planning, preferably with the assistance of cone beam computed tomography, considerable skill, and a good working knowledge of anatomy and bone biology. Feeling comfortable with doing localized, indirect sinus floor elevations as originally proposed by Robert Summers[3,4] is also a prerequisite with undertaking maxillary molar IMIs. And, of course, using minimally invasive surgery and knowing when and how to use particulate bone graft materials and barriers and/or to undertake immediate nonocclusal loading are also critical.

There is no one way to do immediate molar implantation, as will be seen in this book. Differences among experts do exist, and those experts who have contributed to this book have made this clear. However, all agree that a molar implant should be placed ideally into the tooth's interradicular septal bone and initially stabilized by contact with the buccal and linguopalatal buttresses of bone. Gaps should always be left buccally to avoid any contact with the buccal plate, especially if the latter is thin, and while gap grafting may not be essential, the clinician must know when grafting is necessary to avoid unwanted local buccolingual/palatal shrinkage of the alveolar ridge, leading to crestal bone loss, gingival recession, unfavorable soft tissue coloration, and eventually implant hardware exposure.

I personally have learned a great deal from interacting with the experts who contributed to this book, as I believe you will as well. All of them were forthcoming and generous in sharing their experiences and knowledge, and all are still undertaking pioneering work on a day-to-day basis. Let's keep the dream going strong!

References

1. Ketabi M, Deporter D, Atenafu EG. A systematic review of outcomes following immediate molar implant placement based on recently published studies. Clin Implant Dent Relat Res 2016; 18:1084–1094.
2. Deporter D, Ketabi M. Guidelines for optimizing outcomes with immediate molar implant placement. J Periodontal Implant Dent 2017;9:37–44.
3. Summers RB. The osteotome technique: Part 3—Less invasive methods of elevating the sinus floor. Compendium 1994;15: 698–710.
4. Summers RB. The osteotome technique: Part 4—Future site development. Compend Contin Educ Dent 1995;16:1090–1099.

ACKNOWLEDGMENTS

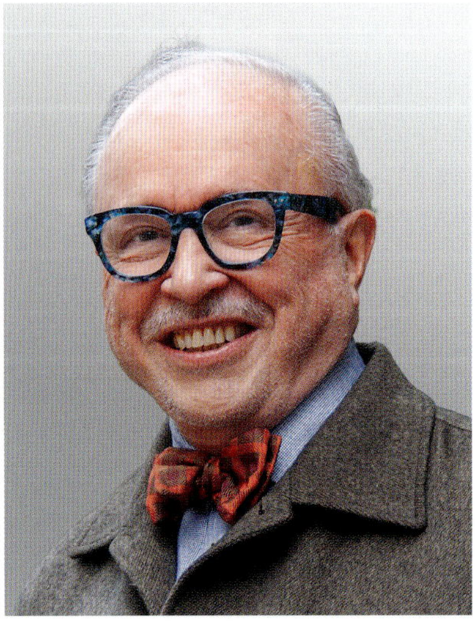

Compiling and editing a book for a highly regarded publisher like Quintessence is no small task, but their team made this second book with them a pleasant and rewarding experience. Despite delays due to COVID-19, the book Publishing Director, Bryn Grisham, was always supportive and understanding. In the end, this book project has kept me focused and (for the most part) sane during the coinciding unbelievably stressful pandemic that has interrupted all of our lives.

I also am truly grateful for the enthusiasm and support provided by our international group of contributors, each one a bright star helping us to unravel all the mysteries of immediate implant placement with or without immediate function. They have taken what seemed impossible and made it become reality. Everyone has been a privilege to work with, so generous with their knowledge and expertise and humble in their accomplishments. Thanks too to the graduate periodontic residents in our program at University of Toronto who were always keen to help, especially Drs Quang Nguyen and Ryan Noh. During the project, Ryan revealed that in addition to being a talented clinician, he is also a budding but already accomplished medical illustrator and offered his time and talent to do most of the illustrations in the book. The young people who we now receive in our training programs are truly gifted and a pleasure and honor to teach. I anticipate that many of them will contribute in a major way to the future of periodontics and implant dentistry.

Douglas Deporter

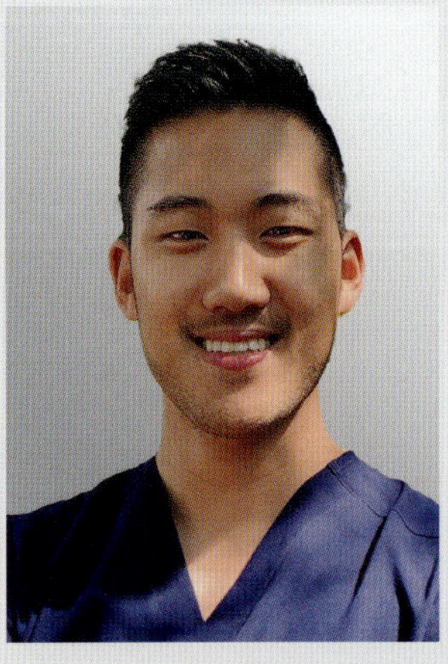

Special Thanks to Ryan Noh

Ryan Noh is currently enrolled in the Graduate Periodontic Program, Faculty of Dentistry, University of Toronto. Having been raised by parents who were both artists, he found a love of drawing at an early age. He worked selflessly and enthusiastically to create the majority of the artwork in this book, for which we are forever grateful. Hopefully, he learned a lot about immediate molar implants in the process.

During the past 20 years of my career as an academic, teacher, and practicing clinician, I have devoted much effort toward understanding, investigating, and applying the principles of implant dentistry. During this time, there have been so many changes and improvements in the field, but none more interesting and intellectually challenging for me and my colleagues and students than working toward the simplification and predictability of immediate molar implant (IMI) treatment.

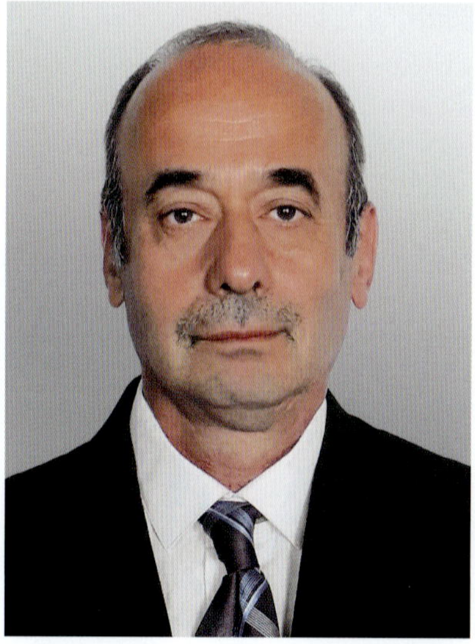

From a patient's point of view, immediate implantation of any condemned tooth is perceived to be the most desirable treatment approach, as it requires the least time and least number of surgical interventions. As has been reported in multiple recent literature reviews, IMIs can have high survival rates, at least in the hands of experienced clinicians using well-defined protocols, and this book was conceived to bring together many of these internationally respected and acclaimed experts to share their hard-earned knowledge in using IMIs successfully.

Firstly, I especially want to thank my dear mentor, Prof Ali Akbar Khoshkhounejad, for his ongoing astute advice and generosity in sharing his extensive experiences with IMIs. Seeing and discussing with him his many remarkable clinical accomplishments was always an encouragement to me in bringing this book to completion. I also would like to thank Prof Moeintaghavi, Dr Ayobian, and Dr Nadaf for their ongoing encouragement and support.

I must confess that much of the work and difficulties encountered with this book project over the last 3 years of necessity had to fall on the shoulders of my coeditor, Prof Douglas Deporter, without whose diligence, hard work, expertise, and international connections, the task would have been impossible. In fact, our scientific collaborations and stimulating conversations over the past two decades have been for me a real privilege, pleasure, and treasure.

I present this book to all students, practicing clinicians, and dental academics interested in learning to excel in dental implant treatments, but especially to all the young, talented, and enthusiastic periodontic residents who have studied with me at the Islamic Azad University Dental School (Isfahan Branch), where I spent nearly 25 years of my life in different administrative and academic positions.

Last but not least, I dedicate this book to my wonderful family, Saeedeh, Shiva, Sara, and Mahdi, for their continuous support, encouragement, and understanding.

Mohammad Ketabi

CONTRIBUTORS

Andrew Ackermann, BChD, MChD
Private Practice Limited to Prosthodontics
Johannesburg, South Africa

Tanatorn Asvaplungprohm, DDS
Implant Dentistry Resident
Department of Periodontology and Implant Dentistry
New York University College of Dentistry
New York, New York

Ehsan Birang, DDS, MS
Assistant Professor
Department of Periodontics
Faculty of Dentistry
Iran University of Medical Sciences
Tehran, Iran

Samvel Bleyan, DDS, MS
Practice Limited to Periodontics and Prosthodontics
Moscow, Russia

Sang-Choon Cho, DDS
Clinical Associate Professor
Director of Advanced Program for International Dentists in Implant Dentistry
Department of Periodontology and Implant Dentistry
New York University College of Dentistry
New York, New York

Shadi Daher, DMD
Clinical Assistant Professor
Department of Oral and Maxillofacial Surgery
Boston University School of Dental Medicine

Private Practice Limited to Oral and Maxillofacial Surgery
Boston, Massachusetts

Maziar Ebrahimi Dastgurdi, DDS, MS
Private Practice
Toronto, Ontario

Massimo Del Fabbro, MsC, PhD
Professor
Department of Biomedical, Surgical, and Dental Sciences
University of Milan
Milan, Italy

Douglas Deporter, DDS, Dipl Perio, PhD
Professor
Discipline of Periodontology and Oral Reconstruction Center
Faculty of Dentistry
University of Toronto
Toronto, Ontario

Vahid Esfahanian, DDS, MS
Associate Professor
Department of Periodontology and Implant Dentistry
Faculty of Dentistry
Islamic Azad University, Isfahan Branch
Isfahan, Iran

Nasim Farkhani, DDS, MS
Assistant Professor
Department of Periodontology and Implant Dentistry
Faculty of Dentistry
Islamic Azad University, Isfahan Branch
Isfahan, Iran

Marcello Ferrer, DMD, MS
National Director of Periodontics and Implantology
San Sebastián University

Private Practice in Esthetics, Periodontics, and Implantology
Santiago, Chile

Stuart J. Froum, DDS
Adjunct Clinical Professor
Director of Clinical Research
Department of Periodontology and Implant Dentistry
New York University College of Dentistry

Private Practice
New York, New York

Howard Gluckman, BDS, MChD, PhD
Private Practice in Oral Medicine and Periodontics
Director of the Implant and Aesthetic Academy
Cape Town, South Africa

Adjunct Assistant Professor
Department of Periodontics
University of Pennsylvania School of Dental Medicine
Philadelphia, Pennsylvania

Andre Hattingh, BChD, MChD
Private Practice Limited to Periodontics
Sevenoaks, United Kingdom

Salah Huwais, MChD
Private Practice Limited to Periodontics and Implantology
Jackson, Michigan

Adjunct Assistant Professor
Department of Periodontics
University of Pennsylvania School of Dental Medicine
Philadelphia, Pennsylvania

Adjunct Assistant Professor
Department of Periodontics
University of Illinois at Chicago College of Dentistry
Chicago, Illinois

Jaffer Kermalli, BsC, DDS, MsC
Clinical Instructor
Graduate Periodontics Program
Faculty of Dentistry
University of Toronto

Private Practice Limited to Periodontics
Toronto, Ontario

Mohammad Ketabi, BDS, DDS, MS
Professor
Department of Periodontology and Implant Dentistry
Faculty of Dentistry
Islamic Azad University, Isfahan Branch
Isfahan, Iran

Ali Akbar Khoshkhounejad, DDS, MSc
Professor
Department of Periodontology
Tehran University of Medical Sciences

Private Practice
Tehran, Iran

Nikfam Khoshkhounejad, DDS, MSc
Assistant Professor
Department of Prosthodontics
Tehran Universtiy of Medical Sciences
Tehran, Iran

Hyongsup Kimm, DDS
Implant Dentistry Resident
Department of Periodontology and Implant Dentistry
New York University College of Dentistry
New York, New York

Martin Leung, BDS
Implant Dentistry Resident
Department of Periodontology and Implant Dentistry
New York University College of Dentistry
New York, New York

Maryse Manasse, DMD, MEd
Clinical Assistant Professor
Department of Periodontology and Implant Dentistry
New York University College of Dentistry
New York, New York

Mauro Marincola, DDS, MSD
Professor and Clinical Director
Dental Implant Unit
Faculty of Dentistry
University of Cartagena
Cartagena, Colombia

Rodrigo Neiva, DDS, MS
Chair
Department of Periodontics
University of Pennsylvania School of Dental Medicine
Philadelphia, Pennsylvania

Sourav Panda, MDS
Doctoral Candidate
Department of Biomedical, Surgical, and Dental Sciences
University of Milan
Milan, Italy

Associate Professor
Institute of Dental Science and SUM Hospital
Siksha O Anusandhan University
Bhubaneswar, India

Klenise Paranhos, DDS, MS
Adjunct Clinical Assistant Professor
Department of Periodontology and Implant Dentistry
New York University College of Dentistry

Clinical Assistant Professor
Touro College of Dental Medicine
New York Medical College
New York, New York

Viraj Patel, BDS
Implant Dentistry Resident
Department of Periodontology and Implant Dentistry
New York University College of Dentistry
New York, New York

Adriano Piattelli, MD, DDS, DrHC, DrHC
Full Professor
School of Dentistry
Saint Camillus International University for Health Sciences
Rome, Italy

Azadeh Rahmati, DDS, MS
Private Practice Limited to Oral Maxillofacial Radiology
Lahijan, Iran

Charles Schwimer, DMD
Adjunct Professor
Department of Periodontics
University of Pennsylvania School of Dental Medicine
Philadelphia, Pennsylvania

Clinical Professor
Department of Periodontics
University of Pittsburgh School of Dental Medicine

Private Practice
Pittsburg, Pennsylvania

Miguel Simancas-Pallares, DDS, MS, MSc
Associate Professor
Division of Pediatric and Public Health
Adams School of Dentistry
University of North Carolina School of Dentistry
Chapel Hill, North Carolina

Richard Smith, DDS
Associate Clinical Professor
Department of Prosthodontics
Columbia University College of Dental Medicine

Private Practice
New York, New York

Dong-Seok Sohn, DDS, PhD
Professor and Chair
Department of Oral and Maxillofacial Surgery
Catholic University Hospital
Daegu, South Korea

Silvio Taschieri, MD, DDS
Academic Researcher
Department of Biomedical, Surgical, and Dental Sciences
University of Milan

Associate Professor
Department of Odontostomatology
IRCCS Orthopedic Institute Galeazzi
Milan, Italy

Professor
Department of Surgical Dentistry
First Moscow State Medical University
Moscow, Russia

Margherita Tumedei, DDS, PhD
Researcher
Department of Biomedical, Surgical, and Dental Sciences
University of Milan
Milan, Italy

Buddhapoom Wangsrimongkol, DDS
Implant Dentistry Resident
Department of Periodontology and Implant Dentistry
New York University College of Dentistry
New York, New York

Yung Cheng Paul Yu, DDS
Clinical Assistant Professor
Department of Periodontology and Implant Dentistry
New York University College of Dentistry
New York, New York

1

INTRODUCTION TO IMMEDIATE MOLAR TREATMENT OPTIONS

Douglas Deporter

The use of endosseous dental implants to replace missing or hopeless teeth has become routine practice in contemporary patient treatment. Indeed, implant-supported or implant-retained prostheses often are considered the treatment of first choice in both partial and complete edentulism because of their reported excellent long-term performance and patient satisfaction. Nevertheless, while treatment costs for a single implant-supported molar crown can be comparable to a three-unit, tooth-supported fixed partial denture, the longer treatment times and multiple interventions needed to complete the implant-based treatment do remain hurdles in gaining patient acceptance.[1,2] The original and well-tested principles of implant placement in healed extraction sites with a submerged initial healing interval continue to be used, and certainly molar replacement with single implants using this approach is reported to be predictably successful in the long term, particularly in the mandible and when natural teeth are present on either side of the implant.[3–8] However, the public is now aware of accelerated treatment approaches such as All-on-4 and "Teeth in a day" that provide immediate implant placement and immediate implant function. This awareness has fed the need to develop faster but equally successful treatment protocols for molar replacement. One such protocol is the replacement of condemned molar teeth using immediate implant placement with or without immediate function, and this book reviews the history, current status, technique prerequisites, and recent advances for this approach using a variety of implant types.

Timing of Implant Placement

Several classifications have been proposed to specify the timing of implant placement in relation to tooth extraction.[9–12] We have chosen the classification of Hämmerle et al,[11] which is based on the extent of both soft and hard

TABLE 1-1 Classification of timing of implant placement*

CLASSIFICATION	DEFINITION	ADVANTAGES	DISADVANTAGES
Type 1	Implant placement immediately following tooth extraction and as part of the same surgical procedure	• Reduced number of surgical procedures • Reduced overall treatment time • Optimal availability of existing bone	• Site morphology may complicate optimal placement and anchorage • Thin tissue biotype may compromise optimal outcome • Potential lack of keratinized mucosa for flap adaptation • Adjunctive surgical procedures may be required • Procedure is technique sensitive
Type 2	Complete soft tissue coverage of the socket (4–8 weeks)	• Increased soft tissue area and volume facilitates soft tissue flap management • Resolution of local pathology can be assessed	• Site morphology may complicate optimal placement and anchorage • Treatment time is increased • Socket walls exhibit varying amounts of resorption • Adjunctive surgical procedures may be required • Procedure is technique sensitive
Type 3	Substantial clinical and/or radiographic bone fill of the socket (12–16 weeks)	• Substantial bone fill of the socket facilitates implant placement • Mature soft tissues facilitate flap management	• Treatment time is increased • Adjunctive surgical procedures may be required • Socket walls exhibit varying amounts of resorption
Type 4	Healed site (> 16 weeks)	• Clinically healed ridge • Mature soft tissues facilitate flap management	• Treatment time is increased • Adjunctive surgical procedures may be required • Large variations are present in available bone volume

*Reprinted with permission from Hämmerle et al.[11]

tissue healing after tooth extraction. Hämmerle's type 1 sites are those where an implant is placed into a fresh extraction socket. Type 2 sites are referred to as *early* placement sites, ie, those where an implant is delayed until soft tissue closure over the extraction site has been achieved (typically 4 to 8 weeks). Type 3 sites are referred to as *delayed* implant placement sites, meaning those sites where substantial new bone formation has been allowed to happen before implant placement (typically 12 to 16 weeks). Finally, type 4 sites are those where the extraction sites have healed fully (ie, longer than 16 weeks), the tooth having been removed at some point in the distant past. The suggested advantages and disadvantages of the four types are summarized in Table 1-1.[11]

From the patient's point of view, type 1 implantation, ie, truly immediate, is the most desirable as it takes the least time and least number of surgical interventions to achieve. There are, however, technical challenges for the surgeon, such as avoiding bur chatter, controlling the final implant position, gaining sufficient primary stability, and maintaining and/or manipulating adequate soft tissue for appropriate site closure.[13] If the site has a thin gingival biotype preoperatively (ie, < 2-mm soft tissue thickness) and/or minimal keratinized gingival tissue (< 2-mm width), even if it is possible to stabilize an immediate molar implant (IMI), its health in the long term may be compromised because of an increased risk of peri-implant crestal bone loss needed to reestablish biologic width relative to implant type and placement depth.[14–20] Thus, van Eekeren et al[19] recently reported that gingival biotype had an impact on bone-level implant placement but not on tissue-level implant placement or when the implant-abutment connection was at least 2.5 mm above the crestal bone level. They suggested that when treating patients with initial mucosal thicknesses of 2 mm or less, choosing a tissue-level implant with the implant-abutment connection 2.5 mm above the crestal bone level for a posterior site (ie, esthetically less demanding) could help to minimize crestal bone loss. These considerations help to explain why IMIs are classified as being difficult and requiring considerable experience and ability of the surgeon.[21]

The decision to undertake early implantation (type 2, after 4 to 8 weeks of site healing) could be made for a variety of reasons, such as an existing acute local infection at extraction or a desire to permit some soft tissue healing and increases in amount and thickness of keratinized tissue before implant insertion. However, it needs to be remembered that some loss of alveolar ridge width and height will certainly have occurred, especially if a flap had been raised for the extraction, as most alveolar remodeling happens within the first 3 to 6 months postextraction.[22] Outcomes following early placement in various tooth sites can be comparable with those following immediate or delayed implant placement.[23,24] Early implant placement after a ridge preservation grafting procedure done at the time of extraction also may be a helpful protocol,[25] although it would add at least one extra surgical procedure. Most recently, however, it has been reported that early placement after extraction can give success rates similar to ridge preservation grafting and implant placement after 4 months of healing, at least at nonmolar sites.[26]

The benefits of waiting 12 to 16 weeks postextraction (type 3 sites) are that substantial new bone formation will have occurred within the socket and that the state of maturity of the gingival tissues will facilitate their manipulation. The disadvantages of this approach are again the loss in alveolar ridge dimensions, the longer treatment times, and the fact that additional surgical costs may be incurred. For example, it may become necessary to use commercial graft and barrier materials to thicken thin cortical bone buccally after osteotomy preparation, manage bony dehiscences, and/or regain local ridge anatomy to optimize patient comfort and prosthetic emergence profiles.

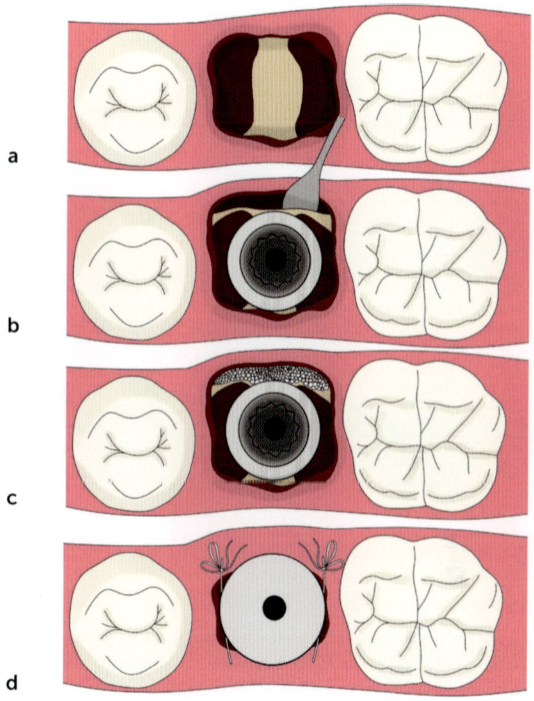

FIG 1-1 Buccal onlay grafting with xenograft can help to maintain alveolar ridge width. *(a)* Flapless surgery is used to remove a mandibular first molar revealing a type B interradicular septum (IRS) and an intact but thin (< 1.5 mm) buccal bone plate (see Box 1-1 for IRS classification). *(b)* A buccal full-thickness "pouch" was created using a small periosteal elevator. *(c)* Xenograft particles were packed into the pouch to reinforce the buccal bone. *(d)* The soft tissues were stabilized with sutures after placing a wide-diameter healing abutment.

Rationale and Early Work with IMIs

One of the original goals with immediate implant placement was that it would avoid or at least minimize the rapid alveolar ridge shrinkage that occurs both vertically and horizontally during normal extraction site healing. The greatest loss in alveolar ridge dimensions happens within the first 3 months postextraction, and by 1 year, buccolingual or buccopalatal ridge width shrinkage can be as high as 50%.[22,27] Worse still is the fact that the greatest loss in width happens midbuccally at the extraction socket, ie, exactly where the clinician wishes to locate an implant.[28] Looking at available human data, however, while losses in alveolar dimension can be reduced following immediate implant placement, they cannot be eliminated because many factors contribute to the losses.[29–33] Even when marginal bone gaps around immediate implants placed in molar extraction sites completely fill with new bone, resorption will still be seen on the external aspects of the associated ridge, particularly on the buccal.[29,34,35] Nevertheless, appropriate clinical management such as buccal particulate bone onlay/contour grafting can compensate for this thinning of buccal bone, provided that all socket walls remain intact following IMI placement[36,37] (Fig 1-1). If, as commonly happens, the buccal bony wall is missing or

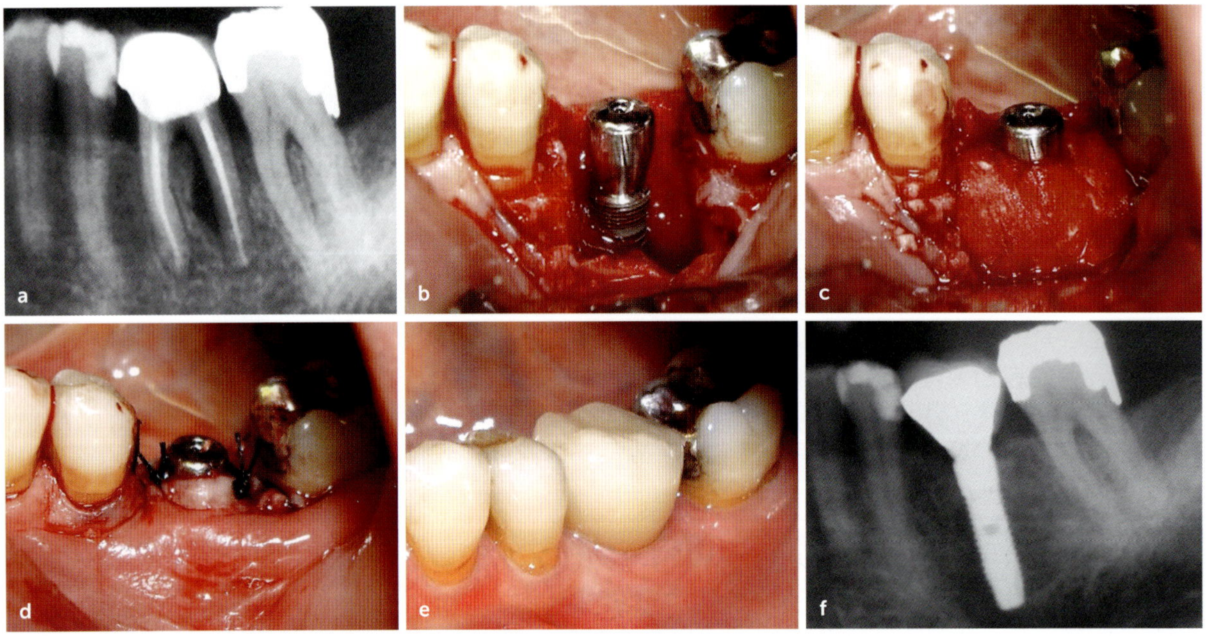

FIG 1-2 *(a)* The mandibular left first molar suffered failure of previous endodontic treatment and required extraction. *(b)* Flap elevation was needed to place this IMI, as the endodontic infection had caused considerable loss of buccal bone. However, the other three socket walls were intact and their crestal bone levels of sufficient height to suggest that GBR could be successful in restoring the lost buccal bone. *(c)* Because the IMI was well-stabilized, GBR (particulate allograft and collagen barrier) was used to promote regeneration of lost bone. *(d)* The immediate postoperative image of the implant site. *(e)* The clinical status of the restored IMI after 12 months in function. *(f)* The radiographic status of the IMI 12 months after the GBR procedure was performed. Note the excellent regeneration and stable crestal bone.

deficient, other treatment options can be chosen, the most common one being socket preservation grafting and delayed implant placement.[38]

Alternatively, if an IMI can be adequately stabilized, the deficiency often may be corrected with traditional guided bone regeneration (GBR) techniques[39] (Fig 1-2). One recent report claimed that—provided that flapless surgery was used to place IMIs at sites with buccal bone dehiscences (Elian type II sockets)—outcomes could have success similar to those with implants placed into intact sockets (Elian type I).[40] This was achieved by trimming and inserting a collagen membrane under the buccal soft tissue and densely packing xenograft into all defects around the seated implant, followed by placement of a healing abutment with a diameter corresponding to that of the extraction socket. The wide healing abutment will help to simulate primary soft tissue closure, sheltering the graft. Another group of investigators have since reported that densely packed xenograft alone can give the same benefit.[41] It was noted, however, that a healing interval of at least 6 months is needed to achieve favorable outcomes because xenograft has no known osteoinductive properties, and healing would be dependent on the response of osteoprogenitor cells of the periosteal layer of the buccal soft tissue.

While immediate implants were first used in the replacement of single-rooted teeth, innovators in implant dentistry were fast to translate the methodology to molar sites.[8,42–47] For example, Fugazzotto[45] described in detail an approach for placing immediate implants into the interradicular septum (IRS) bone of mandibular molars, focusing on ways to avoid bur chatter and drift (see chapter 3). He also reviewed the healing sequence following tooth extraction starting from clot formation. By 14 to 16 days, newly formed granulation tissue is replaced by connective tissue that subsequently converts to osteoid with calcification so that by 6 weeks, the socket is almost entirely filled with new trabecular bone. Fortunately, the placement of an immediate implant does not affect this normal healing sequence provided that the implant is sufficiently stable to avoid early micromovements.[48]

Fugazzotto further described protocols for maxillary IMIs[46] (see chapter 4). Osteotomy site location was first established in the IRS bone using a guide

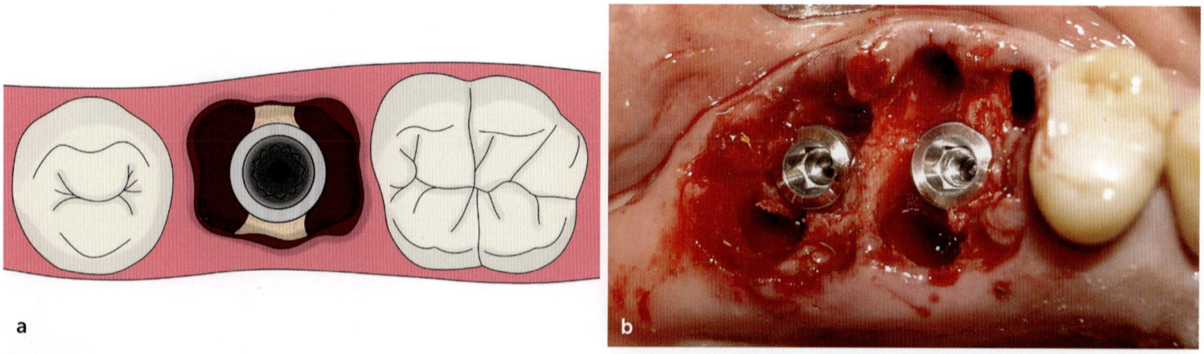

FIG 1-3 *(a)* An illustration of a site where an IMI could not be contained within IRS but was nevertheless stabilized by contact with the remaining lingual and buccal buttresses of the IRS. There is no actual contact between implant and buccal cortex, and the remaining peri-implant gaps have filled with blood and should heal with new bone fill provided that a large-diameter healing abutment will be added. *(b)* This first molar IMI was stabilized by the remaining buccal and palatal buttresses of a type B IRS.

drill, round bur, or narrow-diameter trephine, depending on the quantity of remaining apical bone. Thereafter, a series of handheld osteotomes of increasing diameter and a surgical mallet were used to finalize the osteotomy shape and depth as originally described by Summers.[49,50] Initial localization using a trephine was selected when there was insufficient remaining IRS bone height apically to receive the implant without disturbing the maxillary sinus. The trephine was used to create a core of IRS bone, taking care to stop short of the cortical sinus floor by about 1 mm. Thereafter, the core of bone released by the trephine was impacted apically with osteotomes to elevate the sinus floor. The safe insertion of a threaded implant could then be achieved. Others described a similar approach for maxillary first molars with 98% survival of implants at 3 years.[51] However, the recent introduction of the concept of osseodensification using Densah burs (Versah) for use in similar situations has eliminated the need for hammering on osteotomes, making placement of maxillary IMIs more patient-friendly[52] (see chapters 7 and 11).

Ideally, IMIs will be stabilized primarily either by being contained completely in IRS bone, or by contact with the remaining furcal bone buttresses located buccally and lingual/palatally without direct contact with the buccal and lingual/palatal socket walls (Fig 1-3). Unless these walls are very thick, insertion torque forces received by them could cause microfractures and early crestal bone loss. Any remaining gaps between the socket walls and implant periphery need not necessarily be grafted[34] (see also chapter 11) as long as the blood clots that have filled them can be sheltered by the repositioned flap margins in conjunction with appropriately sized healing abutments that can act as prosthetic sealing devices. More will be said of this later in this book.

When Immediate Molar Replacement Is Not Feasible

Before IMI therapy is proposed to a potential patient, the patient should be advised that the final decision on the feasibility of the approach cannot be made until after the tooth has been extracted. Factors such as root ankylosis, fracture of the buccal plate, unintended socket expansion during extraction, unexpected difficulty in tooth removal, or acute infection might make immediate implant placement impossible or less predictable. For example, if the extraction ends up being more traumatic than expected, requires elevation of a large mucoperiosteal flap, and/or results in significant loss of IRS and/or bone buccally or lingually/palatally, it may be necessary to delay implant placement and instead regain some of this lost bone using the techniques of socket preservation grafting.[53–56] There will always be value in using a flapless procedure to avoid disruption of the periosteal blood supply, but generally only if the original buccal bone at the crest has been determined to be intact.[55,57,58] Noteworthy is the fact that buccal bone loss after extraction has been reported to be significantly less if its original postextraction thickness was 3 mm rather than 1 mm.[59]

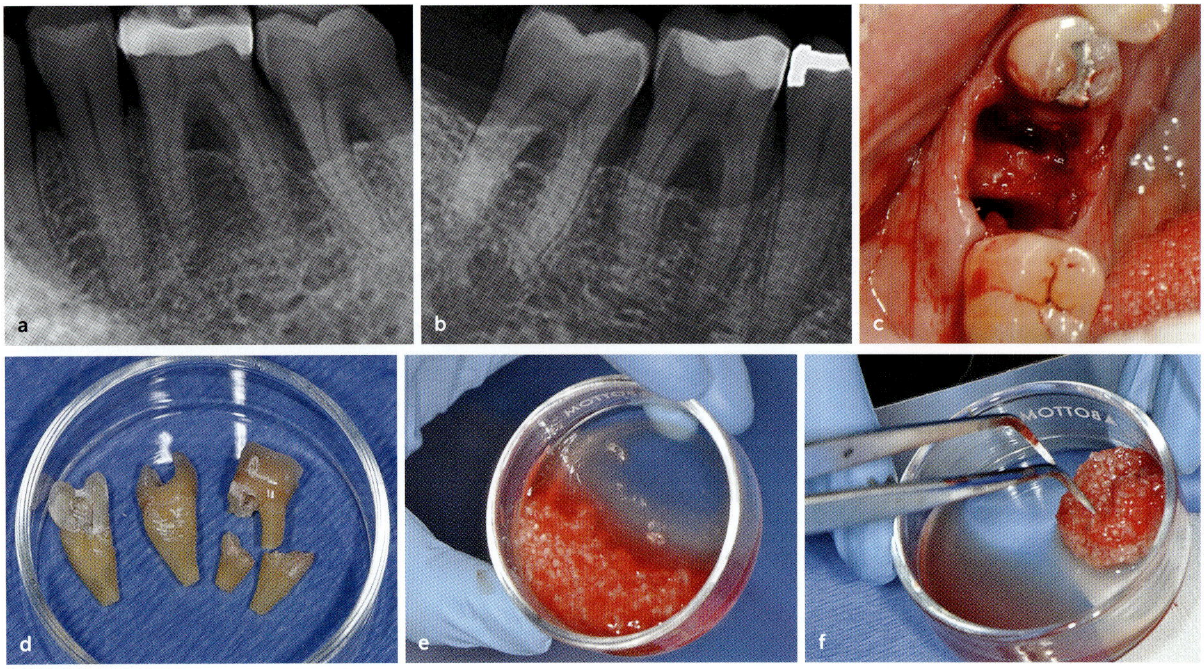

FIG 1-4 *(a)* The mandibular left first molar had a grade III furcation defect and was deemed hopeless in this man in his 50s who had insulin-dependent diabetes. *(b)* The mandibular right first molar in the same patient also required extraction. *(c)* The teeth were removed atraumatically without flap elevation after sectioning the roots through the furcation. The IRS for each of the teeth was classified as type B according to Smith and Tarnow.[67] (Surgery performed by Dr Suzette Guo, University of Toronto.) *(d)* The extracted tooth fragments are seen here after removal of all restorative materials as well as the pulpal and periodontal ligament soft tissues. *(e)* Once the tooth-derived particulate graft material was prepared using a dedicated processing machine, it was mixed with the liquid phase of platelet-rich concentrated growth factors (ie, autologous fibrin glue) obtained after centrifugation of a sample of the patient's venous blood in citrate-coated, white-capped plastic tubes as described by others.[63] *(f)* Mixing the patient's platelet growth factors and tooth graft particles resulted in a sticky pellet of tooth autograft biomaterial that could be easily used to fill the tooth sockets. →

If a flap is raised for tooth extraction and the socket deemed unsuitable for an IMI, the principles of GBR are followed for socket preservation, commonly using a particulate graft material (generally a mineralized allograft or xenograft) isolated and covered with a protective membrane and/or autologous platelet-rich fibrin (PRF) clots.[60–64] While the particulate graft material may delay socket healing somewhat,[38] it has generally been accepted that *(1)* grafting is beneficial in reducing alveolar ridge shrinkage, and *(2)* a mineralized slowly resorbing particulate graft material is preferred.[56] Ideally, a barrier material that can be left exposed crestally is preferred, as this will not deleteriously affect the anatomy of the buccal vestibule in any attempt to gain primary flap closure and will promote an increase in the quantity of keratinized tissue.[65,66] Examples of socket preservation using two different barrier approaches in a single patient can be seen in Fig 1-4.

Case report

As can be seen in Figs 1-4a and 1-4b, both the left and right mandibular first molars had grade III furcation defects and required extraction. The remaining IRS bone for both was classified as type B (ie, sufficient to stabilize an IMI),[67] which, under other circumstances, would have been favorable for IMI placement (Fig 1-4c). However, the patient had insulin-dependent diabetes with a history of severe periodontitis, and the clinician cautiously opted for socket preservation and delayed implant placement. Rather than using a commercially available allograft or xenograft, it was decided to process the extracted tooth fragments to form a genetically compatible particulate dentin graft (Fig 1-4d; see chapter 6). This was prepared using a dedicated processing machine (TOP Graft VacuaSonic System, CosmoBioMedicare). The more traditional approach would have been to use a mineralized particulate allograft or a xenograft like Bio-Oss (Geistlich).

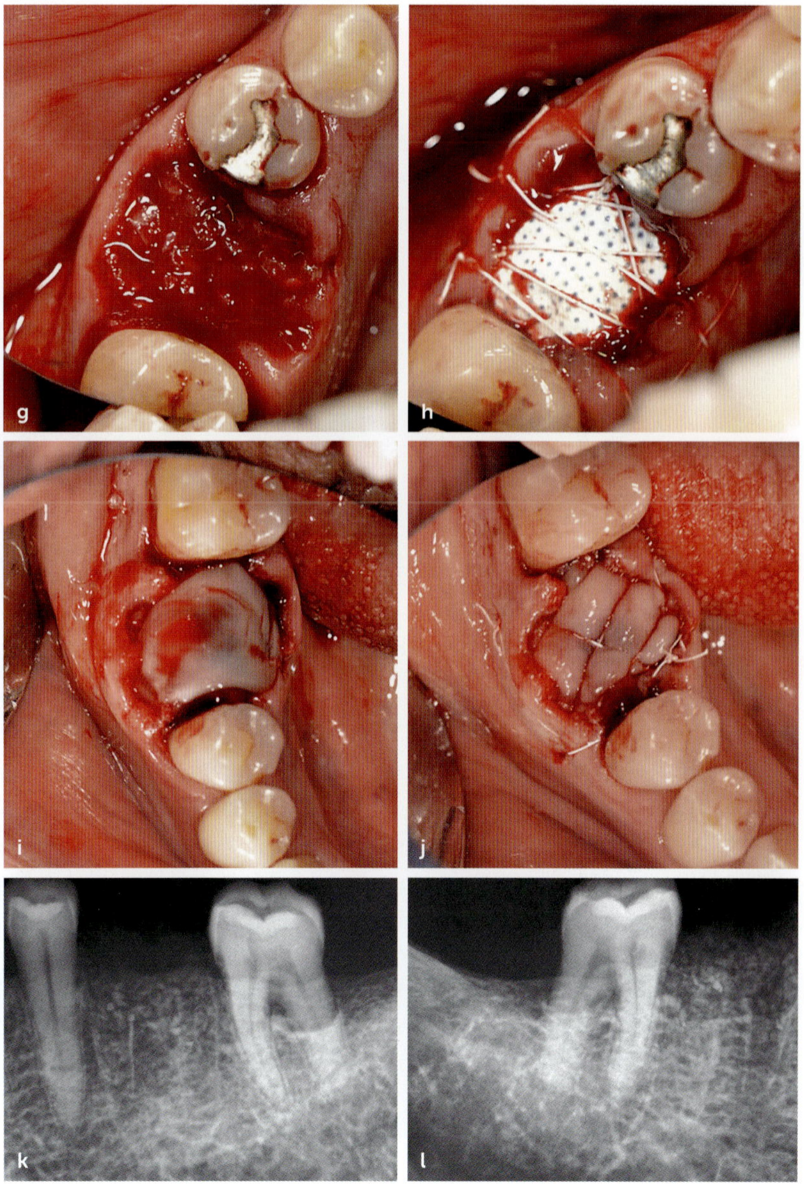

FIG 1-4 *(cont) (g)* The sticky particulate tooth autograft was packed into the extraction site. *(h)* A double-barrier technique[68] was used at the left site to protect the particulate graft material: After first using a collagen barrier (Bio-Gide, Geistlich), a dense PTFE barrier (Cytoplast, Osteogenics) was trimmed appropriately, placed over the first barrier, and secured with sutures. *(i)* After atraumatic extraction and placement of the tooth-derived particulate autograft, the right site was covered with two autologous PRF clots[63] as the only barrier. *(j)* The right site covered with autologous fibrin clots was sutured, leaving the clots exposed. *(k)* The immediate postoperative radiograph of the grafted left molar site. *(l)* The immediate postoperative radiograph of the grafted right molar site.

After preparation, the dentin graft particles were mixed with autologous liquid fibrinogen isolated by centrifugation from the patient's venous blood to form the equivalent of "sticky bone"[63] (Figs 1-4e and 1-4f). Both sockets were filled with this graft preparation enriched by addition of the liquid fibrinogen and its platelet-derived growth factors (Fig 1-4g). The left grafted socket was covered with two barrier materials, first a resorbable collagen membrane and then a dense polytetrafluoroethylene (PTFE) nonresorbable barrier that was left exposed to the oral cavity[65,68] (Fig 1-4h). On the patient's right side, the grafted socket was covered with two PRF clots prepared from the patient's own blood[63] and again left exposed (Figs 1-4i and 1-4j). Immediate postoperative radiographs of the grafted sockets can be seen in Figs 1-4k and 1-4l.

Both sites healed well, resulting in sufficient bone at 4 months to allow single implant placement using a nonsubmerged technique and later restoration with single metal-ceramic crowns (Figs 1-4m to 1-4q). Because all particulate bone graft materials are known to interfere somewhat with normal extraction socket healing,[69] some clinicians have suggested an alternative approach using only autologous PRF clots to fill

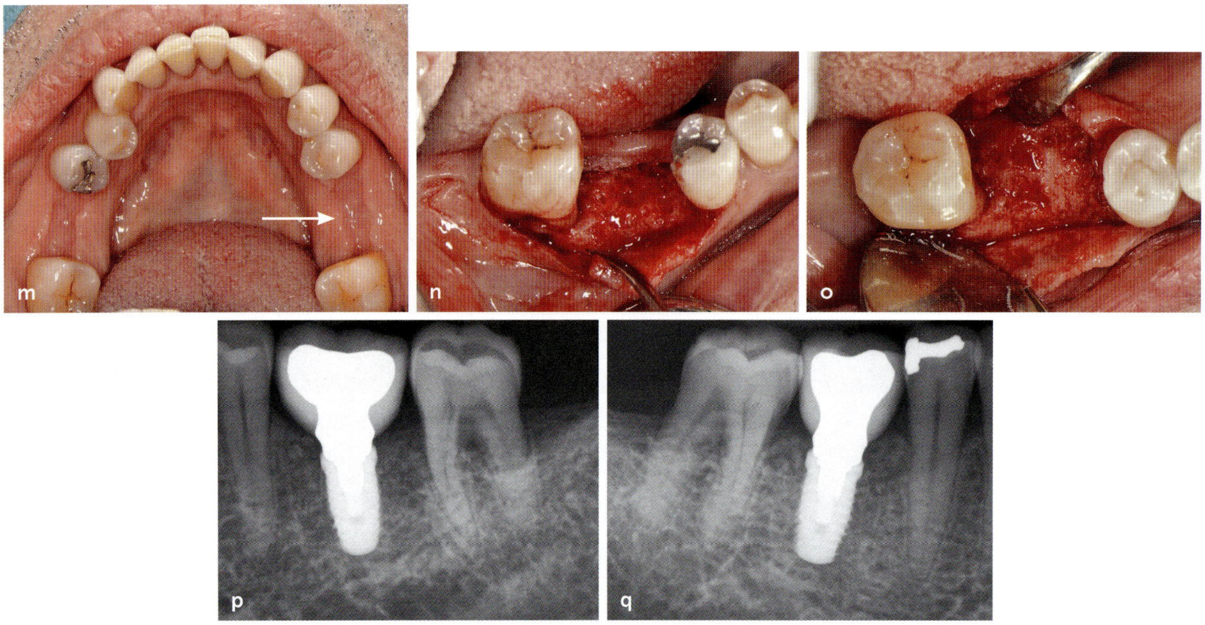

FIG 1-4 *(cont) (m)* A clinical photograph taken at the 6-week postoperative visit. Both molar sites appear to be healing well, but the patient reported having less discomfort at the side managed with the autologous fibrin clot barrier *(arrow)*. *(n)* A clinical photograph taken of the right side after 4 months of healing showing excellent new bone formation. *(o)* The contralateral site showing good site healing immediately before implant placement. *(p)* The restored left molar implant. *(q)* The restored right molar implant.

the socket.[70–72] One recent systematic review assessing the healing potential of a wide variety of grafting materials suggested that PRF was the most effective in promoting new vital bone formation.[73] However, another recent literature review with meta-analysis of published data using the latter approach suggested that more study is needed before routine usage can be prescribed.[74]

History of Immediate Molar Replacement

Early protocols for IMI placement provided scant details on procedural steps but led to acceptable outcomes for the time. In a small study published in 2000, Schwartz-Arad et al[75] reported outcomes for 56 IMIs placed in 43 patients during the period from 1989 to 1996. One implant was placed in 1989 and another 2 years later. This led to three IMIs being placed in 1993, 10 in 1994, 16 in 1995, and finally 23 in 1996, all by a single surgeon. In total, 17 IMIs were placed in maxillas and the remaining 39 in mandibles. If and how the procedure was modified over these 8 years was not indicated. Likewise, it was not stated whether there had been failed attempts in other patients. No criteria for patient selection were given, but it was reported that the majority of the implants had somehow been placed centrally in the molar sockets, while five molars had been replaced using two implants each, ie, one into each molar root socket. Implant lengths (10 to 14 mm) were chosen to engage as much apical bone as possible. Grafting of any peri-implant defects was done only at some sites, but indications were not given. The graft preferred was autogenous bone collected from implant burs or adjacent bone. Likewise, barriers were only occasionally used (six bioabsorbable collagen and two nonresorbable expanded PTFE, GORE-TEX, W. L. Gore) without explanation as to why the operator felt it necessary. Primary flap closure with the aid of releasing incisions was included where bone grafting and membranes had been used, but information was not given on how the remainder of the sites had been handled. Nevertheless, the 5-year cumulative survival rate was reported to be 89% (84% for men and 93.5% for women). Differences in outcomes also were found in maxilla versus mandible (82% vs 92% respectively) and with smoking (90% for nonsmokers vs 83% for smokers).

Fugazzotto[45,46] later described detailed protocols that he had developed for both mandibular and maxillary IMI placement. Osteotomies were created in suitable IRS bone, and all peri-implant gaps were grafted with xenograft particles covered with either titanium-reinforced ePTFE barriers or resorbable collagen barriers secured with tacks and followed by primary, tension-free soft tissue closure. As an aside, the problem with using GORE-TEX ePTFE barrier membranes was that great surgical skills and meticulous patient compliance were needed to achieve and maintain soft tissue closure over the site for the complete submerged implant healing interval. If the membranes became exposed by flap dehiscence at some point after placement, site infection was likely, meaning that the exposed barriers and infected graft material needed to be removed.[76] Depending on how long the barriers had been in place, their removal in itself could be traumatic and damaging to the site, compromising the outcome or resulting in early implant failure.

Wagenburg and Froum[44] presented their private practice outcomes with 261 IMIs in the mandible and 202 in the maxilla. In both arches, after decoronation and root removal, implants were placed slightly to the mesial of the IRS bone, most often utilizing a wide-diameter implant generally not in contact with the buccal and lingual/palatal plates of bone. Implants were placed 1 to 2 mm subcrestally. Mineralized freeze-dried bone allograft (FDBA) was tightly packed into peri-implant gaps, followed by placement of a Vicryl resorbable membrane (Ethicon) tucked under the flap margins. No attempt was made to advance the flaps to cover the membranes. Failure rates after at least 1 year in function were reported to be 4.98% in the mandible and 6.44% in the maxilla.

Recent years have seen publication of many more studies of IMI performance, along with recommended prerequisites for success. Assuming that intact socket walls remain, experts suggest flapless extraction and a thick gingival biotype as preferred, and that good initial implant stability (≥ 35 Ncm) is essential. Gap grafting and barrier materials are often considered optional, and implants can be left nonsubmerged for the initial osseointegration period, simplifying the procedure and shortening operating time. Wide-diameter healing abutments may be all that is needed to support the surrounding soft tissues, avoiding gap grafting and allowing healing by secondary intention (see chapters 3, 4, and 11).

Case Selection and Anatomical Considerations with IMI Placement

Contraindications

There are few patient contraindications when considering IMIs. Naturally, compliance with strict postoperative guidelines is essential, and ideally patients will be nonsmokers or minimal smokers, as smoking will negatively impact site healing.[77,78] Patients with a history of severe periodontitis (even if previously treated with apparent success) also may be at greater risk with immediate implants, especially in maxillary sites and with time in function.[79-82] As well, patients currently taking oral bisphosphonate medications or who have previously taken them for more than a few years will likely be at greater risk of complications and implant failure.[83] One way to reduce risks here is to prepare the extraction sockets with PRF clots immediately before implant insertion.[84] Other patients who may not be appropriate are those with uncontrolled diabetes,[85] those with a history of head and neck radiation in the previous 12 to 24 months,[86] those who are currently taking receptor activator of nuclear factor kappa-B ligand (RANKL)-inhibiting anticancer drugs,[87] and those who have a history of bruxism[88] or other parafunctional habits.

It is also worth determining if the patient is vitamin D and/or magnesium deficient before undertaking treatment, especially in older individuals.[89,90] Kim et al[91] recently reported a link between low serum 25-hydroxyvitamin D [25-(OH)D] levels, tooth loss, and prevalence of severe periodontitis in South Koreans aged 50 years and older. It has been reported that vitamin D deficiency reduces host resistance to infection in orthopedic joint replacement procedures. Serum 25-(OH)D levels of 109 patients scheduled to receive a total prosthesis either of the hip, knee, or shoulder were measured after admission to the hospital.[92] Serum 25-(OH)D levels were also measured for patients presenting with periprosthetic joint infection (n = 50) or aseptic loosening of the prosthesis (n = 31) who were scheduled to undergo revision surgery. Significant differences in 25-(OH)D levels were found when comparing patients with periprosthetic joint infection and patients scheduled for primary arthroplasty ($P < .001$). A significant difference ($P < .001$) was also found when comparing patients with periprosthetic joint infections to those with aseptic prosthesis loosening. Accordingly, investigators suggested single-dose preoperative vitamin D supplementation prior to joint prosthesis surgery.[93]

Others have studied the impact of vitamin D deficiency on the integration of titanium alloy implants in rat femurs.[94] Implants were surface-modified either with double acid etching or with double acid etching followed by discrete crystalline deposition of hydroxyapatite nanoparticles. After 14 days of site healing, implants placed in vitamin D–deficient rats showed significantly weaker integration than those implanted in control animals. Others studied the impact of implant integration in tibias of ovariectomized rats.[95] One group of rats was fed a vitamin D–free diet for 8 weeks, while a second group was fed the same diet for 6 weeks followed by a standard diet containing 2,400 IU/kg of vitamin D for the last 2 weeks of implant site healing. Finally, a control group of normal rats was fed the latter diet for the full 8 weeks. Results showed a significant decrease in cortical bone-to-implant contact in the D-deficient group only. No detectable effect of vitamin D deficiency was observed in cancellous bone.

Site selection

The key to success with IMIs, of course, is careful site selection,[77,96] and more will be said of this in the following chapters. It must be emphasized that the recommended procedures are certainly technique sensitive and—like short implants—may not be appropriate for clinicians who attempt the procedures infrequently.[97] Local hard and soft tissue conditions including gingival biotype and socket anatomy must always be considered. For example, sites with a thin gingival biotype (ie, a periodontal probe inserted into the gingival crevice can been seen through the overlying tissue) and/or a thin (< 1.5 mm) and/or compromised buccal bone plate may not be good candidates or may require more complicated procedures, including GBR. A pretreatment CBCT scan is essential to allow assessment of root positions and shapes, the anatomy of remaining IRS, and the presence of intact buccal and lingual/palatal cortical plates along with their thicknesses (see chapter 2). Pretreatment CBCT scans also allow a risk assessment regarding potential damage to neurovascular structures[96] and/or perforation of the lingual cortical plate in the mandible.[98] In the maxilla, pretreatment CBCT records will provide useful information about sinus proximity, intrusion of maxillary molar roots into the sinus, current alveolar ridge dimensions, and furcal roof distance from the sinus floor.

Extraction technique and osteotomy preparation

Of utmost importance with an IMI procedure is the careful, atraumatic removal of the condemned tooth. The ideal approach is to perform the extraction without raising a mucoperiosteal flap in order to minimize disruption to local blood supply and help to minimize loss in alveolar ridge width.[55,99,100] However, initial buccal bone thickness again comes into play as well because even with flapless surgery, greater buccal bone loss will occur if its initial thickness was less than 1.5 mm.[101] Leaving a significant (> 1 mm) buccal implant-to-bone gap with or without grafting also will help to stabilize the buccal crest as new vital bone forms in this gap[31,102] (Fig 1-5).

If a flapless technique is feasible, after making conservative intrasulcular incisions, the molar is first decoronized using a fissure bur and high-speed handpiece. Thereafter, the roots are sectioned free with the same bur so as to permit their removal individually using small-tipped elevators and/or periotomes[103] (Fig 1-6). A very helpful tool is a thin, long, high-speed diamond bur inserted into the ligament spaces where needed to create narrow channels into which a small elevator or periotome subsequently can be inserted and used to loosen the individual roots (Fig 1-7). This bur should be used to remove tooth structure rather than bone and reach a depth of at least two-thirds the root length, by which time the root fragments should be easily removed. Wang et al[104] discussed the use of periotomes, suggesting that the first step should be to use a 15c blade supracrestally to release the gingival fibers from the tooth. Afterward, a thin periotome can be placed subcrestally to widen the periodontal ligament spaces circumferentially but primarily at proximal surfaces so as to minimize damage to buccal bone. Again, using a thin diamond pencil-type bur and a high-speed handpiece could minimize any

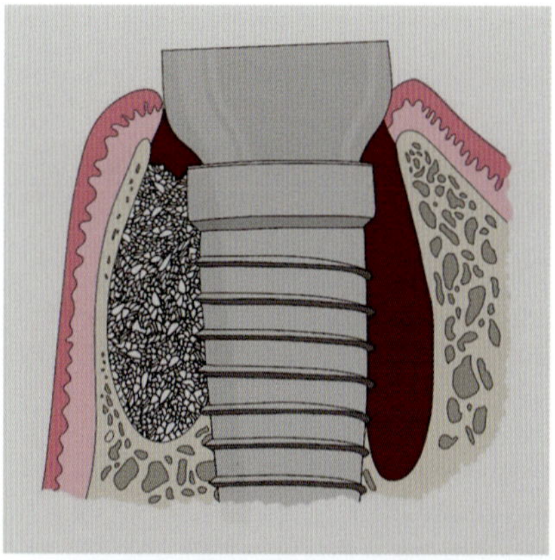

FIG 1-5 If an IMI can be stabilized in IRS of a molar socket having a thin (≤ 1.5 mm) buccal cortical plate of bone, a buccal gap should be left and most likely grafted in order to prevent significant vertical resorption of this cortex and significant loss in buccolingual ridge width. In this illustration, the lingual gap was left ungrafted as it would fill with a blood clot, which, if sheltered by a healing abutment, would lead to new bone formation and gap fill.

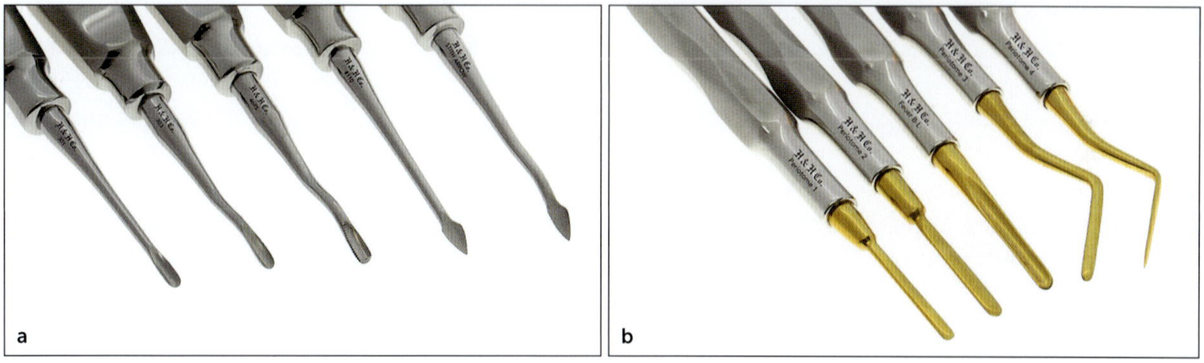

FIG 1-6 *(a)* Examples of fine-tipped surgical elevators useful for loosening molar roots after decoronation and sectioning. *(b)* Samples of periotome tips useful for luxating separated molar roots prior to their removal.

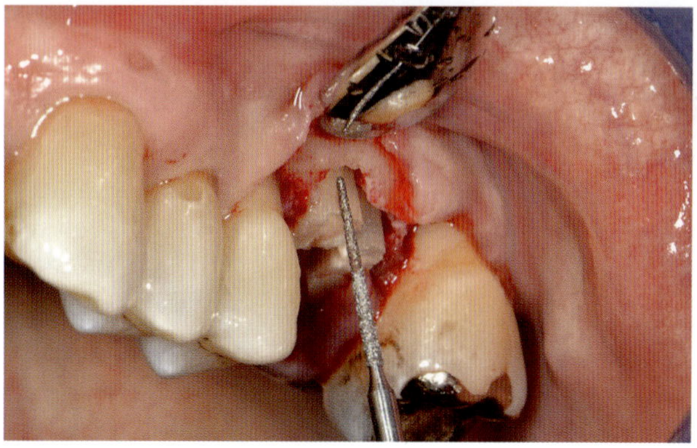

FIG 1-7 A long, small-diameter high-speed diamond bur can be used to create narrow channels in the periodontal ligament spaces of the molar roots prior to using thin luxators/elevators or periotomes to avulse the roots individually. The penetration depth of the bur should be at least two-thirds of the tooth root length to reduce the risk of root fracture during subsequent luxation/removal. Normally, use of this bur should be limited to the proximal root surfaces so as not to damage the IRS or thin cortical plates. The bur shown in this photograph is an FGSurg Medium Needle Diamond bur #859.36.10 (Brasseler).

periotome-related bone damage as well as shorten the time required for the procedure. Progressively larger periotomes are used to further loosen each root and permit its removal with root forceps.

As stated earlier, optimal placement of an IMI generally will be into the IRS. Smith and Tarnow[67] classified molar socket IRS into three groups (Box 1-1). Type A were denoted as those with sufficient volume to contain the whole coronal periphery of the selected implant, while type B were those with sufficient volume to stabilize the implant but with dehiscences in the IRS after osteotomy preparation at one or more aspects of the implant. With either of these IRS situations, it may be wise to leave the osteotomy one size smaller in diameter than the intended final implant bur to ensure adequate implant stability (ie, ≥ 35 Ncm). Achieving adequate implant stability, particularly with type B situations, may require engaging

BOX 1-1 Smith and Tarnow classification of molar extraction sites for immediate implant placement[67]

Type A	Adequate septal bone to circumferentially contain the coronal portion of the implant within the bone completely
Type B	Enough septal bone to stabilize the implant but not fully contain it, leaving gaps between one or more surfaces of the implant and the socket walls
Type C	Not enough bone within the socket to stabilize the implant without engaging the outer walls of the socket

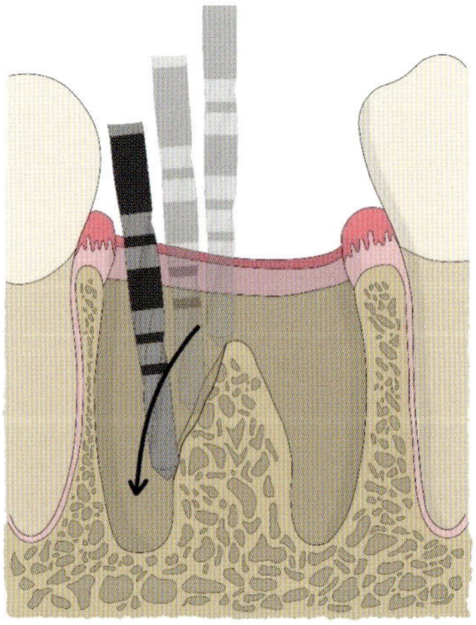

FIG 1-8 If osteotomy preparation is undertaken after removal of both roots, it is often difficult to stabilize the initial burs within the IRS, with the result that bur slippage may damage the IRS.

3 to 5 mm of bone apical to the IRS.[105] Optimal 3D positioning also dictates IMI placement 2 to 3 mm below the gingival margins of adjacent teeth, greater than 2 mm away from the buccal cortical bone plate—particularly if it is thin—and 1.5 to 4 mm away from any adjacent teeth. Subcrestal implant positioning has also been recommended for particular implant designs,[106–109] as this too will help to compensate for any untoward vertical loss in crestal bone height during initial site healing.

The problem with removing tooth roots before starting osteotomy preparation is that it can be difficult to control the burs, which in a type B IRS can easily slip into one or other of the tooth root sockets (Fig 1-8). As a result, most clinicians now agree that initial implant osteotomy preparation for an IMI is best begun before removing the tooth roots. Their recommendation is that after decoronation and before sectioning of the molar roots, a high-speed handpiece and round bur be used to begin the osteotomy directly into the furcation area of the tooth and underlying bone. This will provide anatomical guidance and stability for effective bur function. Once into bone, and provided that the subsequent burs will not be in direct contact with the remaining tooth structure causing chatter, a pilot bur followed by the dedicated implant burs can be used to partly or completely finish the osteotomy before sectioning and removing the individual roots. This technique was pioneered by individuals such as Rodriguez-Tizcareño[110] and others.[111,112] One recent publication compared this approach to the situation where roots were removed before osteotomy preparation, and found the former approach to give better outcomes in terms of ideal implant location and stability.[112]

Specific implant design features for IMIs

The greatest concern with the placement of IMIs is being able to achieve adequate primary stability in a prosthetically favorable location, ie, often centrally in the IRS. Initially, IMI placement relied on modifying existing surgical techniques[45] to accommodate standard implant designs, and certainly the introduction of osseodensification burs to expand and sculpt IRS bone has been an important advancement[113] (see chapter 7). Manufacturers have also introduced implants with more aggressive threads to help with initial implant stabilization.[114] Others have proposed the use of ultra-wide (≥ 6-mm diameter) implants relying on engagement of any buccal and lingual/palatal bone struts for implant stabilization[108] (see Fig 1-3 and chapter 8). Wider-diameter implants offer the advantage of increased bone-to-implant contact, less coronal stress in molar sites with their heavy occlusal loading, and as a result, less crestal bone loss. They also provide prosthetic platforms that permit more natural molar implant crown profiles and emergence profiles. Disadvantages include possible excessive torque in the posterior mandible during insertion and violating the buccal plate if the implant periphery contacts it.

Making a decision regarding appropriate implant diameter should be based on the following considerations:

- Mesiodistal ridge width[115]
- Type of IRS
- Subantral bone height (in the maxilla)

In regard to types A and B IRS, the usual diameter chosen will likely be 4 to 5 mm. Diameters greater than 5 mm may be appropriate for type C septa, large mesiodistal ridge lengths, and limited subantral bone height where sinus floor elevation is contraindicated as part of IMI insertion. Tapered implant shapes also may help to improve initial implant stability.[116]

Managing gingival biotype with IMIs

As already stated, with bone-level implant designs, thin gingival biotype may affect treatment outcomes by predisposing to unwanted crestal bone loss needed for biologic width accommodation and increasing risk of both peri-implant mucositis and peri-implantitis, particularly if buccal bone thickness also is an issue.[15,117–122] Placing implants subcrestally along with the use of longer healing abutments at sites with a thin gingival biotype may help in reducing crestal bone loss.[123] Platform switching also appears to be of benefit in reducing bone loss, while also promoting thicker buccal soft tissues with less likelihood for recession.[124–126] However, if the clinician wishes to minimize untoward effects on crestal bone at sites with a thin gingival biotype, soft tissue grafting to increase the peri-implant keratinized tissues may be the best option. Grafting with autologous connective tissue taken from the patient's palate or tuberosity (or if need be with free gingival grafts) generally has been regarded as the gold standard approach, although commercially available collagen matrix products also have been used.[127–131] Timing for undertaking this grafting appears not to be crucial, as it can be done before or at the time of implant placement or even later if need be.[132]

Gap grafting and wound closure

As discussed earlier, when IMI protocols were originally conceived, it was felt that any socket spaces or gaps that remained after implant insertion needed to be managed with some sort of mineralized particulate graft[56] covered with a resorbable or nonresorbable barrier material and submerged under a mucoperiosteal flap released sufficiently to allow tension-free complete wound closure. This added to the time involved for the procedure, its difficulty and cost, unfavorable alterations of the associated vestibule, and the risk of postoperative complications. Supported by more recent findings, most clinicians now prefer to simplify the procedure by allowing nonsubmerged healing of IMIs, often with little or no gap grafting.[133] Gap grafting at IMI sites may help to protect thin cortical bone, particularly on the crucial buccal aspect[34,134] (see Fig 1-5). However, it is unlikely to totally eliminate vertical crestal bone loss, especially if a flap has been raised for the procedure, making it important to place the implant 1 to 2 mm subcrestally.

Clinicians should avoid the trap of choosing implant diameters that will obliterate any buccal gaps (gap type 2 of Deporter et al[135]) because this could apply unwanted pressure on the buccal wall and likely encourage its resorption. While experts do vary in their choice of a crucial gap size requiring grafting, most feel that, provided the IMI is adequately stabilized, gaps less than 3 mm and certainly less than 2 mm in width should not need grafting. More recently, experienced clinicians have suggested and documented that gaps need no grafting regardless of their size[136] (see chapter 11). Using a wide-diameter healing abutment as sold or customized (see also chapter 12) or placing an immediate provisional crown can be used to support repositioned soft tissues and shield any gaps that have spontaneously filled with blood.[137–140] Using a healing abutment or immediate provisional crown will also provide some early nonocclusal loading, favorably influencing bone healing.[141] Additional advantages here would be the ability to add and subtract material for gingival support and contouring during the osseointegration phase.

Finally is the matter of how to manage the soft tissues following IMI placement without flap elevation if no gap grafting is done. Clinicians have taken

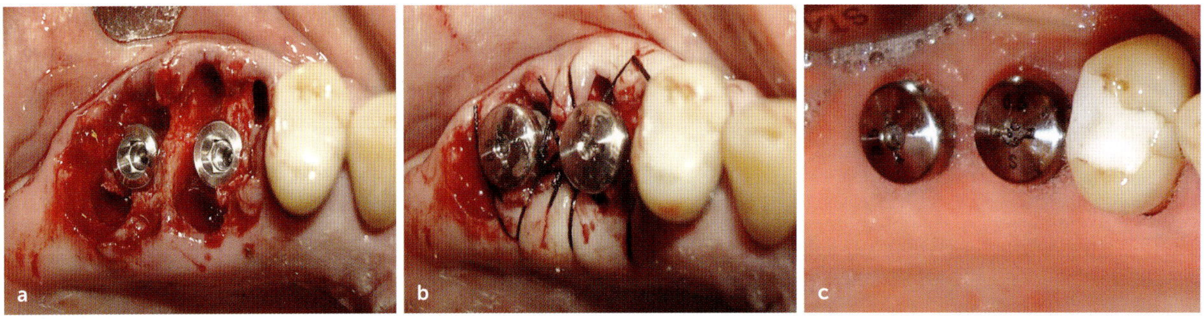

FIG 1-9 *(a)* After placing these two IMIs, large ungrafted gaps remained buccally and palatally. *(b)* Wide-diameter healing abutments were inserted and the soft tissues repositioned and passively sutured. *(c)* The site after 3 months of healing.

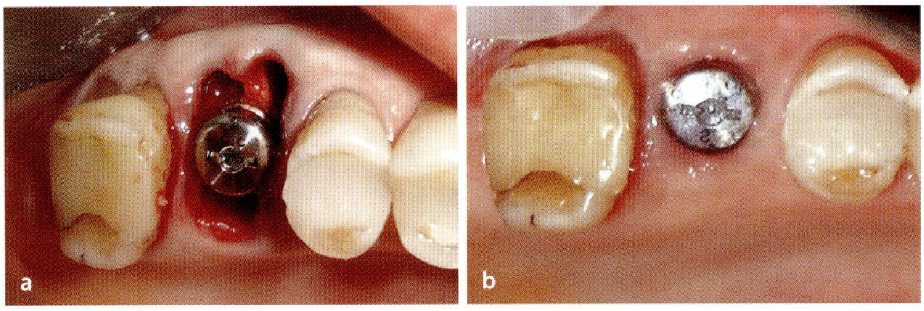

FIG 1-10 *(a)* Following flapless surgery and implant placement, the gaps remaining around this IMI were left without grafting or suturing. *(b)* Spontaneous bone fill and soft tissue healing occurred without complication.

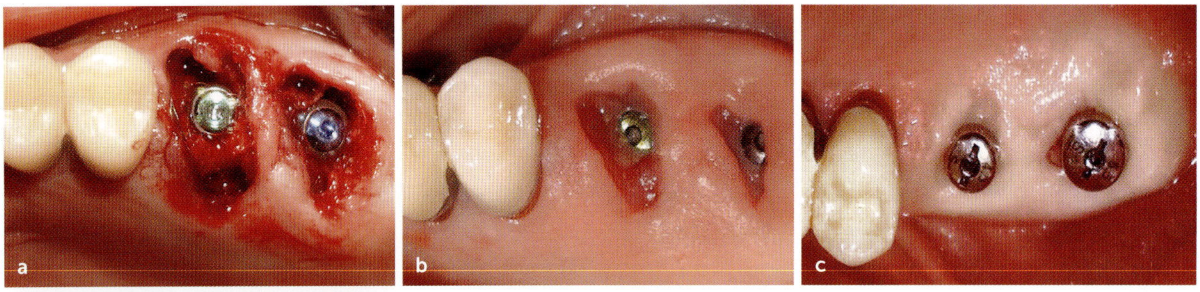

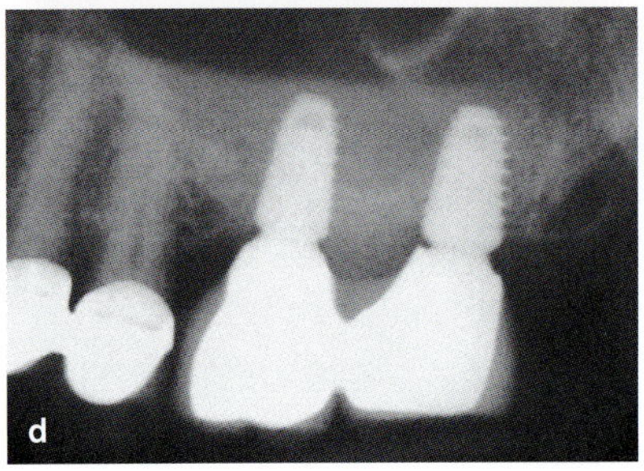

FIG 1-11 *(a)* These two IMIs were left without healing abutments, without grafting, and without suturing after inserting healing caps only. *(b)* The large gaps filled in with granulation tissue. *(c)* After 3 months of healing and re-entry surgery, the implants were ready for restoration. *(d)* The posttreatment radiograph after 12 months of implant function.

various approaches. As already stated, the most common approach is to add a wide-diameter healing abutment and passively suture the soft tissues around it (Fig 1-9). Others prefer not even to suture, leaving the gaps exposed because there are no graft particles that could be lost (Figs 1-10 and 1-11). At the opposite extreme, releasing incisions can be made to help with some flap advancement (Fig 1-12). Some clinicians prefer to cover the whole site with a free gingival graft (previously coined a “socket seal”), a resorbable or nonresorbable barrier or collagen plug, or autologous PRF clots[142–148] (Figs 1-13 to 1-15). In the final analysis, soft tissue coverage following IMI placement without gap grafting seems not to be an issue.

FIG 1-12 *(a and b)* The clinician treating this patient did not graft the defects but opted to make a horizontal releasing incision in the palate to mobilize the soft tissues after placing a large-diameter healing abutment.

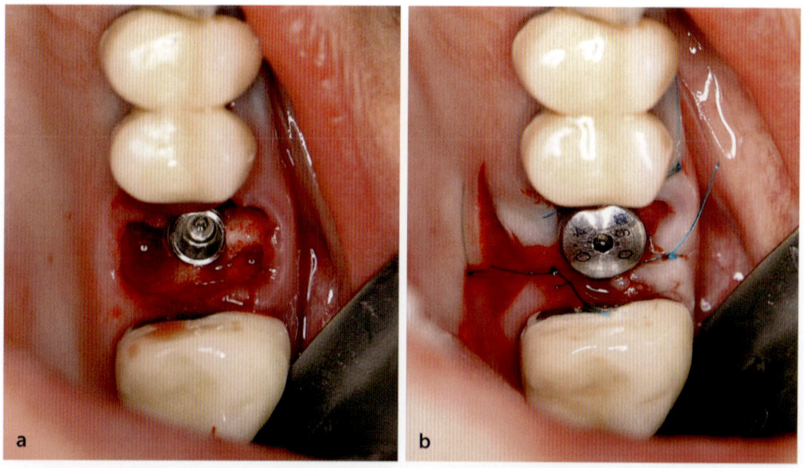

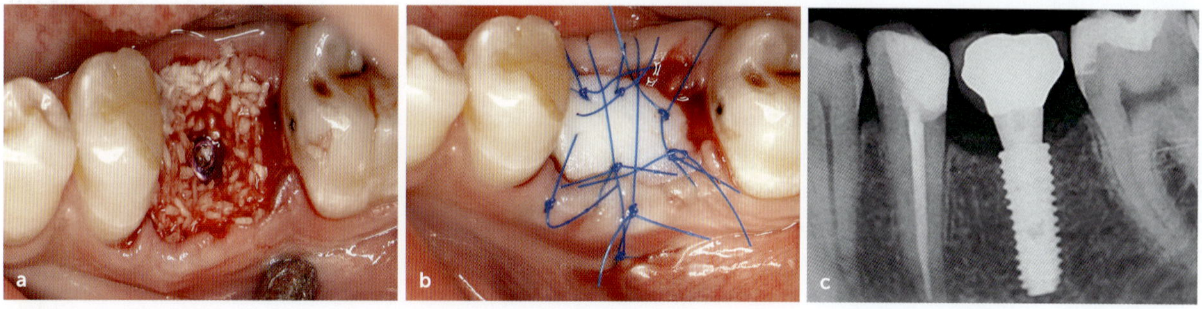

FIG 1-13 *(a)* The gaps around this IMI were filled with a bone substitute before placing a free gingival graft as a protective barrier. *(b)* This free gingival graft served two purposes: protecting the gaps filled with graft material and increasing the thickness of the overlying keratinized tissue. *(c)* Stable crestal bone levels can be seen in this 1-year follow-up postrestoration radiograph. (Courtesy of Dr Omid Nadaf, Tehran, Iran.)

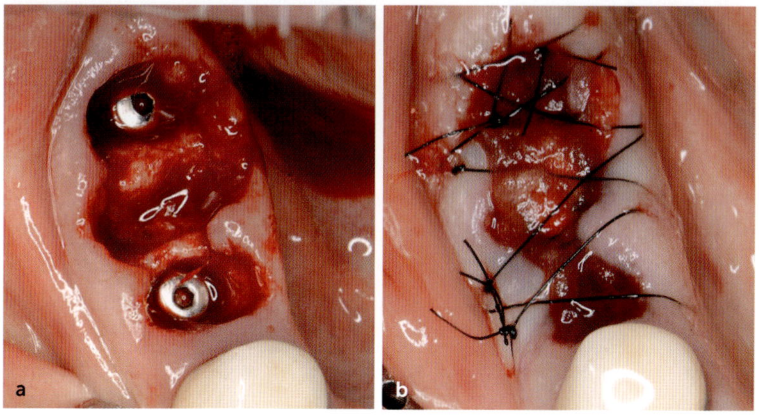

FIG 1-14 *(a)* An IMI was placed in the distal root socket of the first molar and an immediate implant into the socket of the second premolar. The procedure was flapless with allograft material placed into the gaps. *(b)* Allograft material was placed into the gaps, and the surgeon opted to place collagen plugs (Collacone, Botiss) to protect the blood clots that had formed in the gaps. (Courtesy of Dr Amir Moeintaghavi, Mashad, Iran.)

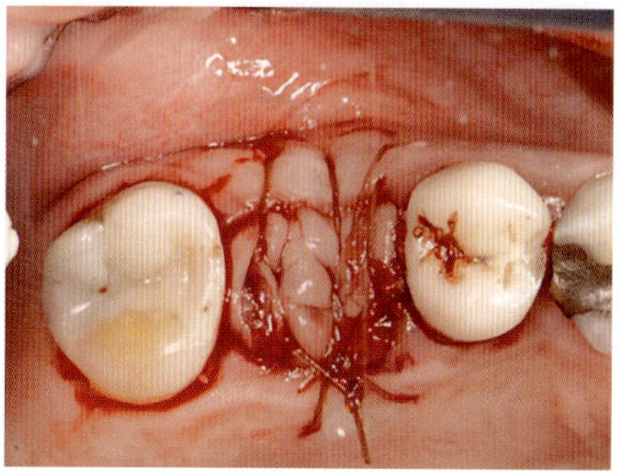

FIG 1-15 Some clinicians prefer to use autologous PRF membranes to fill peri-implant gaps or to cover particulate graft materials.

Performance of IMIs

Atieh et al[149] conducted a systematic review and meta-analysis of the performance of IMIs based on studies published up to and including October 2008. While the results were encouraging (estimated 99% survival rate), the reviewers noted that none of the identified nine relevant publications were randomized, double-blinded, controlled studies, ie, of the best quality. They concluded that further investigations would be needed before immediate molar placement could be adequately scrutinized as a recommended treatment protocol. A limitation of their review was that studies were included if they had a minimal functional period of only 6 months. In a similar review and meta-analysis, Ketabi et al[150] assessed studies of IMIs published from November 2008 to May 2015 and for which a minimum of 1 year in function had been specified. Unfortunately, the quality of the 15 studies identified for inclusion was no better than those reviewed by Atieh et al, there still being no randomized, double-blinded, controlled investigations.

There can be no doubt that placing implants into fresh extraction sockets is a difficult procedure.[151] A recent systematic review of published data by Antetomaso and Kumar[152] compared outcomes with implants placed into fresh extraction sockets to those with delayed implant placement. Their database included 3,049 implants, of which 1,440 had been placed into fresh extraction sites. Ninety-five of the 3,049 implants were classified as failures, giving an overall failure rate of 3.1%. However, 72.6% of the failures had been IMIs. They also concluded that more immediate implants failed in patients with a history of periodontitis, confirming earlier results by others reporting on IMI results.[79]

Atieh et al[149] identified only two IMI studies that had included delayed molar implant placement as controls, and based on these two studies, concluded that there appeared to be no significant differences. Ketabi et al[150] later found five more studies with a total of 316 implants in 243 patients that again compared performance to delayed placement molar implants. Similar high survival rates with controls were found for IMIs (98% for maxilla and 99% for mandible). However, in this latter review,[150] implant survival appeared to be affected by implant diameter, with ultra-wide implants (> 6–9 mm width) in some studies showing significantly higher failure rates than those of lesser diameter (4–6 mm). This finding could have been due to inadequate thickness of buccal and/or lingual/palatal cortical bone remaining after osteotomy preparation, which could easily happen with implant diameters greater than 6 mm,[153–155] inadequate buccal gaps left, inadequate depth of implant insertion relative to crestal bone, and/or the often high insertion torque values needed for wide-diameter IMI placement in the posterior mandible.

The most recent systematic review with meta-analyses of immediate implant placement was published by Canellas et al.[156] Only randomized clinical trials that included delayed implant placement as controls with outcomes of at least 1 year were included, but all tooth sites—not just molar sites—were lumped together. Meta-analysis suggested increased risk of implant failure by 3% using immediate implant protocols. However, subgroup analysis suggested that anterior tooth sites gave better results with immediate implants, while molar sites presented better results with delayed implants, stressing once more that placing IMIs is a challenging endeavor. Other recent authors also supported this conclusion.[151,152]

In addition to survival outcomes, Ketabi and Deporter attempted to estimate IMI success rates based on levels of crestal bone loss. Eight of the 15 qualifying papers in their review had included radiographic data presented as means with standard deviations. Following meta-analysis, the overall mean bone loss after at least 1 year in function was only 0.57 mm. According to established criteria[157] (*success* being defined as bone loss not > 1 mm at 1 year in function and no more than 0.2 mm/year thereafter), this finding suggested not only high survival but also high success rates for IMIs. However, radiographic data presented as group means can be misleading. For example, based on bone loss, Annibali et al[158] reported an IMI success rate of 95% at 1 year. One of 20 implants had developed peri-implantitis, needed surgical intervention as a rescue procedure, and was classified as a failure. However, seven other implants showed greater than 1 mm bone loss (1.3–1.87 mm) at 1 year, and this finding could have reduced the success rate at 1 year to 60%. Other investigators[159–162] have considered the 1-year upper limit for bone loss indicative of successful implants to be not greater than 1.5 or 2 mm, and using these criteria, Annibali et al's success rate would remain at 95%. Nevertheless, high survival/success rates for IMIs in the published literature should not be interpreted to indicate that they represent a straightforward and predictable procedure.[21] Gaining bur stability in IRS bone for IMIs may require unique techniques that are site-specific, while preparing for and inserting ultra-wide implants (see chapter 8) can be extremely challenging and result in too little buccal bone remaining or even loss of buccal bone and an aborted procedure. Experience and skill become very important here.

Conclusion

Installing molar implants on the day of tooth extraction (ie, IMIs) or in the first few weeks of site healing is appealing to patients as it shortens treatment time and possibly treatment costs. However, IMI placement is a difficult procedure that generally needs to be performed by highly skilled and experienced surgeons who have the opportunity to do this type of work on a regular basis. Proper case selection includes considering the reason for tooth extraction; the socket anatomy remaining after extraction; the dimensions of the IRS; the appropriate implant shape, length, and diameter; the depth and 3D positioning of implant insertion; the size of peri-implant gaps and whether or not to graft them; and the appropriateness of including soft tissue grafting at sites with a thin and/or narrow gingival biotype. High initial implant stability is essential for success.

KEY POINTS

- Pretreatment CBCT scans are recommended to assess the suitability of a molar site to receive an IMI (see chapter 2).
- Assuming the existence of an intact buccal cortical plate of bone of thickness greater than 1.5 mm, flapless surgery is recommended for the extraction.
- Instrumentation should begin with decoronation of any remaining crown structure.
- Osteotomy preparation may best be accomplished by beginning to drill through the remaining tooth structure with the intent of achieving the optimal, prosthetically driven 3D implant location.
- Tooth roots are ideally left in situ until the osteotomy is partially or completely finished, after which they should be separated and removed atraumatically.
- Implants ideally should be placed in IRS with no contact of buccal bone, leaving gaps of 2 mm or greater to fill with blood or graft material and ultimately new bone; an exception to this rule is where a wide implant is needed to manage a site with a type C septum.
- Implants are best submerged 1 to 2 mm subcrestally to the lower of the buccal or lingual/palatal cortical plates.
- Peri-implant gaps need not always be grafted, but whether filled with graft or just the patient's blood, gaps should be sheltered by adding large-diameter or custom healing abutments, assuming of course adequate implant stability (> 35 Ncm).

References

1. Scheuber S, Hicklin S, Brägger U. Implants versus short-span fixed bridges: Survival, complications, patients' benefits. A systematic review on economic aspects. Clin Oral Implants Res 2012;23(suppl 6):50–62.
2. Aghaloo TL, Mardirosian M, Delgado B. Controversies in implant surgery. Oral Maxillofac Surg Clin North Am 2017;29:525–535.
3. Grant BT, Pancko FX, Kraut RA. Outcomes of placing short dental implants in the posterior mandible: A retrospective study of 124 cases. J Oral Maxillofac Surg 2009;67:713–717.
4. Levin L, Laviv A, Schwartz-Arad D. Long-term success of implants replacing a single molar. J Periodontol 2006;77:1528–1532.
5. Polizzi G, Rangert B, Lekholm U, Gualini F, Lindström H. Brånemark System Wide Platform implants for single molar replacement: Clinical evaluation of prospective and retrospective materials. Clin Implant Dent Relat Res 2000;2:61–69.
6. Tolstunov L. Implant zones of the jaws: Implant location and related success rate. J Oral Implantol 2007;33:211–220.
7. Crespi R, Capparè P, Crespi G, Gastaldi G, Gherlone EF. Delayed implants outcome in maxillary molar region. Clin Implant Dent Relat Res 2017;19:261–267.
8. Koo KT, Wikesjö UM, Park JY, et al. Evaluation of single-tooth implants in the second molar region: A 5-year life-table analysis of a retrospective study. J Periodontol 2010;81:1242–1249.
9. Wilson TG, Weber HP. Classification of and therapy for areas of deficient bony housing prior to dental implant placement. Int J Periodontics Restorative Dent 1993;13:451–459.
10. Zitzmann NU, Naef R, Schärer P. Resorbable versus nonresorbable membranes in combination with Bio-Oss for guided bone regeneration [published correction appears in Int J Oral Maxillofac Implants 1998;13:576]. Int J Oral Maxillofac Implants 1997;12:844–852.
11. Hämmerle CH, Chen ST, Wilson TG Jr. Consensus statements and recommended clinical procedures regarding the placement of implants in extraction sockets. Int J Oral Maxillofac Implants 2004;19(suppl):26–28.
12. Esposito M, Zucchelli G, Cannizzaro G, et al. Immediate, immediate-delayed (6 weeks) and delayed (4 months) post-extractive single implants: 1-year post-loading data from a randomised controlled trial. Eur J Oral Implantol 2017;10:11–26.
13. Bhola M, Neely AL, Kolhatkar S. Immediate implant placement: Clinical decisions, advantages, and disadvantages. J Prosthodont 2008;17:576–581.
14. Suárez-López Del Amo F, Lin GH, Monje A, Galindo-Moreno P, Wang HL. Influence of soft tissue thickness on peri-implant marginal bone loss: A systematic review and meta-analysis. J Periodontol 2016;87:690–699.
15. Linkevicius T, Apse P, Grybauskas S, Puisys A. The influence of soft tissue thickness on crestal bone changes around implants: A 1-year prospective controlled clinical trial. Int J Oral Maxillofac Implants 2009;24:712–719.
16. Puisys A, Linkevicius T. The influence of mucosal tissue thickening on crestal bone stability around bone-level implants. A prospective controlled clinical trial. Clin Oral Implants Res 2015; 26:123–129.
17. Schmidt JC, Sahrmann P, Weiger R, Schmidlin PR, Walter C. Biologic width dimensions: A systematic review. J Clin Periodontol 2013;40:493–504.
18. Berglundh T, Lindhe J. Dimension of the periimplant mucosa. Biological width revisited. J Clin Periodontol 1996;23:971–973.
19. van Eekeren P, van Elsas P, Tahmaseb A, Wismeijer D. The influence of initial mucosal thickness on crestal bone change in similar macrogeometrical implants: A prospective randomized clinical trial. Clin Oral Implants Res 2017;28:214–218.
20. Garaicoa-Pazmino C, Mendonça G, Ou A, et al. Impact of mucosal phenotype on marginal bone levels around tissue level implants: A prospective controlled trial. J Periodontol 2021;92:771–783.
21. Dawson A, Chen S (eds). The SAC Classification in Implant Dentistry. Berlin: Quintessence, 2009.
22. Tan WL, Wong TL, Wong MC, Lang NP. A systematic review of post-extractional alveolar hard and soft tissue dimensional changes in humans. Clin Oral Implants Res 2012;23(suppl 5): 1–21.
23. Soydan SS, Cubuk S, Oguz Y, Uckan S. Are success and survival rates of early implant placement higher than immediate implant placement? Int J Oral Maxillofac Surg 2013;42:511–515.
24. Sanz I, Garcia-Gargallo M, Herrera D, Martin C, Figuero E, Sanz M. Surgical protocols for early implant placement in post-extraction sockets: A systematic review. Clin Oral Implants Res 2012;23(suppl 5):67–79.
25. Naenni N, Bienz SP, Muñoz F, Hämmerle CHF, Jung RE, Thoma DS. Volumetric changes following ridge preservation or spontaneous healing and early implant placement with simultaneous guided bone regeneration. J Clin Periodontol 2018;45:484–494.
26. Lim HC, Seo S, Thoma DS, Park JC, Hong JY, Shin SY. Late implant placement following ridge preservation versus early implant placement: A pilot randomized clinical trial for periodontally compromised non-molar extraction sites. J Clin Periodontol 2020;47:247–256.
27. Schropp L, Wenzel A, Kostopoulos L, Karring T. Bone healing and soft tissue contour changes following single-tooth extraction: A clinical and radiographic 12-month prospective study. Int J Periodontics Restorative Dent 2003;23:313–323.
28. Covani U, Ricci M, Bozzolo G, Mangano F, Zini A, Barone A. Analysis of the pattern of the alveolar ridge remodelling following single tooth extraction. Clin Oral Implants Res 2011;22:820–825.
29. Matarasso S, Salvi GE, Iorio Siciliano V, Cafiero C, Blasi A, Lang NP. Dimensional ridge alterations following immediate implant placement in molar extraction sites: A six-month prospective cohort study with surgical re-entry. Clin Oral Implants Res 2009;20:1092–1098.
30. Botticelli D, Berglundh T, Lindhe J. Hard-tissue alterations following immediate implant placement in extraction sites. J Clin Periodontol 2004;31:820–828.
31. Ferrus J, Cecchinato D, Pjetursson EB, Lang NP, Sanz M, Lindhe J. Factors influencing ridge alterations following immediate implant placement into extraction sockets. Clin Oral Implants Res 2010;21:22–29.
32. Kinaia BM, Shah M, Neely AL, Goodis HE. Crestal bone level changes around immediately placed implants: A systematic review and meta-analyses with at least 12 months' follow-up after functional loading. J Periodontol 2014;85:1537–1548.
33. Abdelhafez RS, Alhabashneh R, Khader Y, Hijazi M, Jarah M. Dimensional changes in alveolar ridge following extraction of teeth in the maxillary premolar area in subjects with thick and thin gingival biotypes: A pilot study. Int J Periodontics Restorative Dent 2016;36:431–436.
34. Chen Z, Li J, Wang HL, Yu H. Initial bone volume changes after immediate implant placement associated with filling the gap using bovine bone in molar sites. Int J Oral Maxillofac Implants 2019;34:521–528.

35. Covani U, Cornelini R, Barone A. Bucco-lingual bone remodeling around implants placed into immediate extraction sockets: A case series. J Periodontol 2003;74:268–273.
36. Brugnami F, Caiazzo A. Efficacy evaluation of a new buccal bone plate preservation technique: A pilot study. Int J Periodontics Restorative Dent 2011;31:67–73.
37. Naenni N, Bienz SP, Jung RE, Hämmerle CHF, Thoma DS. Histologic analyses of flapless ridge preservation in sockets with buccal dehiscence defects using two alloplastic bone graft substitutes. Clin Oral Investig 2019;23:3589–3599.
38. Vignoletti F, Matesanz P, Rodrigo D, Figuero E, Martin C, Sanz M. Surgical protocols for ridge preservation after tooth extraction. A systematic review. Clin Oral Implants Res 2012; 23(suppl 5):22–38.
39. Werbitt MJ, Goldberg PV. The immediate implant: Bone preservation and bone regeneration. Int J Periodontics Restorative Dent 1992;12:206–217.
40. Elian N, Cho SC, Froum S, Smith RB, Tarnow DP. A simplified socket classification and repair technique. Pract Proced Aesthet Dent 2007;19:99–106.
41. Hu C, Gong T, Lin W, Yuan Q, Man Y. Immediate implant placement into posterior sockets with or without buccal bone dehiscence defects: A retrospective cohort study. J Dent 2017;65:95–100.
42. Krump JL, Barnett BG. The immediate implant: A treatment alternative. Int J Oral Maxillofac Implants 1991;6:19–23.
43. Beagle JR. The immediate placement of endosseous dental implants in fresh extraction sites. Dent Clin North Am 2006;50: 375–389.
44. Wagenberg B, Froum SJ. A retrospective study of 1925 consecutively placed immediate implants from 1988 to 2004. Int J Oral Maxillofac Implants 2006;21:71–80.
45. Fugazzotto PA. Implant placement at the time of mandibular molar extraction: Description of technique and preliminary results of 341 cases. J Periodontol 2008;79:737–747.
46. Fugazzotto PA. Implant placement at the time of maxillary molar extraction: Treatment protocols and report of results. J Periodontol 2008;79:216–223.
47. Becker W, Becker BE. Replacement of maxillary and mandibular molars with single endosseous implant restorations: A retrospective study. J Prosthet Dent 1995;74:51–55.
48. Araújo MG, Sukekava F, Wennström JL, Lindhe J. Tissue modeling following implant placement in fresh extraction sockets. Clin Oral Implants Res 2006;17:615–624.
49. Summers RB. A new concept in maxillary implant surgery: The osteotome technique. Compendium 1994;15:152–162.
50. Summers RB. The osteotome technique: Part 3—Less invasive methods of elevating the sinus floor. Compendium 1994;15: 698–710.
51. Acocella A, Bertolai R, Sacco R. Modified insertion technique for immediate implant placement into fresh extraction socket in the first maxillary molar sites: A 3-year prospective study. Implant Dent 2010;19:220–228.
52. da Rosa JCM, Pértile de Oliveira Rosa AC, Huwais S. Use of the immediate dentoalveolar restoration technique combined with osseodensification in periodontally compromised extraction sites. Int J Periodontics Restorative Dent 2019;39:527–534.
53. Araújo MG, da Silva JCC, de Mendonça AF, Lindhe J. Ridge alterations following grafting of fresh extraction sockets in man. A randomized clinical trial. Clin Oral Implants Res 2015;26:407–412.
54. Avila-Ortiz G, Elangovan S, Kramer KW, Blanchette D, Dawson DV. Effect of alveolar ridge preservation after tooth extraction: A systematic review and meta-analysis. J Dent Res 2014;93:950–958.
55. Barone A, Toti P, Piattelli A, Iezzi G, Derchi G, Covani U. Extraction socket healing in humans after ridge preservation techniques: Comparison between flapless and flapped procedures in a randomized clinical trial. J Periodontol 2014;85:14–23.
56. Hämmerle CH, Araújo MG, Simion M; Osteology Consensus Group 2011. Evidence-based knowledge on the biology and treatment of extraction sockets [published correction appears in Clin Oral Implants Res 2012;23:641]. Clin Oral Implants Res 2012;23(suppl 5):80–82.
57. Lee J, Lee JB, Koo KT, Seol YJ, Lee YM. Flap management in alveolar ridge preservation: A systematic review and meta-analysis. Int J Oral Maxillofac Implants 2018;33:613–621.
58. Tomasi C, Donati M, Cecchinato D, Szathvary I, Corrà E, Lindhe J. Effect of socket grafting with deproteinized bone mineral: An RCT on dimensional alterations after 6 months. Clin Oral Implants Res 2018;29:435–442.
59. Barone A, Ricci M, Tonelli P, Santini S, Covani U. Tissue changes of extraction sockets in humans: A comparison of spontaneous healing vs. ridge preservation with secondary soft tissue healing. Clin Oral Implants Res 2013;24:1231–1237.
60. Dahlin C, Linde A, Gottlow J, Nyman S. Healing of bone defects by guided tissue regeneration. Plast Reconstr Surg 1988;81:672–676.
61. Urban T, Kostopoulos L, Wenzel A. Immediate implant placement in molar regions: A 12-month prospective, randomized follow-up study. Clin Oral Implants Res 2012;23:1389–1397.
62. Natto ZS. Flapless extraction and immediate implant placed into a mandibular molar site: A clinical case report and 5-year follow-up. J Oral Implantol 2019;45:159–164.
63. Sohn DS, Huang B, Kim J, Park I, Park CC. Utilization of autologous concentrated growth factors (CGF) enriched bone graft matrix (sticky bone) and CGF-enriched fibrin membrane in implant dentistry. J Implant Adv Clin Dent 2015;7(10):11–29.
64. Waasdorp J, Feldman S. Bone regeneration around immediate implants utilizing a dense polytetrafluoroethylene membrane without primary closure: A report of 3 cases. J Oral Implantol 2013;39:355–361.
65. Bartee BK. The use of high-density polytetrafluoroethylene membrane to treat osseous defects: Clinical reports. Implant Dent 1995;4:21–26.
66. Barboza EP, Stutz B, Ferreira VF, Carvalho W. Guided bone regeneration using nonexpanded polytetrafluoroethylene membranes in preparation for dental implant placements: A report of 420 cases. Implant Dent 2010;19:2–7.
67. Smith RB, Tarnow DP. Classification of molar extraction sites for immediate dental implant placement: Technical note. Int J Oral Maxillofac Implants 2013;28:911–916.
68. Al-Hezaimi K, Rudek I, Al-Hamdan KS, Javed F, Nooh N, Wang HL. Efficacy of using a dual layer of membrane (dPTFE placed over collagen) for ridge preservation in fresh extraction sites: A micro-computed tomographic study in dogs. Clin Oral Implants Res 2013;24:1152–1157.
69. Santos FA, Pochapski MT, Martins MC, Zenóbio EG, Spolidoro LC, Marcantonio E Jr. Comparison of biomaterial implants in the dental socket: Histological analysis in dogs. Clin Implant Dent Relat Res 2010;12:18–25.
70. Anwandter A, Bohmann S, Nally M, Castro AB, Quirynen M, Pinto N. Dimensional changes of the post extraction alveolar ridge, preserved with leukocyte- and platelet rich fibrin: A clinical pilot study. J Dent 2016;52:23–29.
71. Rutkowski JL, Johnson DA, Radio NM, Fennell JW. Platelet rich plasma to facilitate wound healing following tooth extraction. J Oral Implantol 2010;36:11–23.

72. Temmerman A, Vandessel J, Castro A, et al. The use of leucocyte and platelet-rich fibrin in socket management and ridge preservation: A split-mouth, randomized, controlled clinical trial. J Clin Periodontol 2016;43:990–999.
73. Canellas JVDS, Ritto FG, Figueredo CMDS, et al. Histomorphometric evaluation of different grafting materials used for alveolar ridge preservation: A systematic review and network meta-analysis. Int J Oral Maxillofac Surg 2020;49:797–810.
74. Lin CY, Chen Z, Pan WL, Wang HL. Effect of platelet-rich fibrin on ridge preservation in perspective of bone healing: A systematic review and meta-analysis. Int J Oral Maxillofac Implants 2019;34:845–854.
75. Schwartz-Arad D, Grossman Y, Chaushu G. The clinical effectiveness of implants placed immediately into fresh extraction sites of molar teeth. J Periodontol 2000;71:839–844.
76. Fontana F, Maschera E, Rocchietta I, Simion M. Clinical classification of complications in guided bone regeneration procedures by means of a nonresorbable membrane. Int J Periodontics Restorative Dent 2011;31:265–273.
77. Strietzel FP, Reichart PA, Kale A, Kulkarni M, Wegner B, Küchler I. Smoking interferes with the prognosis of dental implant treatment: A systematic review and meta-analysis. J Clin Periodontol 2007;34:523–544.
78. Bezerra Ferreira JD, Rodrigues JA, Piattelli A, Iezzi G, Gehrke SA, Shibli JA. The effect of cigarette smoking on early osseointegration of dental implants: A prospective controlled study. Clin Oral Implants Res 2016;27:1123–1128.
79. Deng F, Zhang H, Zhang H, Shao H, He Q, Zhang P. A comparison of clinical outcomes for implants placed in fresh extraction sockets versus healed sites in periodontally compromised patients: A 1-year follow-up report. Int J Oral Maxillofac Implants 2010;25:1036–1040.
80. Sgolastra F, Petrucci A, Severino M, Gatto R, Monaco A. Periodontitis, implant loss and peri-implantitis. A meta-analysis. Clin Oral Implants Res 2015;26:e8–e16.
81. Lin CY, Chen Z, Pan WL, Wang HL. Is history of periodontal disease still a negative risk indicator for peri-implant health under supportive post-implant treatment coverage? A systematic review and meta-analysis. Int J Oral Maxillofac Implants 2020; 35:52–62.
82. Pandolfi A, Rinaldo F, Pasqualotto D, Sorrentino F, La Torre G, Guerra F. A retrospective cohort study on peri-implant complications in implants up to 10 years of functional loading in periodontally compromised patients [published online ahead of print, 2019 Dec 20]. J Periodontol 2019.
83. Yip JK, Borrell LN, Cho SC, Francisco H, Tarnow DP. Association between oral bisphosphonate use and dental implant failure among middle-aged women. J Clin Periodontol 2012;39:408–414.
84. Mozzati M, Arata V, Giacomello M, et al. Failure risk estimates after dental implants placement associated with plasma rich in growth factor-Endoret in osteoporotic women under bisphosphonate therapy. J Craniofac Surg 2015;26:749–755.
85. Naujokat H, Kunzendorf B, Wiltfang J. Dental implants and diabetes mellitus: A systematic review. Int J Implant Dent 2016;2:5.
86. Claudy MP, Miguens SA Jr, Celeste RK, Camara Parente R, Hernandez PA, da Silva AN Jr. Time interval after radiotherapy and dental implant failure: Systematic review of observational studies and meta-analysis. Clin Implant Dent Relat Res 2015;17:402–411.
87. Aragon-Ching JB, Ning YM, Chen CC, et al. Higher incidence of osteonecrosis of the jaw (ONJ) in patients with metastatic castration resistant prostate cancer treated with anti-angiogenic agents. Cancer Invest 2009;27:221–226.
88. Chrcanovic BR, Kisch J, Albrektsson T, Wennerberg A. Bruxism and dental implant failures: A multilevel mixed effects parametric survival analysis approach. J Oral Rehabil 2016;43:813–823.
89. Choukroun J, Khoury G, Khoury F, et al. Two neglected biologic risk factors in bone grafting and implantology: High low-density lipoprotein cholesterol and low serum vitamin D. J Oral Implantol 2014;40:110–114.
90. Belluci MM, Giro G, Del Barrio RAL, Pereira RMR, Marcantonio E Jr, Orrico SRP. Effects of magnesium intake deficiency on bone metabolism and bone tissue around osseointegrated implants. Clin Oral Implants Res 2011;22:716–721.
91. Kim H, Shin MH, Yoon SJ, et al. Low serum 25-hydroxyvitamin D levels, tooth loss, and the prevalence of severe periodontitis in Koreans aged 50 years and older. J Periodontal Implant Sci 2020;50:368–378.
92. Maier GS, Horas K, Seeger JB, Roth KE, Kurth AA, Maus U. Is there an association between periprosthetic joint infection and low vitamin D levels? Int Orthop 2014;38:1499–1504.
93. Hegde V, Dworsky EM, Stavrakis AI, et al. Single-dose, preoperative vitamin-D supplementation decreases infection in a mouse model of periprosthetic joint infection. J Bone Joint Surg Am 2017;99:1737–1744.
94. Kelly J, Lin A, Wang CJ, Park S, Nishimura I. Vitamin D and bone physiology: Demonstration of vitamin D deficiency in an implant osseointegration rat model. J Prosthodont 2009;18: 473–478.
95. Dvorak G, Fügl A, Watzek G, Tangl S, Pokorny P, Gruber R. Impact of dietary vitamin D on osseointegration in the ovariectomized rat. Clin Oral Implants Res 2012;23:1308–1313.
96. Froum S, Casanova L, Byrne S, Cho SC. Risk assessment before extraction for immediate implant placement in the posterior mandible: A computerized tomographic scan study. J Periodontol 2011;82:395–402.
97. Renouard F, Amalberti R, Renouard E. Are "human factors" the primary cause of complications in the field of implant dentistry? Int J Oral Maxillofac Implants 2017;32:e55–e61.
98. Huang RY, Cochran DL, Cheng WC, et al. Risk of lingual plate perforation for virtual immediate implant placement in the posterior mandible: A computer simulation study. J Am Dent Assoc 2015;146:735–742.
99. Rao W, Benzi R. Single mandibular first molar implants with flapless guided surgery and immediate function: Preliminary clinical and radiographic results of a prospective study [published correction appears in J Prosthet Dent 2008;99:167]. J Prosthet Dent 2007;97(6 suppl):S3–S14.
100. Rousseau P. Flapless and traditional dental implant surgery: An open, retrospective comparative study. J Oral Maxillofac Surg 2010;68:2299–2306.
101. Maia LP, Reino DM, Novaes Junior AB, et al. Influence of periodontal biotype on buccal bone remodeling after tooth extraction using the flapless approach with a xenograft: A histomorphometric and fluorescence study in small dogs. Clin Implant Dent Relat Res 2015;17(suppl 1):e221–e235.
102. Pluemsakunthai W, Le B, Kasugai S. Effect of buccal gap distance on alveolar ridge alteration after immediate implant placement: A microcomputed tomographic and morphometric analysis in dogs. Implant Dent 2015;24:70–76.
103. Sharma SD, Vidya B, Alexander M, Deshmukh S. Periotome as an aid to atraumatic extraction: A comparative double blind randomized controlled trial. J Maxillofac Oral Surg 2015;14:611–615.
104. Wang HL, Kiyonobu K, Neiva RF. Socket augmentation: Rationale and technique. Implant Dent 2004;13:286–296.
105. Lazzara RJ. Immediate implant placement into extraction sites: Surgical and restorative advantages. Int J Periodontics Restorative Dent 1989;9:332–343.

106. Vandeweghe S, Ferreira D, Vermeersch L, Mariën M, De Bruyn H. Long-term retrospective follow-up of turned and moderately rough implants in the edentulous jaw. Clin Oral Implants Res 2016;27:421–426.
107. Madani E, Smeets R, Freiwald E, et al. Impact of different placement depths on the crestal bone level of immediate versus delayed placed platform-switched implants. J Craniomaxillofac Surg 2018;46:1139–1146.
108. Hattingh AC, De Bruyn H, Ackermann A, Vandeweghe S. Immediate placement of ultrawide-diameter implants in molar sockets: Description of a recommended technique. Int J Periodontics Restorative Dent 2018;38:17–23.
109. Froum SJ, Cho SC, Suzuki T, Yu P, Corby P, Khouly I. Epicrestal and subcrestal placement of platform-switched implants: 18 month-result of a randomized, controlled, split-mouth, prospective clinical trial. Clin Oral Implants Res 2018;29:353–366.
110. Rodriguez-Tizcareño MH, Bravo-Flores C. Anatomically guided implant site preparation technique at molar sites. Implant Dent 2009;18:393–401.
111. Rebele SF, Zuhr O, Hürzeler MB. Pre-extractive interradicular implant bed preparation: Case presentations of a novel approach to immediate implant placement at multirooted molar sites. Int J Periodontics Restorative Dent 2013;33:89–96.
112. Scarano A. Traditional postextractive implant site preparation compared with pre-extractive interradicular implant bed preparation in the mandibular molar region, using an ultrasonic device: A randomized pilot study. Int J Oral Maxillofac Implants 2017;32:655–660.
113. Huwais S, Meyer EG. A novel osseous densification approach in implant osteotomy preparation to increase biomechanical primary stability, bone mineral density, and bone-to-implant contact. Int J Oral Maxillofac Implants 2017;32:27–36.
114. Chu SJ. Implant designs in 2020: Current state of the art addresses primary stability. Compend Contin Educ Dent 2020;41: 432–434.
115. Malkoç S, Basçiftçi FA, Nur M, Catalbas B. Maxillary and mandibular mesiodistal tooth sizes among different malocclusions in a sample of the Turkish population. Eur J Orthod 2011;33: 592–596.
116. Atieh MA, Alsabeeha N, Duncan WJ. Stability of tapered and parallel-walled dental implants: A systematic review and meta-analysis. Clin Implant Dent Relat Res 2018;20:634–645.
117. Vervaeke S, Dierens M, Besseler J, De Bruyn H. The influence of initial soft tissue thickness on peri-implant bone remodeling. Clin Implant Dent Relat Res 2014;16:238–247.
118. Schrott AR, Jimenez M, Hwang JW, Fiorellini J, Weber HP. Five-year evaluation of the influence of keratinized mucosa on peri-implant soft-tissue health and stability around implants supporting full-arch mandibular fixed prostheses. Clin Oral Implants Res 2009;20:1170–1177.
119. Adibrad M, Shahabuei M, Sahabi M. Significance of the width of keratinized mucosa on the health status of the supporting tissue around implants supporting overdentures. J Oral Implantol 2009;35:232–237.
120. Bouri A Jr, Bissada N, Al-Zahrani MS, Faddoul F, Nouneh I. Width of keratinized gingiva and the health status of the supporting tissues around dental implants. Int J Oral Maxillofac Implants 2008;23:323–326.
121. Lindhe J, Berglundh T. The interface between the mucosa and the implant. Periodontol 2000 1998;17:47–54.
122. Gharpure AS, Latimer JM, Aljofi FE, Kahng JH, Daubert DM. Role of thin gingival phenotype and inadequate keratinized mucosa width (<2 mm) as risk indicators for peri-implantitis and peri-implant mucositis. J Periodontol 2021;92:1687–1696.
123. Pico A, Martín-Lancharro P, Caneiro L, Nóvoa L, Batalla P, Blanco J. Influence of abutment height and implant depth position on interproximal peri-implant bone in sites with thin mucosa: A 1-year randomized clinical trial. Clin Oral Implants Res 2019;30:595–602.
124. Lazzara RJ, Porter SS. Platform switching: A new concept in implant dentistry for controlling postrestorative crestal bone levels. Int J Periodontics Restorative Dent 2006;26:9–17.
125. Linkevicius T, Apse P, Grybauskas S, Puisys A. Influence of thin mucosal tissues on crestal bone stability around implants with platform switching: A 1-year pilot study. J Oral Maxillofac Surg 2010;68:2272–2277.
126. Saito H, Chu SJ, Zamzok J, et al. Flapless postextraction socket implant placement: The effects of a platform switch-designed implant on peri-implant soft tissue thickness—A prospective study. Int J Periodontics Restorative Dent 2018;38(suppl):s9–s15.
127. Rojo E, Stroppa G, Sanz-Martin I, Gonzalez-Martín O, Alemany AS, Nart J. Soft tissue volume gain around dental implants using autogenous subepithelial connective tissue grafts harvested from the lateral palate or tuberosity area. A randomized controlled clinical study. J Clin Periodontol 2018;45:495–503.
128. Puisys A, Vindasiute E, Linkevciene L, Linkevicius T. The use of acellular dermal matrix membrane for vertical soft tissue augmentation during submerged implant placement: A case series. Clin Oral Implants Res 2015;26:465–470.
129. Oh SL, Masri RM, Williams DA, Ji C, Romberg E. Free gingival grafts for implants exhibiting lack of keratinized mucosa: A prospective controlled randomized clinical study. J Clin Periodontol 2017;44:195–203.
130. Cairo F, Barbato L, Tonelli P, Batalocco G, Pagavino G, Nieri M. Xenogeneic collagen matrix versus connective tissue graft for buccal soft tissue augmentation at implant site. A randomized, controlled clinical trial. J Clin Periodontol 2017;44:769–776.
131. Zeltner M, Jung RE, Hämmerle CH, Hüsler J, Thoma DS. Randomized controlled clinical study comparing a volume-stable collagen matrix to autogenous connective tissue grafts for soft tissue augmentation at implant sites: Linear volumetric soft tissue changes up to 3 months. J Clin Periodontol 2017;44:446–453.
132. Lin CY, Chen Z, Pan WL, Wang HL. Impact of timing on soft tissue augmentation during implant treatment: A systematic review and meta-analysis. Clin Oral Implants Res 2018;29:508–521.
133. Cafiero C, Annibali S, Gherlone E, et al. Immediate transmucosal implant placement in molar extraction sites: A 12-month prospective multicenter cohort study. Clin Oral Implants Res 2008;19:476–482.
134. Araújo MG, Linder E, Lindhe J. Bio-Oss collagen in the buccal gap at immediate implants: A 6-month study in the dog. Clin Oral Implants Res 2011;22:1–8.
135. Deporter D, Khoshkhounejad AA, Khoshkhounejad N, Ketabi M. A new classification of peri implant gaps based on gap location (a case series of 210 immediate implants). Dent Res J (Isfahan) 2021;18:29–39.
136. Smith RB, Tarnow DP, Sarnachiaro G. Immediate placement of dental implants in molar extraction sockets: An 11-year retrospective analysis. Compend Contin Educ Dent 2019;40:166–170.
137. Gober DD, Fien MJ. Flapless extraction socket healing around an immediate implant placed into a mandibular molar site without the use of regenerative materials: A case report. Int J Periodontics Restorative Dent 2016;36:e26–e32.

138. Amato F, Polara G. Immediate implant placement in single-tooth molar extraction sockets: A 1- to 6-year retrospective clinical study. Int J Periodontics Restorative Dent 2018;38:495–501.
139. Akin R. A new concept in maintaining the emergence profile in immediate posterior implant placement: The anatomic harmony abutment. J Oral Maxillofac Surg 2016;74:2385–2392.
140. Bersani E, Coppede AR, de Paula Pinto Prata HH. Immediate loading of implants placed in fresh extraction sockets in the molar area with flapless and graftless procedures: A case series. Int J Periodontics Restorative Dent 2010;30:291–299.
141. Barndt P, Zhang H, Liu F. Immediate loading: From biology to biomechanics. Report of the Committee on Research in Fixed Prosthodontics of the American Academy of Fixed Prosthodontics. J Prosthet Dent 2015;113:96–107.
142. Landsberg CJ. Implementing socket seal surgery as a socket preservation technique for pontic site development: Surgical steps revisited: A report of two cases. J Periodontol 2008;79:945–954.
143. Johnson TM, Berridge JP, Baron D. Protocol for maintaining alveolar ridge volume in molar immediate implant sites. Clin Adv Periodontics 2017;7:207–214.
144. Zafiropoulos GG, Kasaj A, Hoffmann O. Immediate implant placement in fresh mandibular molar extraction socket: 8-year results. A case report. J Oral Implantol 2010;36:145–151.
145. Taschieri S, Lolato A, Ofer M, Testori T, Francetti L, Del Fabbro M. Immediate post-extraction implants with or without pure platelet-rich plasma: A 5-year follow-up study. Oral Maxillofac Surg 2017;21:147–157.
146. Al Nashar A, Yakoob H. Evaluation of the use of plasma rich in growth factors with immediate implant placement in periodontally compromised extraction sites: A controlled prospective study. Int J Oral Maxillofac Surg 2015;44:507–512.
147. S Medikeri R, Meharwade V, M Wate P, V Lele S. Effect of PRF and allograft use on immediate implants at extraction sockets with periapical infection: Clinical and cone beam CT findings. Bull Tokyo Dent Coll 2018;59:97–109.
148. Zhou J, Li X, Sun X, et al. Bone regeneration around immediate placed implant of molar teeth with autologous platelet-rich fibrin: Two case reports. Medicine (Baltimore) 2018;97(44):e13058.
149. Atieh MA, Payne AG, Duncan WJ, de Silva RK, Cullinan MP. Immediate placement or immediate restoration/loading of single implants for molar tooth replacement: A systematic review and meta-analysis. Int J Oral Maxillofac Implants 2010;25:401–415.
150. Ketabi M, Deporter D, Atenafu EG. A systematic review of outcomes following immediate molar implant placement based on recently published studies. Clin Implant Dent Relat Res 2016;18:1084–1094.
151. Mello CC, Lemos CAA, Verri FR, Dos Santos DM, Goiato MC, Pellizzer EP. Immediate implant placement into fresh extraction sockets versus delayed implants into healed sockets: A systematic review and meta-analysis. Int J Oral Maxillofac Surg 2017;46:1162–1177.
152. Antetomaso J, Kumar S. Survival rate of delayed implants placed in healed extraction sockets is significantly higher than that of immediate implants placed in fresh extraction sockets. J Evid Based Dent Pract 2018;18:76–78.
153. Spray JR, Black CG, Morris HF, Ochi S. The influence of bone thickness on facial marginal bone response: Stage 1 placement through stage 2 uncovering. Ann Periodontol 2000;5:119–128.
154. Qahash M, Susin C, Polimeni G, Hall J, Wikesjö UM. Bone healing dynamics at buccal peri-implant sites. Clin Oral Implants Res 2008;19:166–172.
155. Ormianer Z, Palti A, Demiralp B, Heller G, Lewinstein I, Khayat PG. Implant-supported first molar restorations: Correlation of finite element analysis with clinical outcomes. Int J Oral Maxillofac Implants 2012;27:e1–e12.
156. Canellas JVDS, Medeiros PJD, Figueredo CMDS, Fischer RG, Ritto FG. Which is the best choice after tooth extraction, immediate implant placement or delayed placement with alveolar ridge preservation? A systematic review and meta-analysis. J Craniomaxillofac Surg 2019;47:1793–1802.
157. Lekholm U, Zarb G. Patient selection and preparation. In: Branemark P-I, Zarb G, Albrektsson T (eds). Tissue-Integrated Prostheses: Osseointegration in Clinical Dentistry. Chicago: Quintessence, 1985:199–209.
158. Annibali S, Bignozzi I, Iacovazzi L, La Monaca G, Cristalli MP. Immediate, early, and late implant placement in first-molar sites: A retrospective case series. Int J Oral Maxillofac Implants 2011;26:1108–1122.
159. Smith DE, Zarb GA. Criteria for success of osseointegrated endosseous implants. J Prosthet Dent 1989;62:567–572.
160. Roos-Jansåker AM, Lindahl C, Renvert H, Renvert S. Nine- to fourteen-year follow-up of implant treatment. Part II: Presence of peri-implant lesions. J Clin Periodontol 2006;33:290–295.
161. Papaspyridakos P, Chen CJ, Singh M, Weber HP, Gallucci GO. Success criteria in implant dentistry: A systematic review. J Dent Res 2012;91:242–248.
162. Galindo-Moreno P, León-Cano A, Ortega-Oller I, Monje A, O Valle F, Catena A. Marginal bone loss as success criterion in implant dentistry: Beyond 2 mm. Clin Oral Implants Res 2015;26:e28–e34.

2

RADIOGRAPHIC SCREENING FOR IMMEDIATE MOLAR IMPLANT PLACEMENT

Stuart J. Froum
Viraj Patel
Martin Leung
Buddhapoom Wangsrimongkol
Klenise Paranhos
Maryse Manasse

Immediate implant placement at fresh extraction sites of single-rooted teeth was first described in 1989, and subsequently shown to be an effective means to replace hopeless teeth with implant-supported restorations.[1,2] Others took the leap to placing immediate molar implants (IMIs) with similarly good results.[3–7] Indeed, systematic literature reviews with meta-analyses suggested that IMIs can have cumulative survival rates similar to those with implants placed in healed molar sites.[8,9] Most recently, an 11-year retrospective report for IMIs showed an overall survival rate of 97.3% for 300 such implants.[10] Clearly, this is good news for clinicians and patients alike with the obvious advantages of reducing the number of surgical procedures, patient visits, and time required for treatment.[11] Naturally, the general and oral health of the patient will be important for a successful outcome, but local factors need attention as well. The initial stability of the implant is crucial, and this will depend on the bone quantity and quality as well as the condition and amount of interradicular septum (IRS) bone remaining. The feasibility and success of treatment also will hinge on the height of native bone remaining between an intended mandibular IMI apex and the inferior mandibular neurovascular canal. Similarly, in the maxilla, outcomes will depend on the proximity and height of the bone in relation to the maxillary sinus.

Without exception, radiographs are essential in helping to evaluate the above factors prior to surgery. Traditional imaging modalities can include periapical, bitewing, occlusal, cephalometric, and panoramic radiography as well as transtomography and digital radiography. Advanced technologies include magnetic resonance imaging (MRI), conventional tomography, computed tomography (CT), and cone beam computed tomography (CBCT). Radiographs most commonly used in current practice include periapical, panoramic, CT, and CBCT, all of which are evaluated in Table 2-1.[11–22] These diagnostic images will allow the clinician to assess bone volume, structure, and density; topography; and the relationships to important anatomical structures such as nerves, vessels,

TABLE 2-1 Accuracy, advantages, and limitations of conventional and advanced imaging techniques[11–22]

TYPE OF RADIOGRAPH	ACCURACY	ADVANTAGES	LIMITATIONS
Periapical	• Accuracy can vary according to exposure and angle, with variations up to 20 degrees[12]	• Good resolution[13] • Limited radiation (0.5–2 μSv)[13]; mean: 1 μSv • Evaluation of dental disease (including caries and periodontal disease), bone levels, fractures in teeth, and possible internal/external resorption[14]	• 2D image; no bone width evaluation and no ability to locate vital anatomical structures in 3D[15] • No bone density evaluation[13] • Technique sensitive (superimposition of structures)[13] • Limited field of view[15]
Panoramic	• Mean horizontal magnification error: 31.4%[11] • Mean vertical magnification error: 30.6%[11]	• Good overview for screening of patients[14] • Lower radiation (5–20 μSv)[13]; mean: 9 μSv[16] • Demonstrates presence/absence of pathology[14]	• Distortion/error of ~30%[11] • 2D image; no bone width evaluation and no ability to locate vital anatomical structures in 3D[11] • Limited use in bone density evaluation[13] • Technique sensitive (patient positioning/movement)[14,17]
CT scans	• Mean horizontal magnification error: 0%–6%[11] • Mean vertical magnification error: 0%–4%[11]	• Increased accuracy compared with periapical and panoramic radiographs[11] • Higher resolution and better contrast sensitivity[14] • Ability to produce 3D reconstructions, simulate implant placement, and localize anatomy (IAN/sinus membrane) with additional software[14] • Can aid in fabricating surgical guides[18]	• Higher radiation (80–1,600 μSv)[13]; mean: 300 μSv • Equipment space requirements and cost[14] • Production of image artifacts (ie, motion and beam hardening)[14]
CBCT scans	• 98%–99% accuracy[19]	• Increased accuracy[20] • High resolution[13,20] • Quantitative assessment of bone quality and density[21] • Decreased scan time and radiation compared with CT[15] • Diagnostic quality images to help identify pathology[20–22] • Ability to produce 3D reconstructions, simulate implant placement, and localize anatomy (IAN/sinus membrane) with additional software[22] • Can aid in fabricating surgical guides[18]	• Higher radiation than intraoral imaging (10–1,200 μSv)[13]; mean: 100 μSv • Equipment space requirements and cost[14]

IAN = inferior alveolar nerve.

roots of adjacent teeth, the nasal floor, the maxillary sinus cavities, and any clinically relevant pathology. Surgical techniques and implant choice might even be altered based on the findings with these images.

The current consensus is that 3D imaging, including CBCT and CT scans, will generally be superior to conventional radiography in the planning and execution of dental implant surgery,[14,20,23] especially with challenging situations like IMIs. CBCT scans are now universally considered the gold standard for implant site assessment and treatment planning. This is largely because the 3D cross-sectional images they provide help the surgeon to avoid complications. However, despite their obvious benefits, CBCT and CT scans are not without risk. Incorrect imaging protocols and poor prior clinical evaluation may cause x-ray exposure of unnecessary structures or even the need to rescan patients, thereby increasing the risks of stochastic effects.[24] However, with the current ability to obtain sectional views using CBCT, these risks are now considered minimal in comparison to patient exposure with previous forms of CT scans.[13] The evaluation parameters for preoperative screening of IMIs using CBCT or CT scans differ for mandible versus maxilla, and are discussed in the following sections.

TABLE 2-2 Risk assessment of anatomical, site-specific, and pathologic considerations for IMI placement in mandibular molar areas

	FAVORABLE	UNFAVORABLE
Anatomical parameters		
Lingual concavity measurements	Type I (< 2 mm concavity)	Types II and III (> 2 mm concavity)
Mandibular cross-sectional morphology	Types C and P	Type U
Thickness of facial and lingual cortical bone in interdental region	Buccal cortical plate thickness > lingual cortical plate thickness	Lingual cortical plate thickness > buccal cortical plate thickness
Cross section of roots	In presence of no septal bone, distal placement of the implant will provide better stability due to more available bone.	Due to the larger surface area of the mesial roots and proximity of the mesial tooth, this is a more unfavorable position for immediate implantation.
Site-specific parameters		
Septal bone presence	Type A	Types B and C
Root apices to canal	Distance > 2 mm from IAC	Distance < 2 mm from IAC
Thickness of facial and lingual alveolar plates at each root surface	Two separate flat convergent roots with > 2 mm cortical bone thickness	Fused or divergent roots with < 2 mm cortical bone thickness
Interroot distance between adjacent teeth	Distance > 1.5 mm between adjacent teeth	Distance < 1.5 mm between adjacent teeth
Pathologic parameters		
Presence of PA pathology	No PA pathology or after removal of chronic PA pathology	Acute PA pathology

IAC = inferior alveolar canal; PA = periapical.

Radiographic Screening for Mandibular IMI Placement

When screening for immediate mandibular molar implant treatment, a number of anatomical, site-specific, and pathologic considerations need to be evaluated to determine whether the outcome should be considered to have a good/favorable or poor/unfavorable prognosis (Table 2-2).

Anatomical considerations

Mandibular cross-sectional morphology

Chan et al[25] described different types of cross-sectional morphology based on assessment of coronal slices in 103 CBCT scans of mandibular ridges. The three classifications included undercut, convergent, and parallel (Fig 2-1). U-type ridges were defined as those with undercuts, ie, a narrow base but widening coronally in buccolingual dimension. This ridge morphology was noted in 13.6% of cases. Type C and P ridges were without obvious lingual undercuts and were termed convergent or parallel, having prevalence rates of 20.4% and 66% respectively. Undercut ridges were considered to be at the greatest risk of experiencing lingual plate perforations. In another study of CBCT scans collected from 237 patients, Lin et al[26] reported somewhat different findings, with undercut ridges having the highest prevalence (46.7%). Parallel jaws were seen in 32.3% and convergent in 21% of the

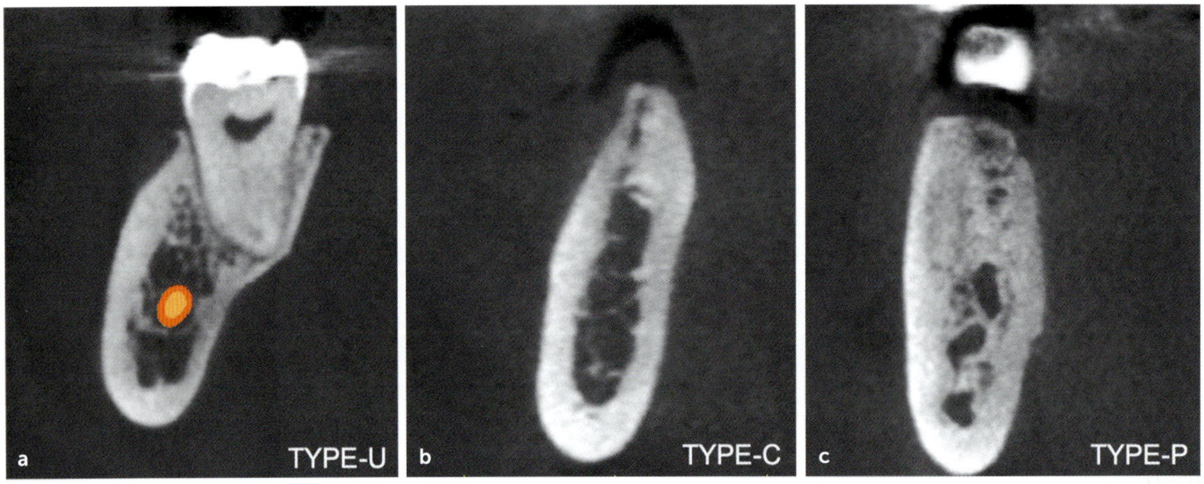

FIG 2-1 These images depict the three types of mandibular ridge morphology in the sagittal plane. *(a)* Undercut. *(b)* Convergent. *(c)* Parallel.

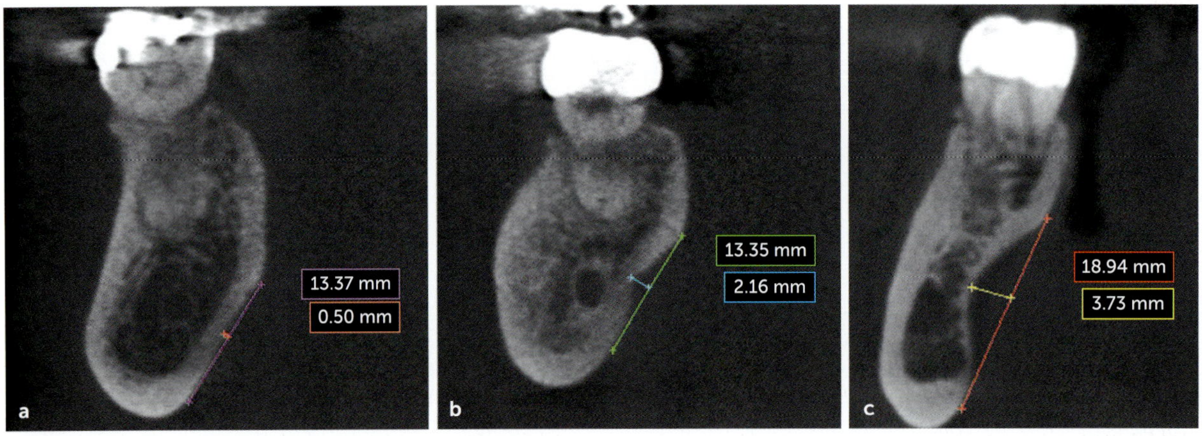

FIG 2-2 *(a)* Type I concavities have < 2 mm in depth. *(b)* Type II concavities have depths of 2 to 3 mm. *(c)* Type III concavities have depths > 3 mm, presenting the greatest risk of lingual plate perforation.

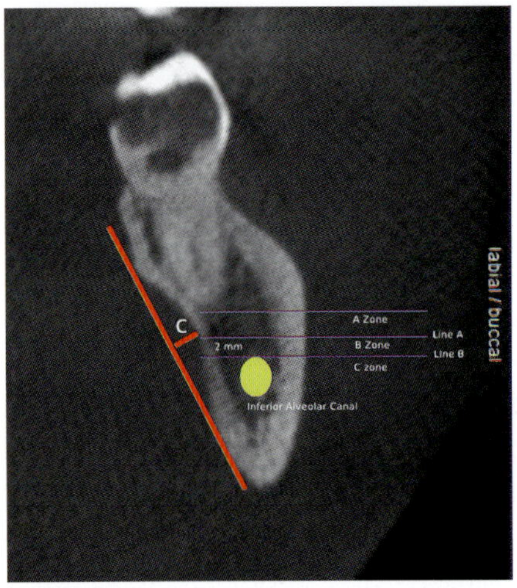

FIG 2-3 Lin et al[26] classified the vertical position of the deepest point in lingual concavity relative to the mandibular canal. Zone A was noted as a line crossing the level of the molar roots and was suggested to be at higher risk.

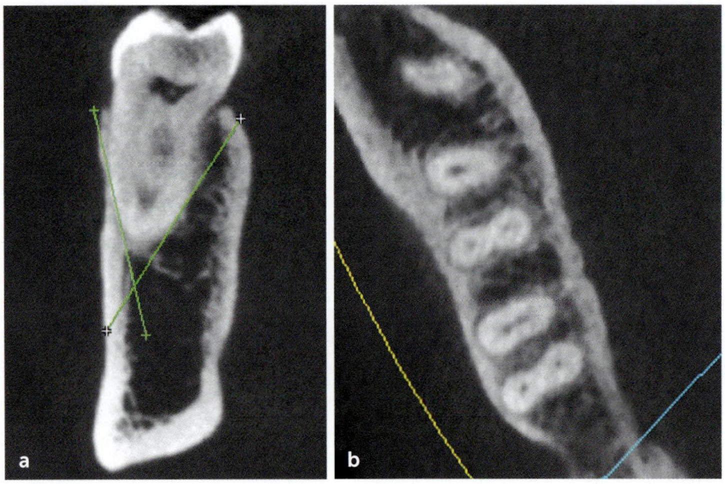

FIG 2-4 *(a)* Both buccal and lingual plates of mandibular molars increase in thickness from their coronal to apical aspects. *(b)* Both mandibular first and second molars commonly show flat root morphologies, leaving favorable IRS for IMI placement.

patient sample. Clearly, undercut ridges are fairly common. In a recent paper, Ho et al showed that the prevalent mandibular ridge shape at the first and second molars were parallel and undercut, respectively.[27]

Lingual concavity measurements

Examination of the lingual concavity or submandibular fossa in the mandible is important for IMI placement as its depth influences the risk of perforation of the lingual cortical plate with possible damage to branches of the submental/lingual artery. Using 100 spiral preoperative CT examinations of patients, Parnia et al[28] classified submandibular fossae according to their depths (Fig 2-2). Type I concavities were classified as those with depth of less than 2 mm and were found in 20% of the patient sample. Type II concavities had a depth of 2 to 3 mm and occurred in 52% of patients, while type III concavities were of depths greater than 3 mm, occurring in 28% of the sampled patients. The investigators concluded that type II and III concavities both had increased risk of lingual plate perforation (LPP) during osteotomy preparation.

Others[26] classified lingual concavities in the coronal plane of undercut mandibles according to the vertical positions of their deepest concave points in relation to the inferior alveolar canal (IAC) (Fig 2-3). Three zones (A, B, and C) were established between the molar root apices and inferior alveolar nerve (IAN) to help to localize the deepest point of concavity. Horizontal lines were traced on relevant CBCT images, the lowest of which (line B) being parallel to the inferior border of the mandible but at the level of the top of the IAC. A second line (line A) was traced parallel to line B but 2 mm coronal to the superior border of the IAC. *Zone A* was defined as the distance from the root apices to line A, while the zone between lines A and line B was defined as *zone B*. Finally, the zone beneath line B was termed *zone C*. The deepest concave point was found to be located in zone C in 48.8% of the images analyzed. When the deepest concave point was located in zone A or B, the risk of IAN damage was higher by 7.82 and 3.52 times respectively compared with when it was located in zone C.

Most recently, Demircan[29] showed that the risk of LPP was significantly higher for second molars (P = .0001), and that the risk increased with age (P = .039). There was a strong relationship between the risk of LPP and undercut mandibles (P = .0001). Also, there was a significant relationship between the risk of IAN damage with undercut cross sections (P = .0001).

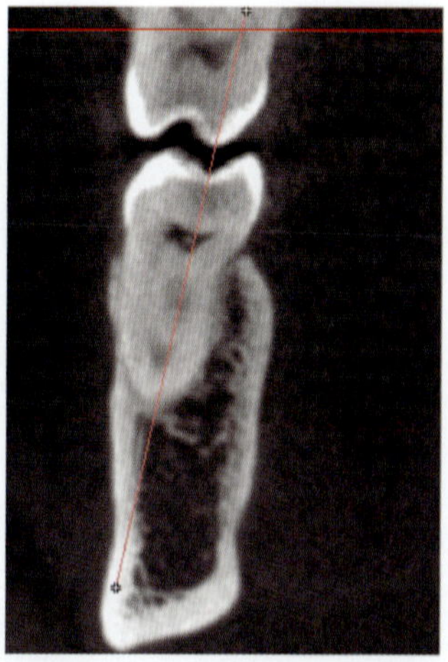

FIG 2-5 A typical buccolingual inclination of a mandibular molar, leaving more bone lingually for stabilizing an IMI.

Thickness of buccal and lingual alveolar plates at each root surface

For the placement of mandibular IMIs, it is important to be aware of the morphology and thickness of the surrounding dental alveolus. A study by Agostinelli et al[30] reported on a tomographic analysis of the bone morphology at mandibular first and second molar sites. They noted that the mean thicknesses of the buccal plate for mandibular first and second molars were 2.13 ± 0.57 mm and 2.59 ± 0.59 mm respectively. For lingual cortices, they measured means of 2.09 ± 0.50 mm for first molars and 1.94 ± 0.53 mm for second molars. It is important to note that both buccal and lingual plates increase in thickness from their coronal to apical aspects (Fig 2-4a). The most prevalent root morphology for both mandibular first (68%) and second (78%) molars was two separate flat roots,[31] providing the necessary IRS bone to engage the implant in a prosthetically favorable position (Fig 2-4b).

The thicknesses of cortical plates in mandibular molar regions can be greatly influenced by the size and strength of the masticatory muscles, including the buccinator and tongue muscles, and the surrounding anatomy. As a result, the teeth may end up lingually inclined (Fig 2-5). As a result, the root apices tend to be more buccally positioned, leaving more bone to engage lingually during IMI placement. Buccal cortical bone tends to increase in thickness from anterior

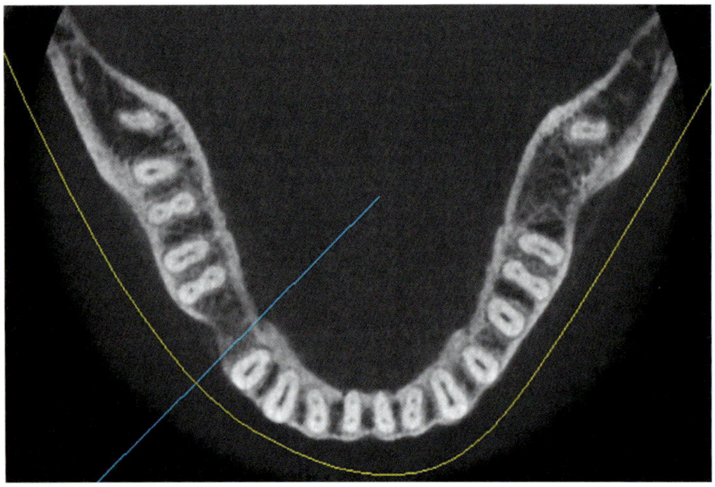

FIG 2-6 The mandibular buccal cortical plate normally thickens from its anterior to posterior aspects.

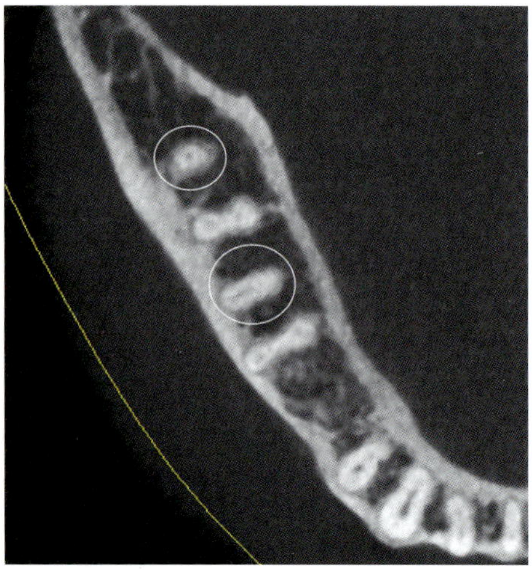

FIG 2-7 The distal roots of mandibular molars generally are smaller in size and surface area than their mesial roots.

to posterior, while lingual cortical plates decrease in thickness from anterior to posterior[31,32] (Fig 2-6). Padhye et al[33] examined CBCT scans of 200 mandibular first molars from patients without radiographic or clinical evidence of periodontal disease, severe root resorption, trauma, or periapical lesions. The mean thicknesses of buccal and lingual buccal bone 2 mm apical to the crest were 0.84 ± 0.39 mm and 2.71 ± 1.17 mm (P = .003). However, it should be noted that others have reported that if buccal bone thickness is 1 mm or less, its measurement can be largely inaccurate.[34] Careful review of every patient's CBCT scan should take these observations into consideration.

Cross-sectional root shapes

Many different root morphologies can present with mandibular molars. However, as already stated, the most common finding is for a mandibular molar to have separate mesial and distal roots with a prevalence of 68% and 78% for mandibular first and second molars respectively.[31] A study by Dunlap and Gher measured the root surface area of mandibular first molars.[35] They reported that the mesial root had a larger surface area than the distal root (Fig 2-7). Therefore, should the operator ever elect to place an IMI into one of the molar root sockets (eg, for a second molar where IMIs are being placed at both the first and second molar sites) to optimize subsequent prosthetic restoration, the distal one would be the preferred.

Site-specific considerations

Septal bone present within the furcation area

Achieving primary stability in mandibular molar extraction sockets can be challenging due to the width of the socket and anatomical limitations beyond the root apices, ie, proximity of the IAC.[10] Therefore, the IRS bone and the peripheral bony walls of the socket offer the safest areas for implant stabilization. Smith and Tarnow classified molar sockets into three types of IRS.[11] Type A sockets are those with wide IRS bone and are anticipated to house the entire coronal body of the IMI (Fig 2-8a). Type B molar sockets are those with sufficient IRS bone to stabilize the implant but not completely encircle its coronal segment (Fig 2-8b). Type C mandibular molar IRS will have little to no septal bone in which to engage the implant (Fig 2-8c), and therefore to achieve initial stability, a wider-diameter implant will likely be needed in order to make contact with the socket walls. Alternatively, a longer implant could be used, but this comes with increased risk because it would need to engage at least 4 mm of native bone apically and runs the risk of damaging the IAN. Of the three categories, type A sockets are the

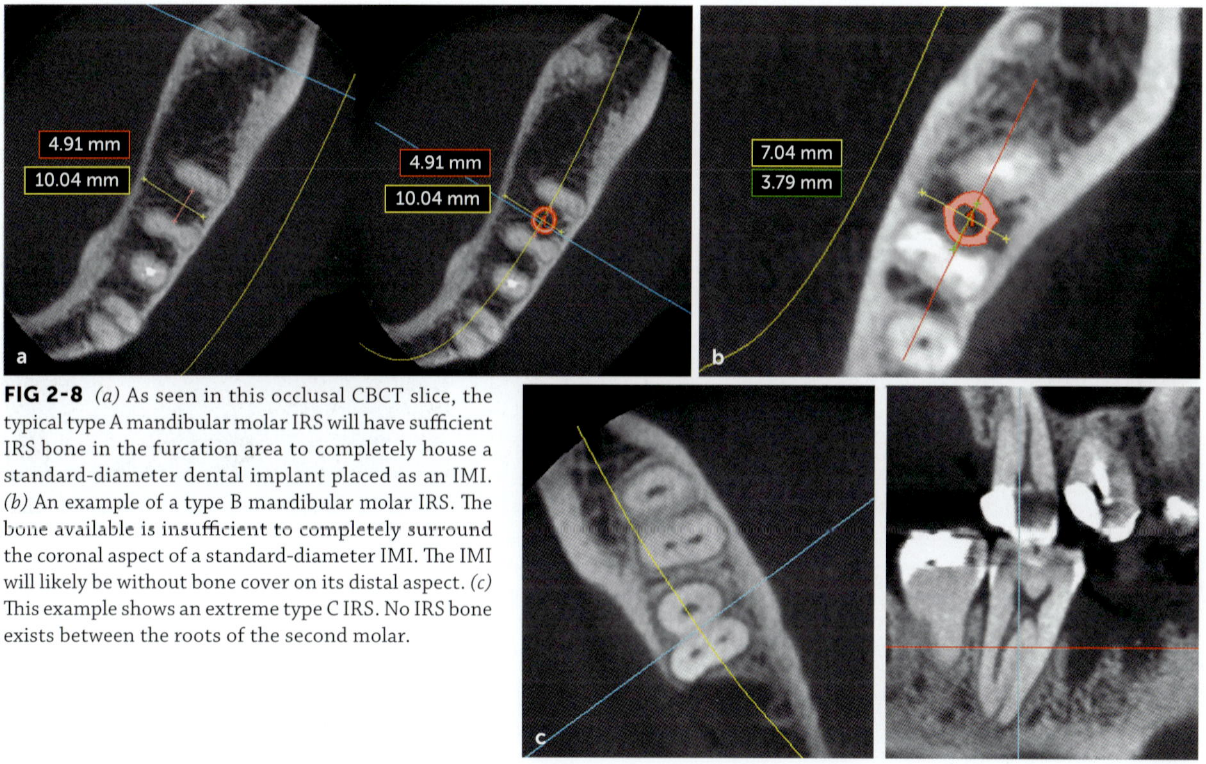

FIG 2-8 *(a)* As seen in this occlusal CBCT slice, the typical type A mandibular molar IRS will have sufficient IRS bone in the furcation area to completely house a standard-diameter dental implant placed as an IMI. *(b)* An example of a type B mandibular molar IRS. The bone available is insufficient to completely surround the coronal aspect of a standard-diameter IMI. The IMI will likely be without bone cover on its distal aspect. *(c)* This example shows an extreme type C IRS. No IRS bone exists between the roots of the second molar.

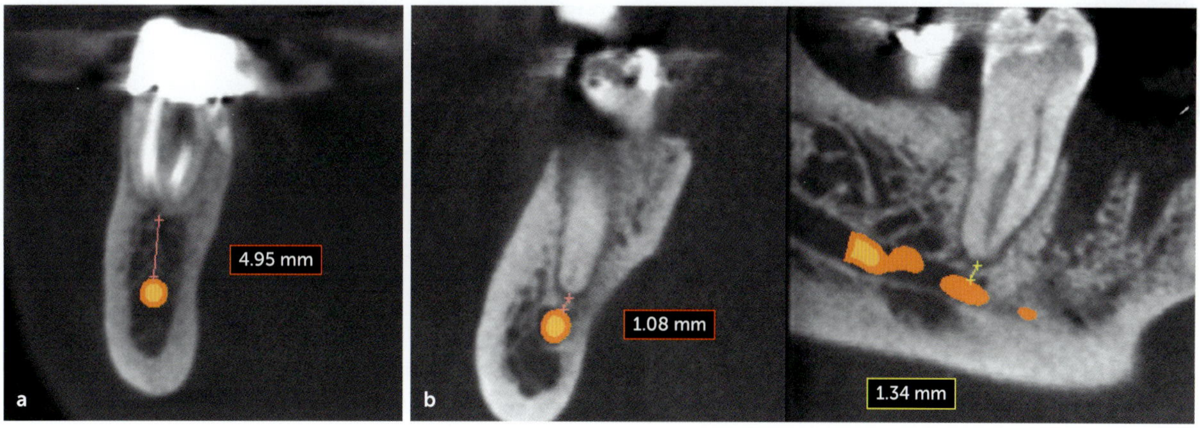

FIG 2-9 *(a)* In this example, the root apices of a mandibular second molar have an RAC of > 2 mm but still possibly insufficient to safely place an IMI secured by 4 mm of apical bone if the implant were to be placed in one of the root sockets instead of the IRS. *(b)* The example shown clearly would be taboo for consideration of IMI placement at this second molar type C socket.

most favorable for IMI placement. However, type B IRS are the most common in the mandible, while type C should be considered the most technique-sensitive and unpredictable if the clinician is inexperienced. Here a better option would be socket preservation grafting and delayed implant placement (see chapter 1). Ho et al recently showed that IRS < 3 mm was found in 76.8% of second and 44.6% of first mandibular molars.[27]

Root apex to canal distance

Root apex to canal (RAC) distance can be defined as the distance from the root tips to the superior border of the IAC[36] (Fig 2-9). IAN damage is the prevalent nerve injury in implant dentistry (64.4%).[37] It can happen during osteotomy preparation (laceration/trauma) or during implant placement (compression).[38] Complications resulting from damage to the IAN

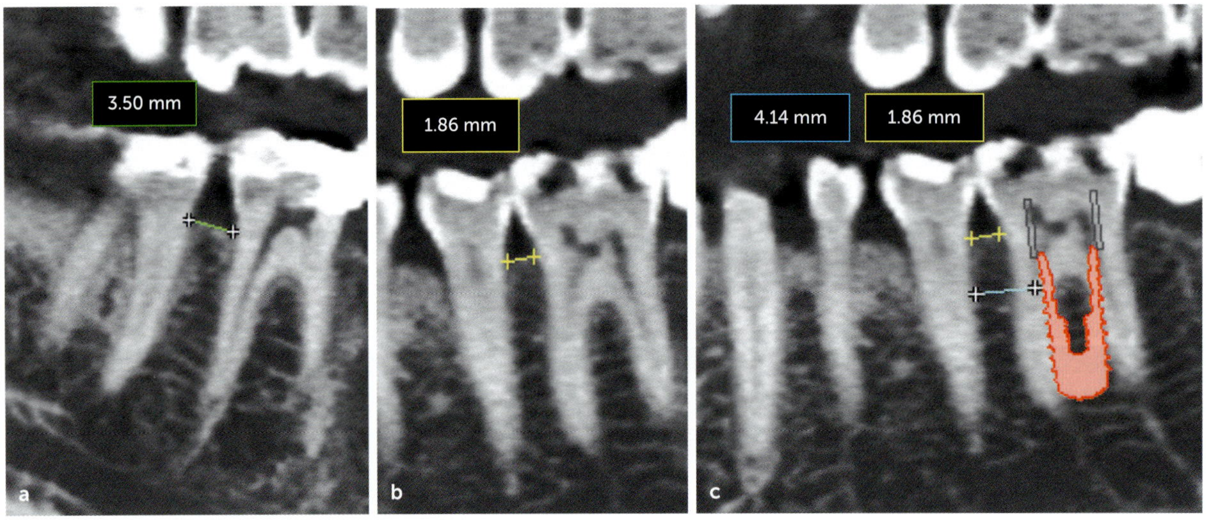

FIG 2-10 *(a)* This patient has a large embrasure between the two molars that fulfill the desired 1.5 mm needed between implant and adjacent tooth. *(b)* This image depicts the typical smaller embrasure space between the mandibular second premolar and first molar. More care is needed here in placing an IMI to prevent interproximal bone loss or impingement of the implant onto the distal of the premolar. *(c)* In this example, placing the IMI into the IRS will help to maintain the interproximal bone between the implant and second premolar.

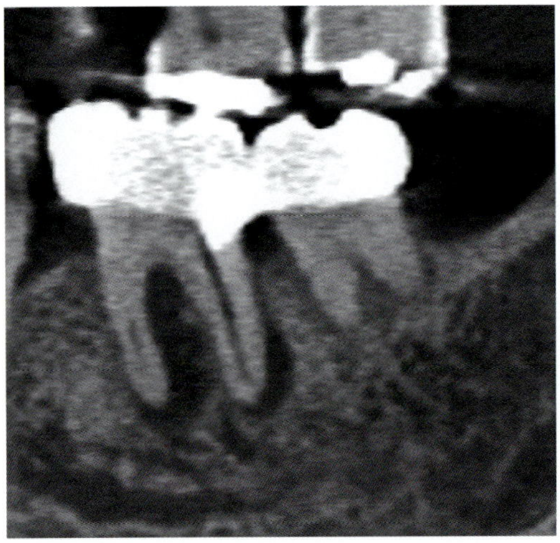

FIG 2-11 This mandibular first molar had acute periapical infection and associated obliteration of the IRS. It was not managed with an IMI.

include temporary or permanent paresthesia or hyperesthesia, which can be debilitating for the patient by affecting daily activities such as speech, eating, drinking, kissing, and shaving.[36–38] Most instances of IAN damage during implant placement have been reported to occur when the RAC distance is less than 2 mm.[39] In their assessment of CBCT scans of mandibular first molar sites, Padhye et al[33] documented that, on average, mesial and distal RACs were 4.31 mm and 4.61 mm, respectively, while Demircan[29] measured these mean RAC distances in males versus females as significantly higher in the former (5.02 mm for males and 3.49 mm for females). Ho et al recently also showed the distances from the root apices of mandibular first molars to be significantly greater that those at second molars. In addition, up to 14.5% of second molar sites had < 10 mm of vertical bone height between the IAC and furcation bone crest.[27]

Interroot distance between adjacent teeth

The distance between roots of adjacent molar teeth is an important consideration when placing implants into fresh extraction sockets. Embrasure spaces between first and second mandibular molars range between 0.8 and 3.2 mm (Fig 2-10a). However, smaller embrasure spaces (0.2–4.5 mm) exist between second premolars and first molars (Fig 2-10b), requiring strict evaluation and measurement when considering immediate implants for first molar sites because 1.5 mm will need to be maintained between the premolar and implant to prevent unwanted interproximal bone resorption.[40] When these distances are less than 1.5 mm, the clinician should consider placing the IMI more distally within the socket in order to avoid the

TABLE 2-3 Risk assessment of anatomical, site-specific, and pathologic considerations for IMI placement in maxillary molar areas

	FAVORABLE	UNFAVORABLE
Anatomical parameters		
Socket measurements in the coronal plane	≥ 5 mm distance between buccal and palatal roots	< 5 mm distance between buccal and palatal roots
Socket measurements in the sagittal plane	≥ 5 mm distance between mesiobuccal and distobuccal roots	< 5 mm distance between mesiobuccal and distobuccal roots
Root apex to sinus floor	> 5 mm distance from root apices to sinus floor	< 5 mm distance from root apices to sinus floor
Position of alveolar recess relative to maxillary first molar roots	Type 2	Type 1, 3, 4
Position of the anterior wall of sinus relative to maxillary first molar roots	Type 2	Type 1, 3
Site-specific parameters		
Septal bone presence	Type A	Type B, C
Root apices intrusion into sinus	Nonintruded	Intruded
Pathologic parameters		
Presence of PA pathology	No PA pathology present or after removal of PA pathology	Acute PA pathology

PA = periapical.

risk of traumatizing adjacent teeth roots (Fig 2-10c). Using an implant that allows platform switching also can assist in situations where the implant-to-tooth distance is only marginally sufficient.[41]

Pathologic considerations

Presence of periapical pathology

Preexisting infection of molars is a common finding and often an indication for extraction. The presence of infection in a fresh extraction socket may have implications for IMIs. Molars with acute infection like that shown in Fig 2-11 are poor candidates. However, Chen et al[42] showed no statistically significant difference when placing implants immediately into sites with chronic infection, as long as the residual infected tissue was removed with the use of degranulating burs. As long as there is sufficient bone remaining to stabilize an IMI, a favorable outcome in chronically infected sites can be anticipated (see also chapter 5). Here the RAC is an important parameter to evaluate.

Radiographic Screening for Maxillary IMI Placement

When screening for IMIs in the maxilla, parameters that need consideration include socket measurements, alveolar recesses in the coronal plane, the relationships between sinus and molar apices in the sagittal plane, IRS bone, distance from molar furcation and alveolar crest to sinus floor, root intrusion into sinus, and pathology (Table 2-3).

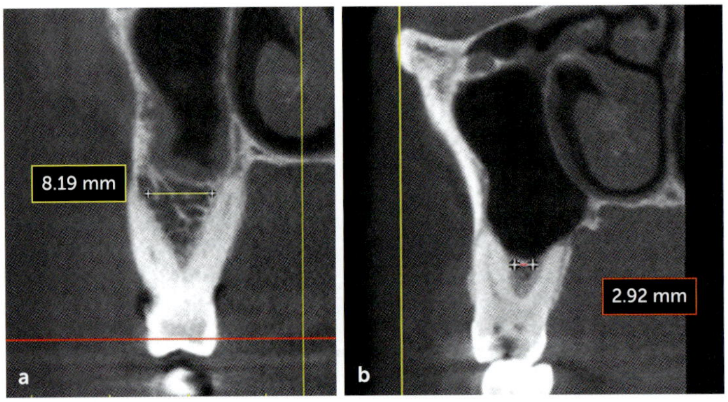

FIG 2-12 *(a)* This CBCT coronal slice reveals there to be 8.19 mm width between the buccal and palatal roots. If the IRS is 5 mm or greater, as it is here, adequate stabilization of an IMI is likely. *(b)* The measurement of IRS width in the coronal plane reveals there to be inadequate bone to stabilize an IMI.

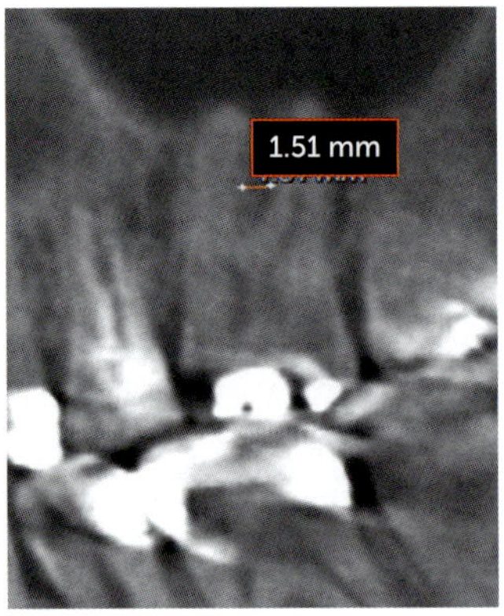

FIG 2-13 The IRS width between the mesiobuccal and distobuccal roots of this maxillary first molar is only 1.51 mm, making the prognosis for an IMI unfavorable.

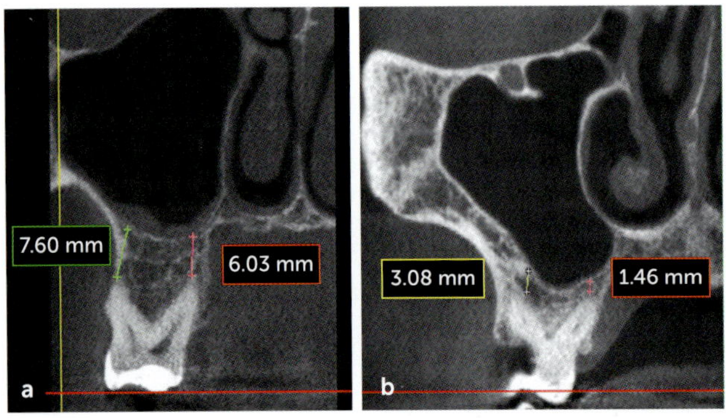

FIG 2-14 *(a)* When the distance from the molar root apices to the sinus floor is greater than 5 mm, adequate stabilization of an IMI is likely achievable. *(b)* In this example, the distances between the molar root apices and the antral floor were less than 5 mm, making IMI placement challenging for the inexperienced clinician, as it would likely require simultaneous indirect sinus floor elevation.

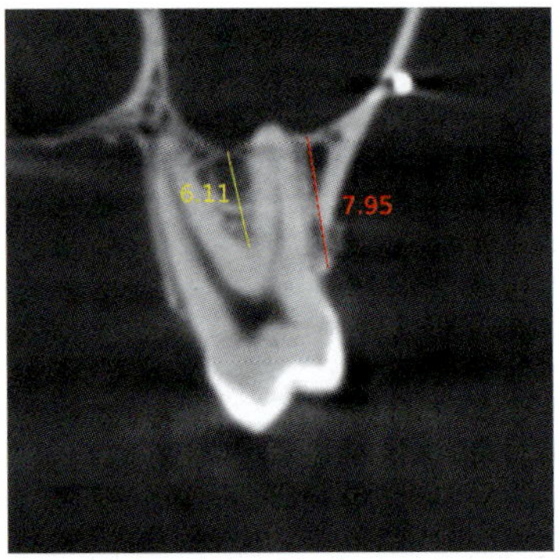

FIG 2-15 Measurements between sinus floor and the alveolar crest and/or the molar furcation can be helpful in planning IMIs. (Courtesy of Dr Maziar Ebrahimi, Toronto, Ontario.)

Anatomical considerations

Socket measurements

Coronal plane. A minimum amount of bone width is required to achieve primary stability of maxillary IMIs. The distance between the buccal and palatal root apices can help to determine whether there is sufficient bone to surround the implant completely. When placing an IMI of standard diameter (4 mm), a minimum of 5 mm of IRS bone width is required[43] (Fig 2-12a). When there is less than 5 mm of bone between the roots, it is difficult to achieve primary stability, and therefore immediate implant placement may be contraindicated (Fig 2-12b).

Sagittal plane. The distance between the mesiobuccal and distobuccal roots of a maxillary molar under consideration for an IMI should also be measured in the sagittal plane. Matsuda et al[43] suggested that a minimum distance of 5 mm of bone width between the two buccal roots of a maxillary molar is required to achieve primary stability using an IMI of standard diameter. When this IRS width is less than 5 mm, the prognosis for IMI placement is likely unfavorable (Fig 2-13).

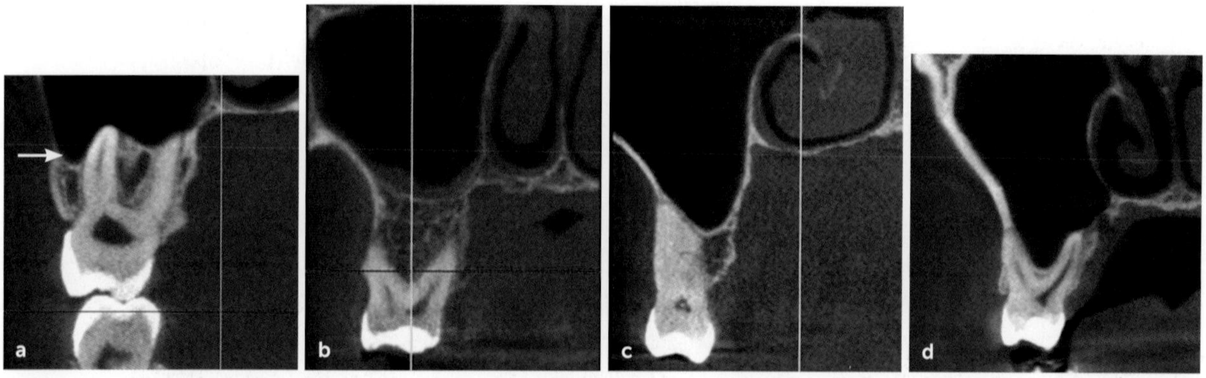

FIG 2-16 *(a)* This coronal view shows the alveolar recess *(arrow)* to be lateral to both molar roots, a favorable situation for an IMI. *(b)* With this molar, the type 2 alveolar recess is located between the buccal and palatal roots, in which case an IMI can be safely placed. *(c)* This type 3 alveolar recess is located medially to both the palatal and buccal roots, indicating a poor prognosis for an IMI because of inadequate bone for stabilization. *(d)* Coronal view of a type 4 alveolar recess. The lack of a recess makes IMI placement unfavorable.

Root apex distance to sinus floor. The bone available from the root apices of a maxillary molar to the sinus floor can be utilized to gain primary stability of an IMI. When distance from the root apex to the sinus floor is 5 mm or more, adequate primary stability of an IMI is likely achievable[43] (Fig 2-14a). In situations where there is less than 5 mm of this subantral bone, IMI placement is deemed more technically challenging and may require simultaneous transcrestal sinus floor elevation or augmentation (Fig 2-14b). In another recent study, Deporter et al[44] measured mean distances from sinus floor to mesiobuccal, distobuccal, and palatal root apices to be 2.89 mm, 2.48 mm, and 2.37 mm for maxillary first molars and 0.93 mm, 2.45 mm, and 2.58 mm for second molars. Other useful CBCT measurements for planning IMIs in maxillae include the distance from alveolar ridge crest to sinus floor and distance from molar furcation to sinus floor (Fig 2-15). Demircan and Çankaya[45] reported the mean distances from alveolar crest to sinus floor to be approximately 7.50 mm, while Matsuda et al[43] calculated the mean distance from molar furcation to sinus floor to be 6.51 mm (standard deviation of 2.94 mm).

Alveolar recesses in the coronal plane

The maxillary alveolar recess defines the inferior border of the maxillary sinus and is another important anatomical landmark when IMIs are being considered for the maxillary first molar. Knowing the locations of alveolar recesses relative to the molar apices allows for proper implant positioning.[45] Alveolar recesses are measured in the coronal view and can be categorized into four groups[45]:

- Type 1: The alveolar recess is lateral to both buccal and palatal roots of the first maxillary molar (Fig 2-16a).
- Type 2: The alveolar recess is between the buccal and palatal roots (Fig 2-16b).
- Type 3: The alveolar recess is medial to both buccal and palatal roots (Fig 2-16c).
- Type 4: No alveolar recess is present in the location of the maxillary first molar (Fig 2-16d).

Relationship between sinus and molar apices in the sagittal plane

When planning maxillary IMI placement, the root apices of the molar teeth in the sagittal plane should be away from the maxillary sinus. Demircan and Çankaya[45] classified the relationships between the antrum and the maxillary first molar using the anterior wall of the sinus as the reference point. Three categories were described. With type 1 relationships, the anterior wall of the maxillary sinus was seen to be

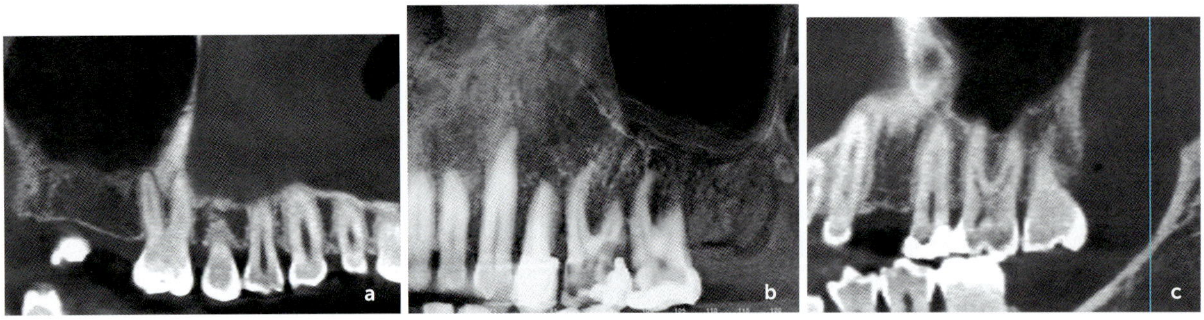

FIG 2-17 *(a)* In the sagittal plane, a type 1 relationship was specified to have the anterior wall of the sinus located between the mesiobuccal and distobuccal roots of the first molar. This relationship is considered too difficult for IMI placement as there is a high risk of sinus floor perforation. *(b)* The anterior wall of the maxillary sinus is posterior to the distobuccal root of the first molar, making the prognosis for an IMI favorable. *(c)* In this type 3 situation, the anterior wall of the antrum is anterior to the mesiobuccal root of the first molar, again making placement of an IMI challenging.

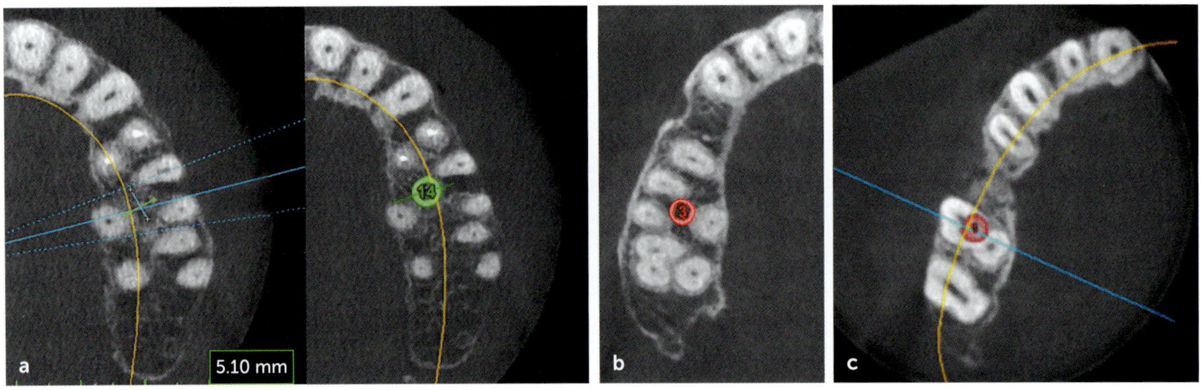

FIG 2-18 *(a)* A type A maxillary socket after Smith and Tarnow.[11] There is adequate IRS to completely house a standard-diameter implant. Implant simulation is depicted in the right-hand occlusal CBCT view. *(b)* With a type B socket, there will be sufficient IRS to stabilize an IMI but not enough to totally house its coronal aspect. Implant simulation predicts the IMI to be contacting all three roots, resulting in significant IRS dehiscences. *(c)* Type C sockets have too little to no IRS for implant stabilization.

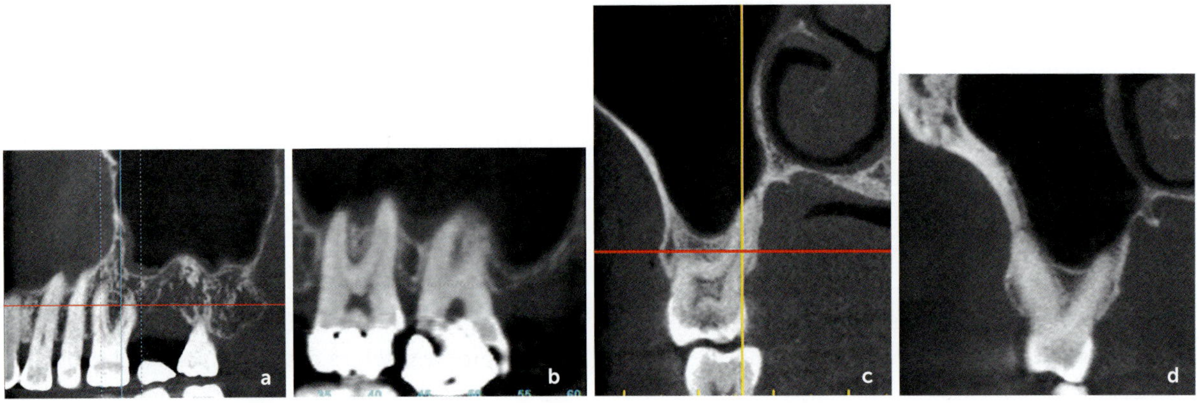

FIG 2-19 *(a)* No root intrusion into the sinus domain makes IMI placement into the IRS favorable. *(b)* Intrusion of both buccal roots into the sinus domain can be a contraindication for IMI placement at this first molar site. *(c)* The palatal root intrusion would make IMI placement challenging for the novice implant surgeon. *(d)* Both buccal and palatal roots intrude into the sinus domain, making this site unfavorable for IMI placement.

between the mesiobuccal and distobuccal roots (Fig 2-17a). With type 2, the anterior wall of the maxillary sinus was described to be posterior to the distobuccal root (Fig 2-17b), while with type 3, the anterior antral wall was anterior to the mesiobuccal root (Fig 2-17c).

Site-specific considerations

IRS bone

Smith and Tarnow[11] categorized molar socket IRS into three types, depending on the degree of difficulty in manipulating them. As stated earlier, type A sockets are those having adequate IRS bone to contain circumferentially the entire coronal portion of an IMI, and are the most favorable sites for IMIs (Fig 2-18a). In contrast, type B sockets were classified as those with enough septal bone to stabilize an IMI but insufficient to encase its coronal portion fully (Fig 2-18b). Finally, type C sockets were classified as those with insufficient septal bone to stabilize an IMI. As a result, achieving stability of an IMI with a type C socket requires that either a wider-diameter implant be used in order to contact the socket walls, or a longer implant be used to go beyond the previous root apices for stability (Fig 2-18c). Deporter et al[44] recently reported on the dimensions of IRS in maxillary molars. Mean coronal-most buccopalatal/mesiodistal IRS widths were 6.52 mm/7.33 mm for first molars and 5.85 mm/6.86 mm at second molar sites. In their patient sample, 61.7% of first molars and 34.0% of second molars had sufficiently broad IRS to encase completely a 5-mm-diameter IMI.

Root intrusion into sinus

When roots intrude into the maxillary sinus, there is an increased risk of oroantral communication after tooth extraction. Demircan and Cancaya classified this occurrence into 4 types[45]:

1. No intrusion (Fig 2-19a)
2. Buccal root intrusion (Fig 2-19b)
3. Palatal root intrusion (Fig 2-19c)
4. Buccal and palatal root intrusion (Fig 2-19d)

The recent data from Deporter et al[44] showed that palatal roots of maxillary first molars showed higher intrusion rates (36.74%) than the two buccal roots, while with second molars, the mesiobuccal roots were more likely to be intruding into sinus (40%).

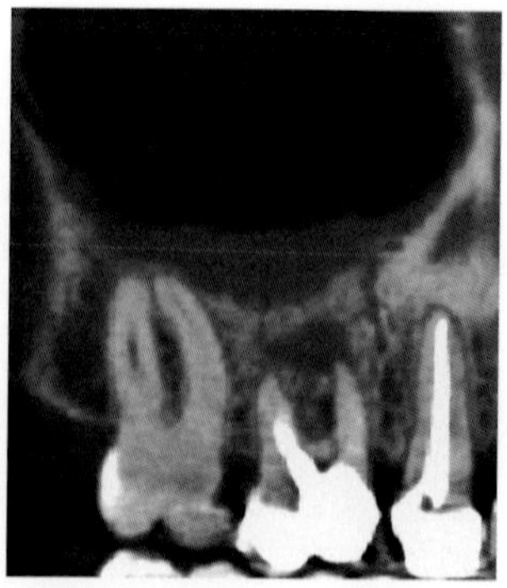

FIG 2-20 Acute periapical infection with sinus penetration at the first molar site precluded IMI placement.

Pathologic considerations

Presence of periapical pathology

Similar to mandibular molar sites, where there is chronic infection in a maxillary molar extraction socket but sufficient bone for implant stabilization after tooth removal and degranulation, IMI placement can be considered favorable.[42] However, as seen in Fig 2-20, where there is acute infection within the socket, IMI placement is contraindicated.

Conclusion

With the increasing demand for faster implant treatment by patients, implant placement into fresh extraction sockets has become a popular treatment modality. However, the IMI approach should be considered a technique-sensitive procedure, one critical factor being the need to achieve adequate initial implant stability. CBCT radiographs are considered the gold standard for initial implant treatment planning, and their benefits over conventional radiographs have been discussed in this chapter. Undertaking thorough assessment of these scans preoperatively with attention being paid to the anatomical, site-specific, and pathologic parameters described here will allow the clinician to predict cases as having either a favorable or unfavorable risk profile. It is important to note that rarely is there an ideal site with all parameters favorable. However, accurate and knowledgeable radiographic screening can be the difference between success and failure.

KEY POINTS

- CBCT pretreatment assessment is considered to be the gold standard for planning IMIs.
- When screening for IMIs, a number of anatomical, site-specific, and pathologic parameters need to be considered.
- For mandibular IMIs, ridge morphology, lingual ridge concavities, thicknesses of buccal and lingual cortices, IRS bone type, and distances from root apices to IAC must be evaluated.
- Mandibular IMIs are ideally placed in IRS if feasible, noting that second molar sites are of greater risk because of local anatomy.
- With maxillary IMIs, socket measurements, alveolar recesses in the coronal plane, relationships between sinus floor and molar root apices in the sagittal plane, IRS type, root intrusions into sinus, and distances from furcation and alveolar crest to sinus floor provide crucial information.

References

1. Lazzara RJ. Immediate implant placement into extraction sites: Surgical and restorative advantages. Int J Periodontics Restorative Dent 1989;9:332–343.
2. Schwartz-Arad D, Chaushu G. The ways and wherefores of immediate placement of implants into fresh extraction sites: A literature review. J Periodontol 1997;68:915–923.
3. Becker W, Becker BE. Replacement of maxillary and mandibular molars with single endosseous implant restorations: A retrospective study. J Prosthet Dent 1995;74:51–55.
4. Schwartz-Arad D, Grossman Y, Chaushu G. The clinical effectiveness of implants placed immediately into fresh extraction sites of molar teeth. J Periodontol 2000;71:839–844.
5. Fugazzotto PA. Implant placement at the time of maxillary molar extraction: Treatment protocols and report of results. J Periodontol 2008;79:216–223.
6. Fugazzotto PA. Implant placement at the time of mandibular molar extraction: Description of technique and preliminary results of 341 cases. J Periodontol 2008;79:737–747.
7. Block MS. Placement of implants into fresh molar sites: Results of 35 cases. J Oral Maxillofac Surg 2011;69:170–174.
8. Atieh MA, Payne AG, Duncan WJ, de Silva RK, Cullinan MP. Immediate placement or immediate restoration/loading of single implants for molar tooth replacement: A systematic review and meta-analysis. Int J Oral Maxillofac Implants 2010;25:401–415.
9. Ketabi M, Deporter D, Atenafu EG. A systematic review of outcomes following immediate molar implant placement based on recently published studies. Clin Implant Dent Relat Res 2016;18:1084–1094.
10. Smith RB, Tarnow DP, Sarnachiaro G. Immediate placement of dental implants in molar extraction sockets: An 11-year retrospective analysis. Compend Contin Educ Dent 2019;40:166–170.
11. Smith RB, Tarnow DP. Classification of molar extraction sites for immediate dental implant placement: Technical note. Int J Oral Maxillofac Implants 2013;28:911–916.
12. Gupta S, Patil N, Solanki J, Singh R, Laller S. Oral implant imaging: A review. Malays J Med Sci 2015;22:7–17.
13. Jacobs R, Quirynen M. Dental cone beam computed tomography: Justification for use in planning oral implant placement. Periodontol 2000 2014;66:203–213.
14. Reddy MS, Mayfield-Donahoo T, Vanderven FJ, Jeffcoat MK. A comparison of the diagnostic advantages of panoramic radiography and computed tomography scanning for placement of root form dental implants. Clin Oral Implants Res 1994;5:229–238.
15. Low KM, Dula K, Bürgin W, von Arx T. Comparison of periapical radiography and limited cone-beam tomography in posterior maxillary teeth referred for apical surgery. J Endod 2008;34:557–562.

16. Vazquez L, Saulacic N, Belser U, Bernard JP. Efficacy of panoramic radiographs in the preoperative planning of posterior mandibular implants: A prospective clinical study of 1527 consecutively treated patients. Clin Oral Implants Res 2008;19:81–85.
17. Rondon RH, Pereira YC, do Nascimento GC. Common positioning errors in panoramic radiography: A review. Imaging Sci Dent 2014;44:1–6.
18. Ganz SD. Presurgical planning with CT-derived fabrication of surgical guides. J Oral Maxillofac Surg 2005;63(9 suppl 2):59–71.
19. Saravanan B, Jayavelu P, Riaz R, Tariqsalam AR. Evaluation of the accuracy of cone beam computed tomography for immediate implant placement: A case report. J Pharm Bioallied Sci 2017;9(suppl 1):S274–S280.
20. Estrela C, Bueno MR, Leles CR, Azevedo B, Azevedo JR. Accuracy of cone beam computed tomography and panoramic and periapical radiography for detection of apical periodontitis. J Endod 2008;34:273–279.
21. Stoppie N, Pattijn V, Van Cleynenbreugel T, Wevers M, Vander Sloten J, Ignace N. Structural and radiological parameters for the characterization of jawbone. Clin Oral Implants Res 2006;17:124–133.
22. Klinge B, Petersson A, Maly P. Location of the mandibular canal: Comparison of macroscopic findings, conventional radiography, and computed tomography. Int J Oral Maxillofac Implants 1989;4:327–332.
23. Wanschitz F, Birkfellner W, Watzinger F, et al. Evaluation of accuracy of computer-aided intraoperative positioning of endosseous oral implants in the edentulous mandible. Clin Oral Implants Res 2002;13:59–64.
24. Harris D, Horner K, Gröndahl K, et al. E.A.O. guidelines for the use of diagnostic imaging in implant dentistry 2011. A consensus workshop organized by the European Association for Osseointegration at the Medical University of Warsaw. Clin Oral Implants Res 2012;23:1243–1253.
25. Chan HL, Benavides E, Yeh CY, Fu JH, Rudek IE, Wang HL. Risk assessment of lingual plate perforation in posterior mandibular region: A virtual implant placement study using cone-beam computed tomography. J Periodontol 2011;82:129–135.
26. Lin MH, Mau LP, Cochran DL, Shieh YS, Huang PH, Huang RY. Risk assessment of inferior alveolar nerve injury for immediate implant placement in the posterior mandible: A virtual implant placement study. J Dent 2014;42:263–270.
27. Ho J, Ngeow W, Lim D, Wong C. Anatomic considerations for immediate implant placement in the mandibular molar region: A cross-sectional study using cone-beam computed tomography. Folia Morphol (Warsz). 2021 Jun 29. Epub ahead of print.
28. Parnia F, Fard EM, Mahboub F, Hafezeqoran A, Gavgani FE. Tomographic volume evaluation of submandibular fossa in patients requiring dental implants. Oral Surg Oral Med Oral Pathol Oral Radiol Endod 2010;109:e32–e36.
29. Demircan S. Prosthetically driven immediate implant placement at lower molar area; An anatomical study. Eur Oral Res 2020; 54:25–30.
30. Agostinelli C, Agostinelli A, Berardini M, Trisi P. Radiological evaluation of the dimensions of lower molar alveoli. Implant Dent 2018;27:271–275.
31. Ahmed HA, Abu-bakr NH, Yahia NA, Ibrahim YE. Root and canal morphology of permanent mandibular molars in a Sudanese population [published correction appears in Int Endod J 2007;40:1008]. Int Endod J 2007;40:766–771.
32. Kunte VR, Bhoosreddy AR, Bhoosreddy SA, Pandharbale AA, Shinde MR, Ahire BS. Alveolar bone dimensions of mandibular posterior teeth using cone beam tomography: A pilot study. J Contemp Dent 2016;6:9–14.
33. Padhye NM, Shirsekar VU, Bhatavadekar NB. Three-dimensional alveolar bone assessment of mandibular first molars with implications for immediate implant placement. Int J Periodontics Restorative Dent 2020;40:e163–e167.
34. Domic D, Bertl K, Ahmad S, Schropp L, Hellén-Halme K, Stavropoulos A. Accuracy of cone-beam computed tomography is limited at implant sites with a thin buccal bone: A laboratory study. J Periodontol 2021;92:592–601.
35. Dunlap RM, Gher ME. Root surface measurements of the mandibular first molar. J Periodontol 1985;56:234–238.
36. Froum S, Casanova L, Byrne S, Cho SC. Risk assessment before extraction for immediate implant placement in the posterior mandible: A computerized tomographic scan study. J Periodontol 2011;82:395–402.
37. Juodzbalys G, Wang HL, Sabalys G, Sidlauskas A, Galindo-Moreno P. Inferior alveolar nerve injury associated with implant surgery. Clin Oral Implants Res 2013;24:183–190.
38. Hillerup S. Iatrogenic injury to the inferior alveolar nerve: Etiology, signs and symptoms, and observations on recovery. Int J Oral Maxillofac Surg 2008;37:704–709.
39. Tufekcioglu S, Delilbasi C, Gurler G, Dilaver E, Ozer N. Is 2 mm a safe distance from the inferior alveolar canal to avoid neurosensory complications in implant surgery? Niger J Clin Pract 2017;20:274–277.
40. Grunder U, Gracis S, Capelli M. Influence of the 3-D bone-to-implant relationship on esthetics. Int J Periodontics Restorative Dent 2005;25:113–119.
41. Gardner DM. Platform switching as a means to achieving implant esthetics. N Y State Dent J 2005;71:34–37.
42. Chen H, Zhang G, Weigl P, Gu X. Immediate placement of dental implants into infected versus noninfected sites in the esthetic zone: A systematic review and meta-analysis. J Prosthet Dent 2018;120:658–667.
43. Matsuda H, Borzabadi-Farahani A, Le BT. Three-dimensional alveolar bone anatomy of the maxillary first molars: A cone-beam computed tomography study with implications for immediate implant placement. Implant Dent 2016;25:367–372.
44. Deporter D, Ketabi M, Dastgurdi M, Rahmati A, Atenafu E. CBCT data relevant in treatment planning for immediate maxillary molar implant placement. J Perio Implant Science 2021; 13(2):49–55.
45. Demircan S, Çankaya AB. Is immediate implant placement possible in the maxillary molar area? An anatomical study. Quintessence Int 2016;47:853–859.

3

IMMEDIATE MANDIBULAR MOLAR IMPLANT PLACEMENT

Douglas Deporter

Ali Akbar Khoshkhounejad

Mohammad Ketabi

Maziar Ebrahimi Dastgurdi

Systematic literature reviews on the topic of immediate replacement of failed mandibular molars using dental implants have suggested this treatment modality to be viable and predictable[1–3] (see also chapter 1). One of the earliest reports of mandibular immediate molar implant (IMI) usage was that of Becker and Becker.[4] These clinicians reported 2-year data on a group of 22 reportedly nonbruxing patients in whom 13 single immediate molar and 11 single delayed molar implants of various lengths and diameters had been used. The IMIs were placed either in one of the tooth root sockets or, if possible, into the interradicular septum (IRS) bone, and submerged for initial site healing for 4 to 5 months. Twenty-one standard-diameter (3.75 mm) Brånemark-type (ie, machine-turned or minimally rough[5]) implants of lengths 10, 13, or 15 mm were used, along with one 10 × 4–mm implant, one 6 × 5–mm, and one 8 × 5–mm implant (length × diameter). While the 6-mm-long implant failed at 6 months in function, the remaining implants survived for the 2-year functional period, certainly an encouraging outcome. Considerable subsequent work by other investigators has now documented that the short- to medium-term survival rates of mandibular IMIs are in the high 90 percents, at least in the hands of talented and experienced clinicians.

However, systematic literature reviews with meta-analyses of the findings have stressed that the quality of most IMI studies published to date should be considered low, as few have been designed as prospective, randomized, double-blinded, and controlled, ie, direct within-study comparisons of IMIs to implants placed in healed molar sites. In fact, the same could be said for much of the published data on dental implant investigations. It is also recognized by experts that the procedures needed for successful IMI placement are definitely technique sensitive and difficult to perform, especially by practitioners who attempt them infrequently.[6] A detailed working knowledge of mandibular anatomy is crucial to avoid failures and serious complications such as inferior alveolar nerve (IAN)

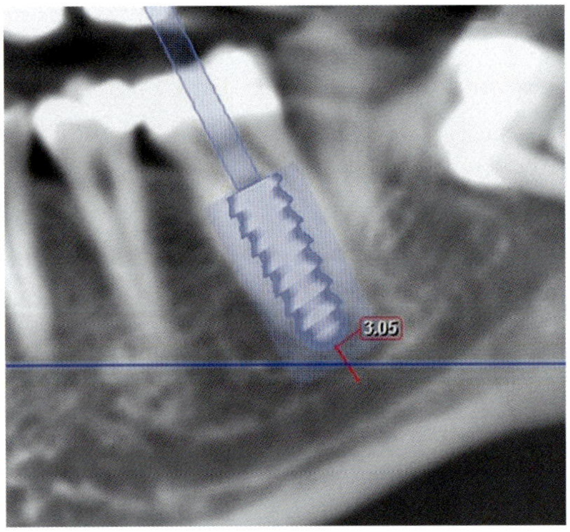

FIG 3-1 If an IMI could be stabilized in the IRS of this molar, a buffer zone of ~ 3 mm apical bone would avoid damage to the IAN.

injury or lingual bone plate perforation at sites with unrecognized mandibular undercuts (see also chapter 2). The purpose of this chapter is to provide key information on the use of mandibular IMIs, including case selection, anatomical considerations, suggested surgical procedures, limitations, and risks.

Case Selection

Given the difficulty and risks of placing mandibular IMIs, case selection and planning are best undertaken with the assistance of CBCT radiographic scans to allow the practitioner to determine the location of the inferior alveolar and mental nerves, the buccolingual alveolar ridge width at the site, the presence of pathology, and the vertical height of available bone, recognizing that a buffer zone of 2 mm from the planned implant apex to the mandibular canal must be maintained to avoid nerve damage (Fig 3-1). Other useful information gleaned from these scans can include the presence or absence of intact buccal and lingual cortical plates and their thicknesses, the dimensions of IRS bone, and the presence and location of any significant mandibular lingual concavities.

If the reason for tooth extraction is advanced periodontal attachment loss, it is important to advise the patient that a history of severe periodontitis does present increased risk of implant failure over the long term compared with patients who have previously been periodontally healthy.[7] Aoki et al[8] reported that implants placed adjacent to teeth with gingival crevices colonized by recognized periodontal pathogens can become infected with the same microorganisms. Even patients who have undergone successful periodontal treatment prior to implant placement can be at increased risk of implant site infection and implant failure following longer times of implant function (≥ 5 years), given the difficulty in preventing periodontal reinfection.[9–11] Determining vitamin D levels in these patients may be helpful in predicting implant outcomes. Regarding patient habits, IMIs are more appropriate in nonsmokers, as smoking has repeatedly been linked to a higher risk for implant failure.[12] Bruxism also has been identified as a risk factor for implant failure,[13] making patients with this condition less suitable for the IMI approach and stressing the need for them to wear nighttime protective occlusal guards should any implant treatment be undertaken.

Anatomical Factors to Consider

IRS and socket anatomy

The IRS represents the ideal position for mandibular IMI placement,[14] and its volume and height should be assessed preoperatively using radiographs.[15] In one survey, IRS was found to be present at 86% of first molar sites and 52% of second molar sites in the mandible.[16] Smith and Tarnow have classified molar socket IRS bone into three categories (A, B, and C) based on quantity (Fig 3-2).[17] Type A IRS sites were designated as those with sufficient bulk of IRS to

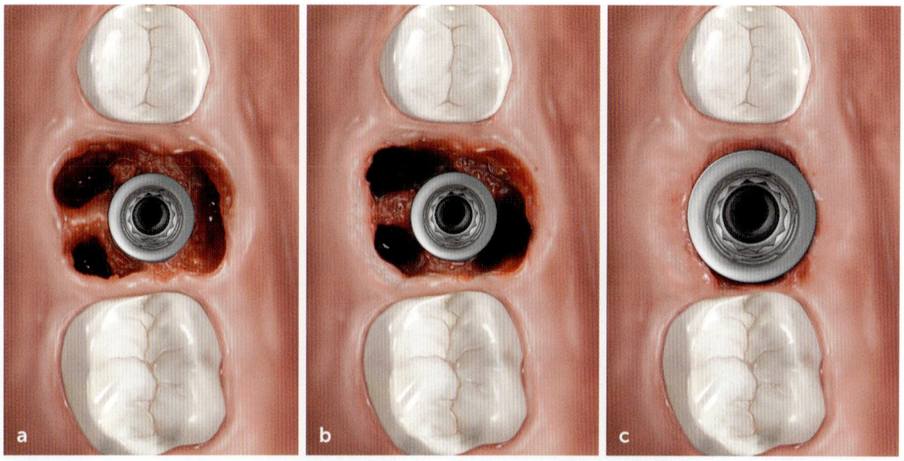

FIG 3-2 An illustration of the classification of molar IRS according to Smith and Tarnow[17] (reprinted with permission). *(a)* Type A socket. The coronal portion of the implant is completely contained within the septal bone. *(b)* Type B socket. The implant is stabilized but not completely contained by the septal bone; a gap is present between the implant and the inner socket walls. *(c)* Type C socket. No septal bone is available for implant stabilization. A wide-diameter implant must engage the inner aspects of the socket walls and/or bone apical to the socket to be stable.

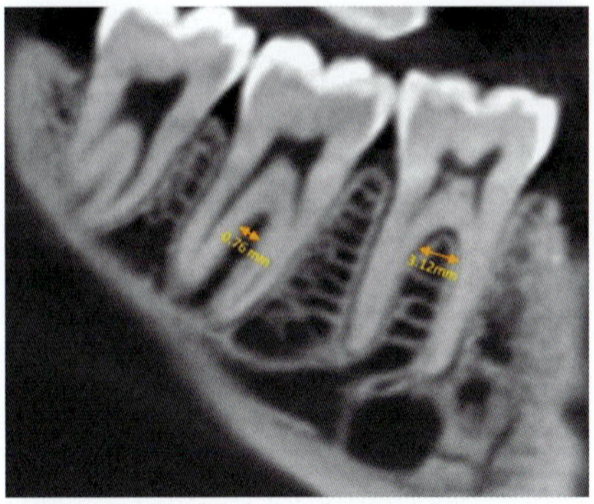

FIG 3-3 Example of a type B IRS at a mandibular first molar and type C at the second molar.

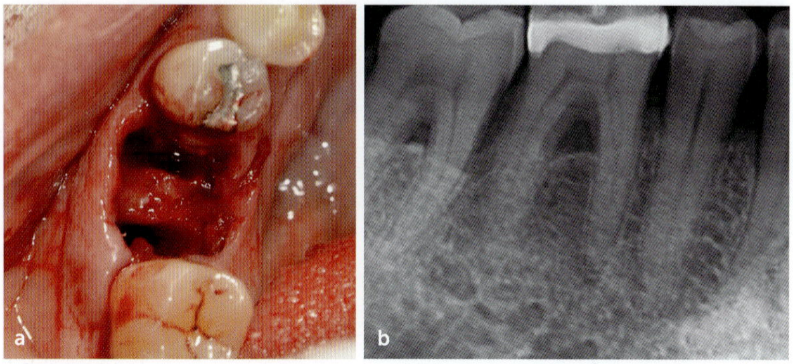

FIG 3-4 *(a)* This patient presented with a favorable type B IRS that could be used to stabilize an IMI. *(b)* The preoperative radiograph shows the favorable apical widening of the first molar IRS.

completely contain the coronal aspect of an osteotomy meant for a standard-diameter (4 to 5 mm) implant, and while they are considered ideal, they rarely occur at mandibular molars. Generally, the best that can be anticipated for a mandibular molar IRS would be type B, defined as one having sufficient bone volume to stabilize but not completely house the coronal aspect of an implant[17] (Fig 3-3). A clinical example of a favorable type B IRS is depicted in Fig 3-4a. With this site, it should be straightforward to initiate an osteotomy. Ideally, a type B IRS like this one will widen apically (Fig 3-4b). In a recent study, Padhye et al[18] examined CBCT scans of 200 mandibular first molars from patients without radiographic or clinical evidence of periodontal disease, severe root resorption, trauma, or periapical lesions. They measured the mean mesiodistal widths of IRS at 2 mm and 4 mm below the molar furcations to be 1.93 ± 0.65 mm and 2.54 ± 0.9 mm respectively, with 38% of sites having widths less than 3 mm, ie, type C.[17]

Type C IRS sites are those sites with insufficient septal bone volume to stabilize an implant (Fig 3-5). In this case, the IRS should be removed and, if feasible, the socket prepared to receive a wider-diameter implant that engages the buccal and lingual furcal bone buttresses if still present[19] (Fig 3-6). Alternatively, but less favored because of poor positioning for the subsequent restoration, the IMI could be placed in one or other of the root sockets (Fig 3-7). The protocol of placing two implants (ie, one into each mandibular molar root socket) to support one molar crown was followed occasionally in the past and may have some benefit in minimizing the risk of root caries of contiguous teeth (see chapter 11). The best option if an IMI is not feasible is to perform socket preservation grafting and delayed implant placement (see chapter 1).

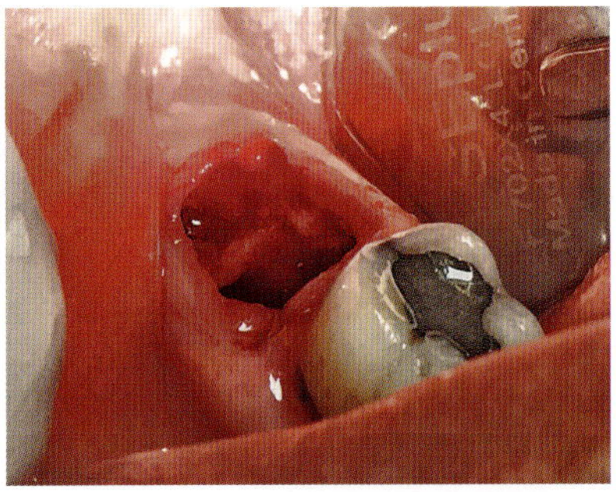

FIG 3-5 If an IMI were to be undertaken with this type C IRS, the middle portion (buccolingually) of the narrow IRS could be removed and an implant wide enough (eg, 5- or 6-mm diameter) to engage the buccal and lingual IRS buttresses could be inserted. Type C IRSs are the most common ones found at mandibular second molar sites. Operator access can make them difficult to prepare for IMIs.

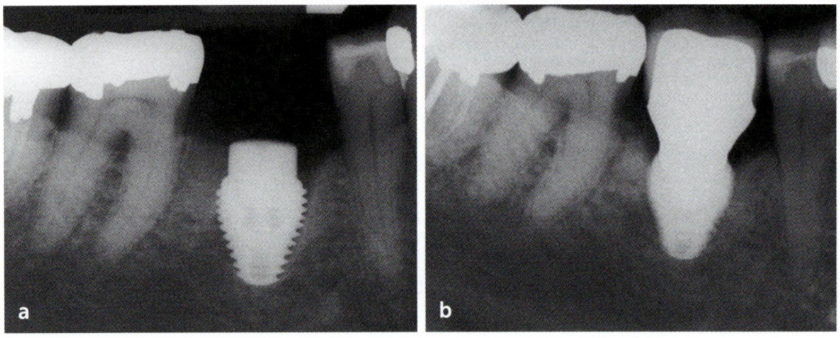

FIG 3-6 *(a)* This mandibular first molar site had a type C IRS that was eliminated to place a wide-diameter implant (9-mm length × 8-mm diameter) stabilized by engaging the buccal and lingual bone buttresses (see also chapter 8). The implant was placed subcrestally as recommended by the manufacturer, and all peri-implant defects were filled with particulate xenograft. A 3-mm-long healing abutment was connected to allow nonsubmerged healing and some nonocclusal loading during site healing. *(b)* The implant has been in function for over 8 years and shows stable crestal bone. (Restoration provided by Dr Reynaldo Todescan, Toronto, Ontario.)

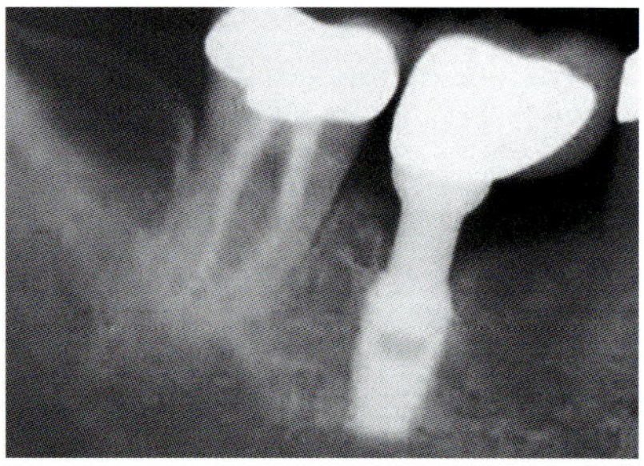

FIG 3-7 In this patient, the operator chose to place an IMI into the distal root socket rather than dealing with a narrow IRS. This choice requires the operator to be aware that a safe distance of 6 mm from tooth root apex to the mandibular canal has to be carefully observed. This will allow up to 4 mm of apical bone to be engaged and leave at least 2 mm between the implant apex and the mandibular canal.

Using the IRS to receive a mandibular IMI generally involves little risk of breaching the inferior alveolar canal (IAC). In contrast, if an IMI were to be placed in a molar root socket rather than in the IRS, Froum et al[15] warned that 53% of mandibular first molars and 73% of mandibular second molars may present high risk for IAN injury with IMI placement (Fig 3-8). If this risk were to be combined with the risk of lingual plate perforation, then the probability of a complication taking place with mandibular IMI placement increased to 57% for first molar and 81% for second molar sites. Obviously then, careful analysis of pretreatment records is crucial for safe insertion of mandibular IMIs.

Available bone at mandibular molar apices

As already stated, the preferred and prosthetically driven location for a mandibular IMI will be the IRS, in which case the implant apex is unlikely to extend significantly beyond the root apices of the extracted tooth. However, if the IRS is type C, as often happens with mandibular second molars, or if a type B IRS has been damaged by chronic infection, it may be necessary to involve bone more apically. In these situations, it is generally held that engagement of up to 4 mm of this bone will be needed to stabilize a standard-diameter implant, and this may risk damaging the IAC.[15,20] The margin for safety is to leave a distance of 2 mm from the osteotomy apex to the IAC. Again, then, it may be more appropriate to perform socket preservation grafting and delayed implant placement.

Mandibular cross-sectional shape

As discussed in chapter 2, three mandibular cross-sectional jaw morphologies have been identified by Chan et al[21,22]: convergent, parallel, and undercut shapes. Convergent jaws widen from the alveolar crest toward the lower border of the mandible (Fig 3-9a), while parallel mandibles have buccal and lingual

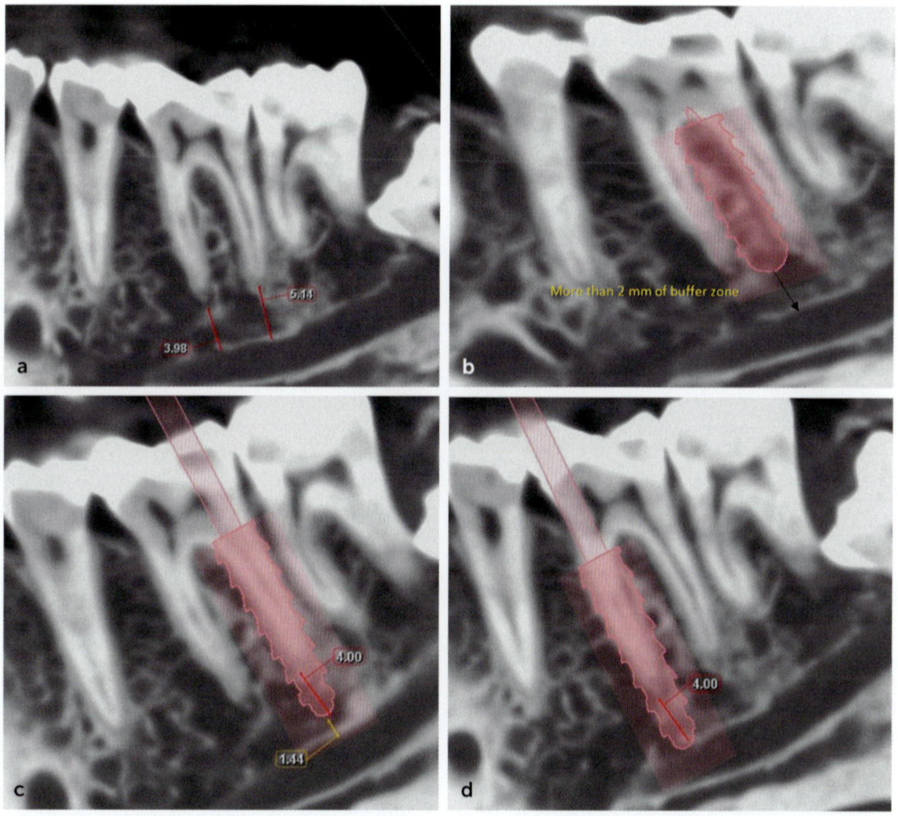

FIG 3-8 *(a)* This first molar shows a type B IRS. The distances from the mesial and distal root apices are 3.98 mm and 5.14 mm, respectively. *(b)* If it were possible to stabilize an IMI in the IRS, there would be no risk of damaging the IAN. *(c)* If an IMI instead were to be placed in the distal root of the same tooth, and 4 mm of apical bone was needed to stabilize the implant, there would be a risk of damaging the IAN as the distance to the latter would be less than 2 mm. *(d)* If an IMI were to be placed in the mesial root socket, allowing for 4 mm of apical bone to stabilize the implant would most certainly damage the IAN.

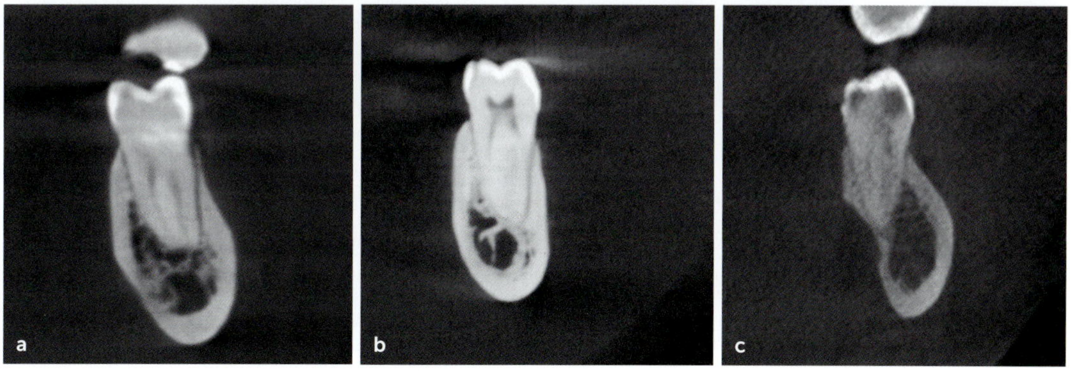

FIG 3-9 *(a)* Convergent jaws widen from the alveolar crest toward the lower border of the mandible. *(b)* Parallel mandibles have buccal and lingual outlines that are largely parallel. *(c)* Undercut jaw shapes are those which are widest at the alveolar crest but narrow toward the base, forming distinct lingual undercuts.

outlines that are largely parallel (Fig 3-9b). Undercut jaw shapes are those which are widest at the alveolar crest but narrow toward the base, forming distinct lingual undercuts (Fig 3-9c). The predicted incidence of lingual plate perforation in mandibular molar sites is generally low (1.1% to 1.2%),[21,23] but undercut mandibles do present a higher risk. In one cross-sectional CBCT study, 66% of mandibles were found to be undercut,[22] with a significantly higher frequency at the mandibular second molar (62.7%) than at first

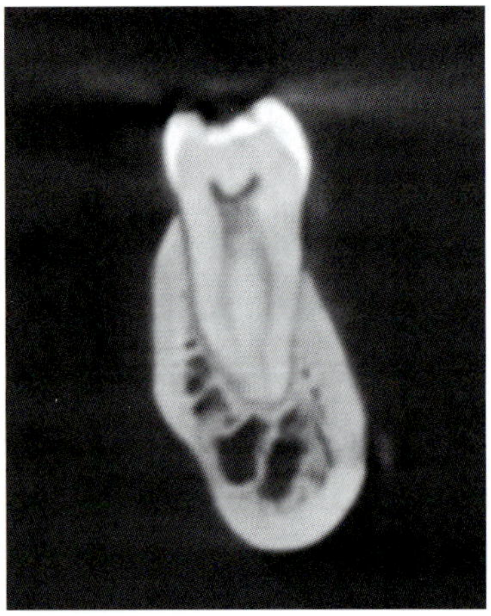

FIG 3-10 The buccal and lingual cortical bone plates tend to thicken with increasing distance from the alveolar crest.

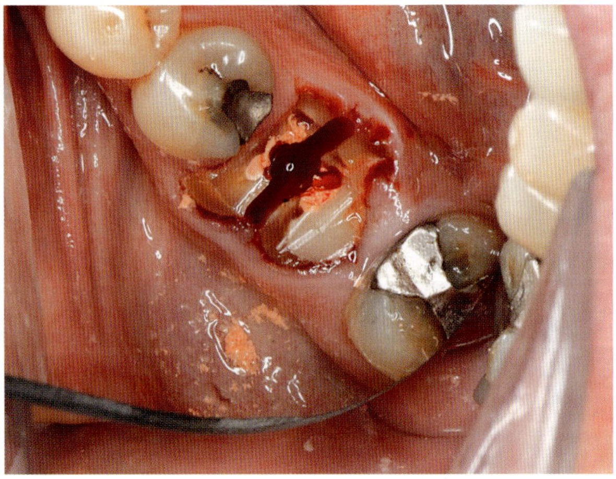

FIG 3-11 This first molar has been decoronated and the two roots separated. A large round bur also was used to establish an entry point to the IRS for osteotomy burs.

molar (56.2%) sites.[21,24,25] Unlike the situation in the anterior mandible where perforations of the lingual plate can result in hemorrhage with potentially life-threatening outcomes, lingual plate perforations in the posterior mandible are less serious unless the perforation is above the mylohyoid ridge where the lingual nerve might be injured, or if the apex of the implant becomes infected somehow at the site of the perforation.[26] Of the sites at which IAC was not the limiting factor for immediate implants, Froum et al[15] noted that while the risk of lingual plate perforation was low at first molar sites (9%), the risk increased to 31% at second molar sites.

Thickness of cortical bone

Other anatomical factors that need to be considered with regard to immediate postextractive mandibular molar implantation are the thicknesses of buccal and lingual cortical bone plates. Theye et al[27] recently provided micro-CT measurements of buccal plate thicknesses and bone densities for maxillary and mandibular molar sites. Crestal buccal plate thickness was found to be less than 1 mm at around 20.8% of mandibular molars, although it can increase to 2 mm or greater at deeper levels[16] (Fig 3-10). In another recent CBCT report, Padhye et al[18] recorded a mean buccal bone thickness at the crest of mandibular first molars as only 0.84 ± 0.39 mm compared with 2.71 ± 1.17 mm lingually. These are important observations because others have shown that if buccal crestal bone thickness is less than 1.5 mm, the risk of postimplantation vertical bone loss is high.[28]

Caution needs to be used, however, in relying on CBCT scans to estimate these bone thicknesses, as a recent report concluded that they are often inaccurate if the real cortical thicknesses are less than 1 mm.[29] With this in mind, ideal 3D positioning of mandibular IMIs should begin slightly toward the lingual and, if possible, the implant should be submerged 1 to 2 mm subcrestally relative to the lower of the buccal or lingual cortical plates.[19,30–33]

Suggested Surgical Protocols

Prior to treatment, patients must receive a thorough oral examination, including assessment of the maximal jaw opening, intra-arch relationships, site-specific buccolingual alveolar ridge width, and specific as well as general maxillomandibular relationships. Panoramic radiographs and CBCT records are needed to evaluate bone quantity and density, buccal cortical bone thickness, proximity of vital structures, adjacent tooth angulations, and an overall 3D volumetric analysis of the alveolar site. Based on the information obtained, diagnostic wax-ups can be made and, if appropriate, surgical templates fabricated. Ideally, during the week before surgery, a full-mouth professional scaling and prophylaxis should be carried out. Use of a systemic antibiotic administered presurgically is also common

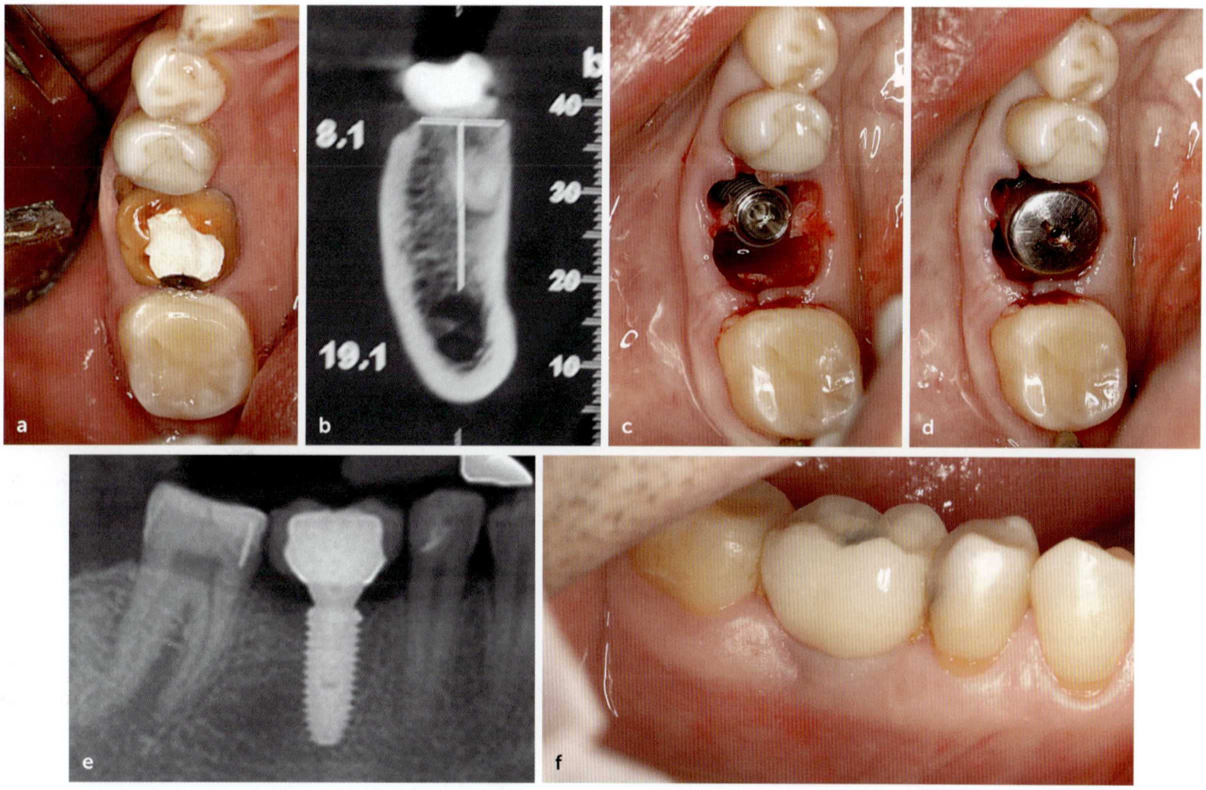

FIG 3-12 *(a)* This mandibular first molar was planned for extraction and replacement with an IMI. *(b)* CBCT images showed plenty of bone height in the region of the IRS. *(c)* Using flapless surgery, the two roots were separated and removed atraumatically, followed by creation of the osteotomy in the type B IRS. An implant of 4.5-mm diameter and 11.5-mm length was placed and secured by the remaining lingual and buccal buttresses of IRS bone. No gap grafting was done. *(d)* A large-diameter healing abutment was added prior to stabilizing the soft tissues with minimal suturing. *(e)* A radiograph of the restored implant after 1 year in function. *(f)* The clinical presentation after 1 year in function. Note the partial buccal collapse of hard and soft tissues distally. (Case provided by Dr Omid Nadaf, Tehran, Iran.)

practice. Some clinicians also prescribe chlorhexidine mouthrinses for use twice daily in the 3 days prior to IMI treatment in order to reduce the intraoral microbial load.

Flap design and atraumatic extraction

Using flapless or minimally elevated flap procedures is preferred with mandibular IMIs, as this will result in minimal disturbance of the periosteal blood supply nourishing buccal bone, leading to less postsurgical crestal bone loss[34,35] and less buccal soft tissue retraction during site healing.[36]

Atraumatic molar extraction with minimal hard and soft tissue damage can be difficult and therefore should begin with molar coronectomy using a high-speed handpiece and fissure bur to allow exposure of the roots at the level of their furcation and subsequent root separation prior to removal[19] (Fig 3-11). The original approach to placing mandibular IMIs was to remove the tooth roots before preparing the osteotomy as in the sample case presented in Fig 3-12. More recent techniques for IMI placement, however, involve leaving the tooth roots in situ until after the osteotomy has been partially or completely developed. A variety of instruments can be used to release each root from bone prior to employing root forceps. These releasing instruments include various periotomes, piezoelectric surgical tips, or even just a high-speed handpiece and long, narrow, tapered diamond bur (eg, FGSurg Medium Needle Diamond bur, Brasseler).[37,38] The latter can be inserted into the periodontal ligament space and used to shave away some of the tooth root substance (generally at the mesial and/or distal surfaces) and/or alveolar bone to a depth of about

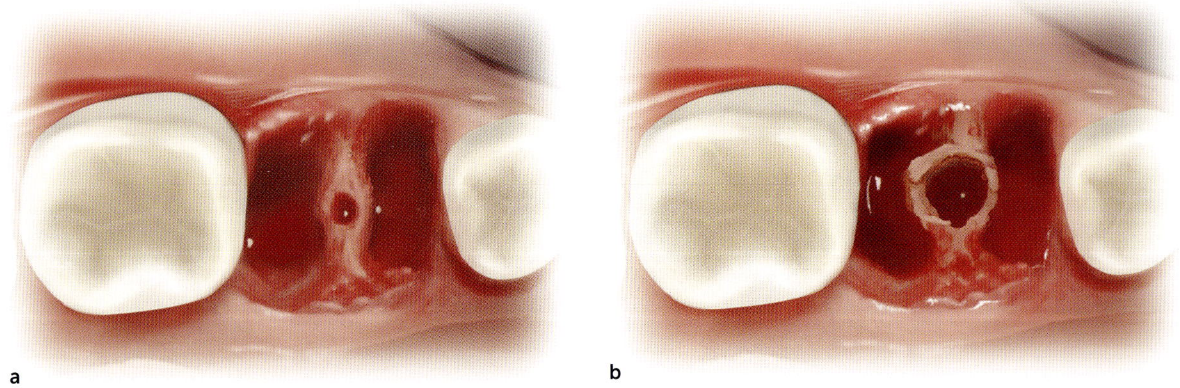

FIG 3-13 Should the molar roots be removed before osteotomy preparation, the IRS may be expanded using densifying burs. *(a)* Narrow IRS. *(b)* Osseodensification to expand the IRS in preparation for osteotomy. (Copyright Versah.)

two-thirds the root length. This will allow the subsequent efficient use of periotomes or narrow-diameter elevators to luxate and remove the individual roots. Keeping the goal of minimizing damage to the buccal bone in mind, buccolingual luxation movements of roots also should be minimized during their removal.

Socket debridement

The need for thorough socket debridement after all tooth fragments have been removed will depend on the health of the surrounding bone tissue and by extension the reason for tooth extraction. If no periapical pathology exists, there is likely little to no need to perform aggressive socket debridement, particularly since remnants of healthy periodontal ligament may be beneficial in achieving osseointegration of immediate implants.[39] However, if the condemned tooth has granulation or cystic tissue related to pulpal or advanced periodontal destruction, most clinicians prefer to remove it meticulously using sharp curettes and even rotary instruments since pathogenic organisms can persist in dormancy in periapical bone, possibly leading to delayed implant failure.[40]

Site preparation

As already stated, the ideal site for mandibular IMI placement is the IRS. Therefore, if suitable IRS exists, the implant osteotomy should be initiated using either a small-diameter round bur, a piezoelectric surgery tip, or a fine, sharp-pointed initial penetration bur positioned at the mesiodistal center of the IRS but slightly toward the lingual in order to compensate for any uncontrollable buccal drifting of any of the subsequent burs needed for completion of the osteotomy.[41] With a type A IRS,[17] the goal would be to develop the osteotomy entirely within it, but as already stated, type A IRSs are rarely found at mandibular molar sites. Most commonly, type B IRSs, ie, those with sufficient bone to stabilize the implant but not completely house it, are encountered with mandibular first molars. If the molar roots are removed before osteotomy preparation, it may be possible to expand and retain most of a type B IRS using osseodensifying burs[42] (Fig 3-13; see also chapter 7). Any dehiscences that may develop in the osteotomy walls during drilling can be managed with bone allografts as long as the implant is stable (ideally ≥ 35 Ncm). As an aside, if both first and second molars are being replaced with IMIs, a useful strategy can be to place the first molar implant in the first molar type B IRS, but to place the second molar implant (most likely with a type C IRS) into the mesial or distal root socket of the extracted tooth (Fig 3-14).

Returning to the difficulty of stabilizing burs in type B IRSs at sites where the molar roots were removed before osteotomy preparation, Fugazzotto[43] suggested a protocol for starting with a narrow-diameter pilot or twist bur first being introduced at an acute angle relative to the base of the IRS (Fig 3-15). Once the entry point had been established here, and in the absence of bur drifting or chatter, he suggested that

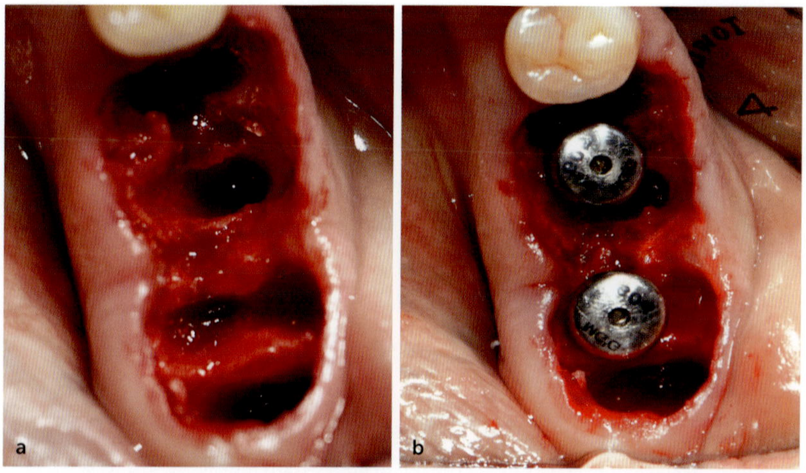

FIG 3-14 *(a)* In this patient, IMIs were planned for both the mandibular first and second molars. *(b)* Two IMIs were placed. The first molar site had a type B IRS, which was used as the osteotomy site, while the second implant was placed into the mesial root socket of the second molar, which had a type C IRS. (Courtesy of Dr Omid Moghadas, Tehran, Iran.)

the bur could then be slowly uprighted. Thereafter, each bur in sequence was made to enter the site at a slightly less acute angle before being straightened up, so that at the end, the preparation would allow implant placement in the correct position stabilized by the buccal and lingual bone buttresses of the IRS. A simpler approach can be to remove only one root, leaving the second root in position to help to stabilize and direct drilling of the osteotomy.

Others have proposed removing all or part of a type B IRS, for example with round burs,[44] trephines,[45] or piezoelectric surgical tips before initiating osteotomy preparation with a pilot bur. However, unless a wider-diameter implant is used (eg, as shown in Fig 3-6), this would require the engagement of up to 4 mm of apical bone and increase the risk of damaging the IAN.

3D positioning of implants

If a planned IMI site has contiguous teeth both mesially and distally, ideally it should be positioned equidistantly around 3 mm from each tooth and certainly no closer than 1.5 mm in order to preserve and restore the interproximal hard and soft tissues. Platform switching (ie, using a healing abutment and subsequently a prosthetic abutment smaller in diameter than the implant platform) can also be used to preserve the interproximal bone and facilitate subsequent soft tissue papilla reformation.[46] Ideal positioning also means placing the implant

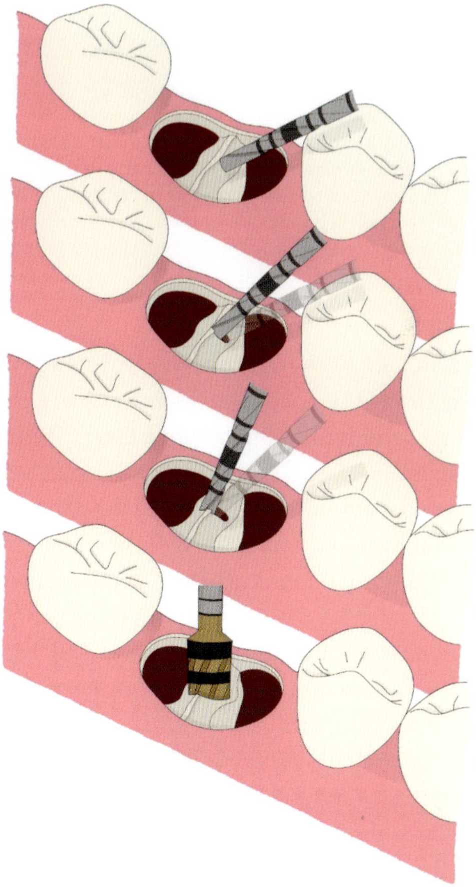

FIG 3-15 A technique proposed in years past by Fugazzotto[43] for dealing with type B mandibular molar IRSs. First, begin osteotomy preparation with the first bur on an angle in order to gain a firm footing. Thereafter, slowly upright each bur sequentially to end up with the correct positioning of the final osteotomy.

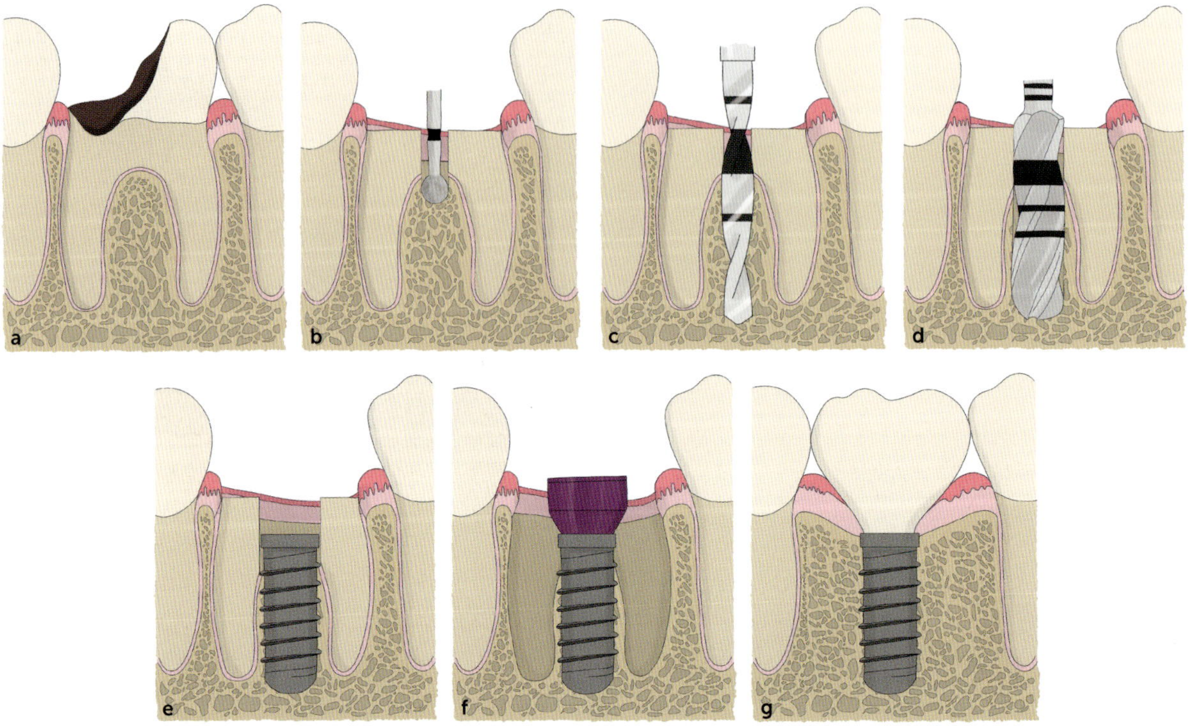

FIG 3-16 *(a)* A hopeless mandibular first molar. *(b)* The tooth is first decoronated and an opening through the furcation created to allow insertion of implant burs. *(c)* A pilot bur is used to establish the required depth of the osteotomy in the type B IRS. *(d)* Subsequent implant burs are used to shape the final osteotomy. *(e)* Ideally, the implant will be placed either before or after removal of the tooth roots and 1 to 2 mm below the lowest bone crest, usually the buccal. *(f)* A large-diameter healing abutment helps to shelter the remaining gaps, whether grafted or not. *(g)* After site healing, a full crown has been added to the prosthetic platform, ideally with a platform-switch feature.

slightly toward the lingual to leave a large buccal gap and thereby minimize buccal bone loss.[47,48] For both bone-level and tissue-level implant designs, vertical implant positioning should ensure that any moderately rough implant surface is fully submerged in bone, ideally to a depth at which the buccal crestal bone is at least 1.5 mm in thickness. Positioning the implant subcrestally by 1 to 2 mm also will contribute to a more pleasing emergence profile of the final molar implant crown.

Mean mesiodistal widths of mandibular first molars have been recorded as 11.5 mm and 10.9 mm in males versus females respectively, while the same measurements for mandibular second molars are 10.9 mm and 10.1 mm.[49] Therefore, with typical mandibular molar sites (mesiodistal width up to 11 mm), having type A or B septa, appropriate implant diameters would be 4.5 to 5 mm. On the other hand, with type C septa or mesiodistal width greater than 11 mm, implants with diameters greater than 5 mm may be the ones to use, as this will help to reduce risk of root caries of the adjacent teeth.

Osteotomy drilling before root removal

As already discussed, placing mandibular IMIs in an ideal position without compromising their primary stability can be difficult if the molar roots are removed before any osteotomy drilling. The best way to minimize these problems is to begin the osteotomy drilling through the molar furcation after decoronation but before removing the tooth roots, leaving the removal of the roots until after the osteotomy is partially or even totally completed[14,50–52] or even until after implant placement (Fig 3-16). In this technique, the retained roots help to guide the osteotomy drills and allow for precise positioning and angulation of the implant, helping to set things up for an ideal emergence profile for the final restoration.

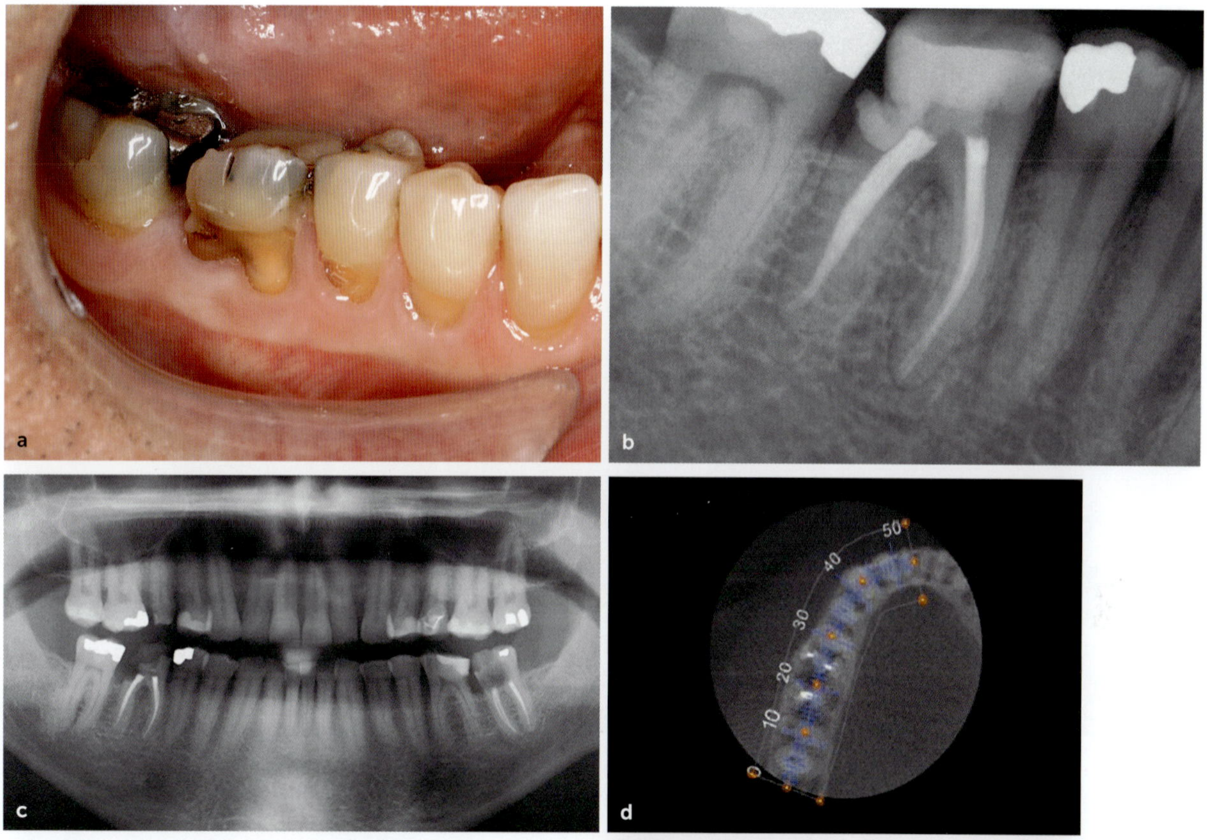

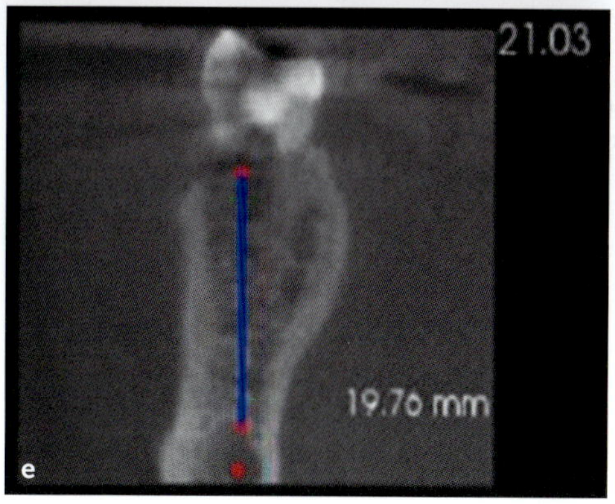

FIG 3-17 *(a)* The mandibular first molar required extraction as it had nonrestorable caries. Note the favorable wide band of keratinized gingiva. *(b)* This radiograph shows deep nonrestorable caries distally at the first molar, which had a type B IRS. *(c)* The patient's preoperative panoramic radiograph indicated that placement of an IMI in the IRS of the right mandibular first molar could be without risk of violating the mandibular canal. *(d)* The axial slices of the CBCT scan showed excellent buccolingual ridge width and a type B IRS at the endodontically treated mandibular right first molar. *(e)* The coronal slices of the CBCT scan through the molar furcation indicated more than adequate bone height to receive a 12-mm-long implant, as there was > 19 mm of bone from the furcation to the mandibular canal.

A sample case is shown in the following images. The patient was a 53-year-old man with a hopeless mandibular first molar (Fig 3-17a). The preoperative radiographs, including periapical (Fig 3-17b) and panoramic (Fig 3-17c) views, showed a type B IRS. The axial slices of the CBCT scans (Fig 3-17d) further confirmed this finding, while a sagittal slice in the furcation area showed sufficient bone height above the mandibular canal (Fig 3-17e). With all of this information, the decision was made to begin osteotomy preparation before removing the tooth roots. The substantial bone above the IAN permitted the choice of a 12-mm-long Straumann bone-level tapered (BLT) implant of standard diameter. It was thought that this implant with its aggressive threads would help to achieve adequate stability for the IMI. Flapless surgery was used following crestal release only. After coronectomy (Fig 3-17f) and creating a stable entry point in the furcation using a large-diameter round bur, a pilot bur was drilled to approximately 12-mm depth and a

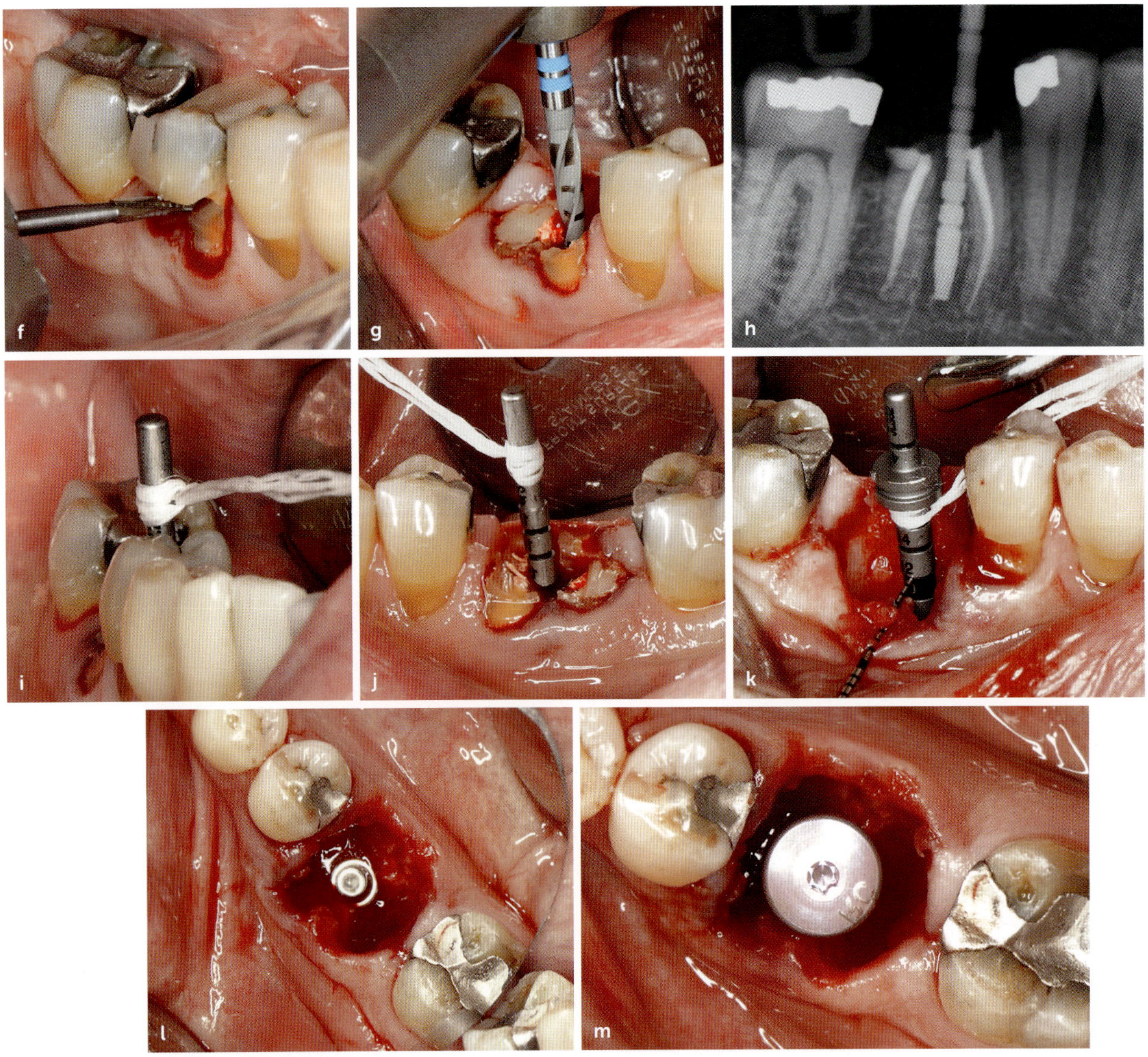

FIG 3-17 *(cont) (f)* The tooth was first decoronated at the level of its furcation. *(g)* The implant pilot bur was used to drill into the IRS via the molar furcation. *(h)* An intraoperative radiograph showing the initial osteotomy depth after using the pilot bur. *(i)* A clinical photograph verifying correct angulation of the osteotomy in the apicocoronal dimension. *(j)* A clinical photograph showing the mesiodistal orientation of the osteotomy after using the pilot drill. *(k)* Following root removal, a depth gauge was inserted into the osteotomy to allow verification of its depth using a periodontal probe positioned horizontally and resting on the buccal plate of bone. At this stage, the osteotomy measured 12 mm in depth in relation to the buccal crestal bone, but since the operator wished to submerge the implant by 2 mm relative to this bone level, the osteotomy was appropriately deepened. *(l)* After using the 3.5-mm-diameter implant bur, a 12-mm-long × 4.1-mm-diameter implant was placed such that the top of the implant was approximately 2 mm subcrestal relative to the buccal bone crest height. *(m)* A large-diameter 6-mm-long healing abutment was connected to the implant to provide some support for the soft tissues once repositioned. Torque testing revealed stability of 35 Ncm.

periapical radiograph taken with a paralleling pin in situ to establish a safe baseline position (Figs 3-17g and 3-17h). The paralleling pin also verified the 3D positioning of the osteotomy (Figs 3-17i and 3-17j). The tooth roots were then removed and a depth gauge inserted to verify the true depth of the osteotomy at this point (Fig 3-17k). The depth was verified to be 12 mm relative to the buccal bone crest, but since the operator wished to place the implant around 2 mm subcrestally, the depth was increased a further 2 mm using the pilot bur. Osteotomy preparation then was continued, finishing with the 3.5-mm-diameter implant bur. At this point, insertion and manual testing of the 3.5-mm-diameter bur showed some move-

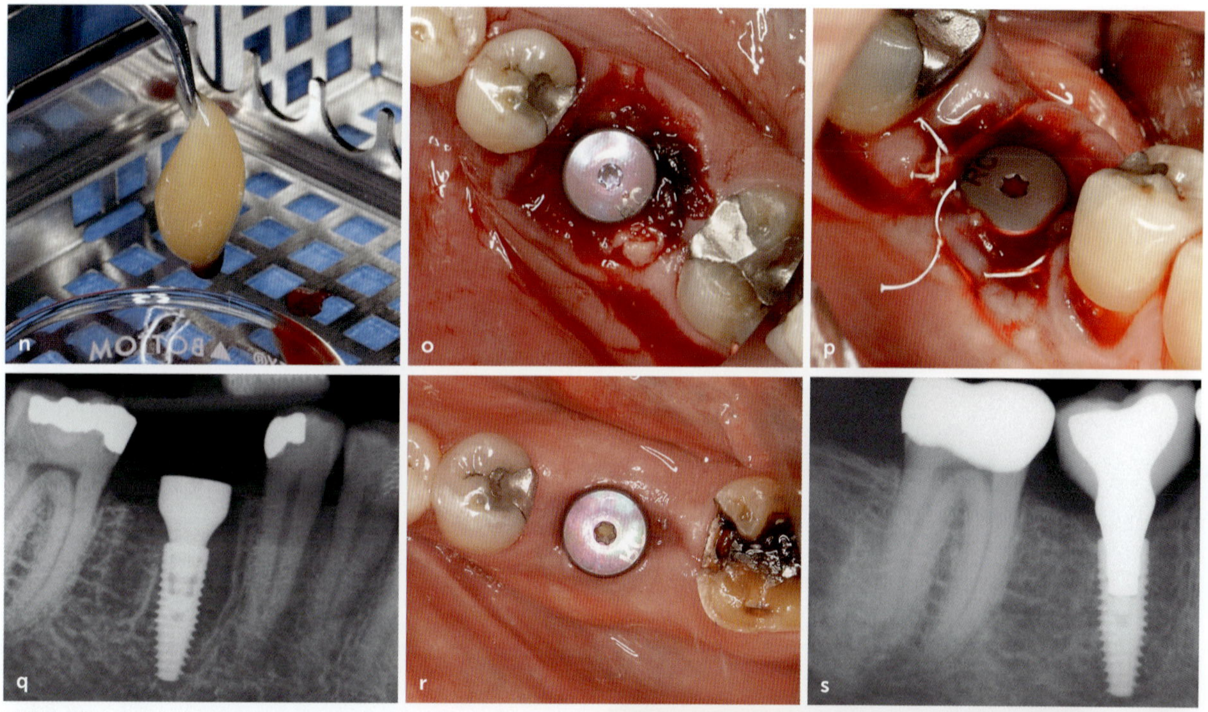

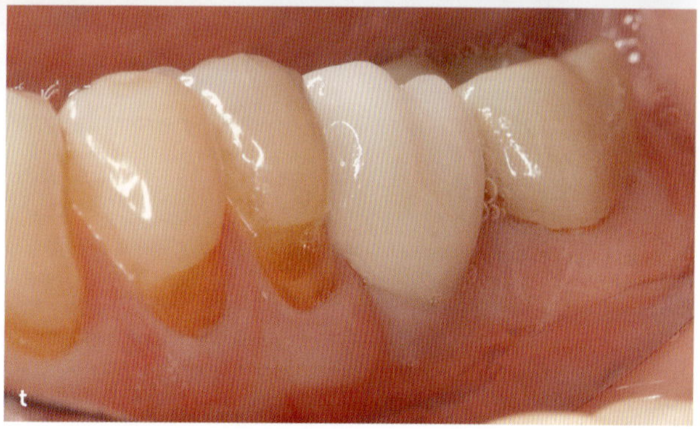

FIG 3-17 *(cont) (n)* Dense growth factor–rich autogenous fibrin clots were prepared from the patient's venous blood.[53] *(o)* The prepared autogenous CGF fibrin clots were used to fill the peri-implant gaps. *(p)* The soft tissues were adapted using PTFE sutures. *(q)* The immediate postoperative radiographic image of the IMI. While the operator needed to engage some of the bone apical to the root apices, no risk had been taken with regard to damaging the mandibular neurovascular bundle. *(r)* A clinical photograph at the 5-week postoperative follow-up confirms healthy soft tissue healing. *(s)* A radiograph of the restored IMI. *(t)* A mirror view of the restored implant. (Surgery performed by Dr Quang Nguyen, University of Toronto.)

ment, and therefore the decision was made to insert the 4.1-mm-diameter implant straightaway rather than performing any more drilling. After placement (Fig 3-17l), the implant was tested with a torque wrench and documented to have 35 Ncm stability. A large-diameter, 6-mm-long healing abutment was connected to the implant and left exposed for the initial integration period (Fig 3-17m).

Prior to the surgery, four red-capped glass blood collection tubes (~9 mL volume each) of the patient's venous blood had been collected and spun in a specially programmed, variable-speed centrifuge (Silfradent Medifuge) for 14 minutes to create autogenous platelet growth factor–enhanced fibrin clots[53] (Fig 3-17n). These concentrated growth factor (CGF) clots were subsequently used to fill all peri-implant gaps (Fig 3-17o), and the soft tissues were stabilized with polytetrafluoroethylene (PTFE) sutures (Fig 3-17p). Others have confirmed that autogenous platelet-rich fibrin clots can be used for this purpose either alone or, if need be (eg, with a three-wall socket), combined with particulate bone allograft or xenograft.[54,55] The immediate postoperative radiograph is shown in Fig 3-17q, while the soft tissue response by 5 weeks is seen in Fig 3-17r. The clinical and radiographic images of the restored implant are shown in Figs 3-17s and 3-17t.

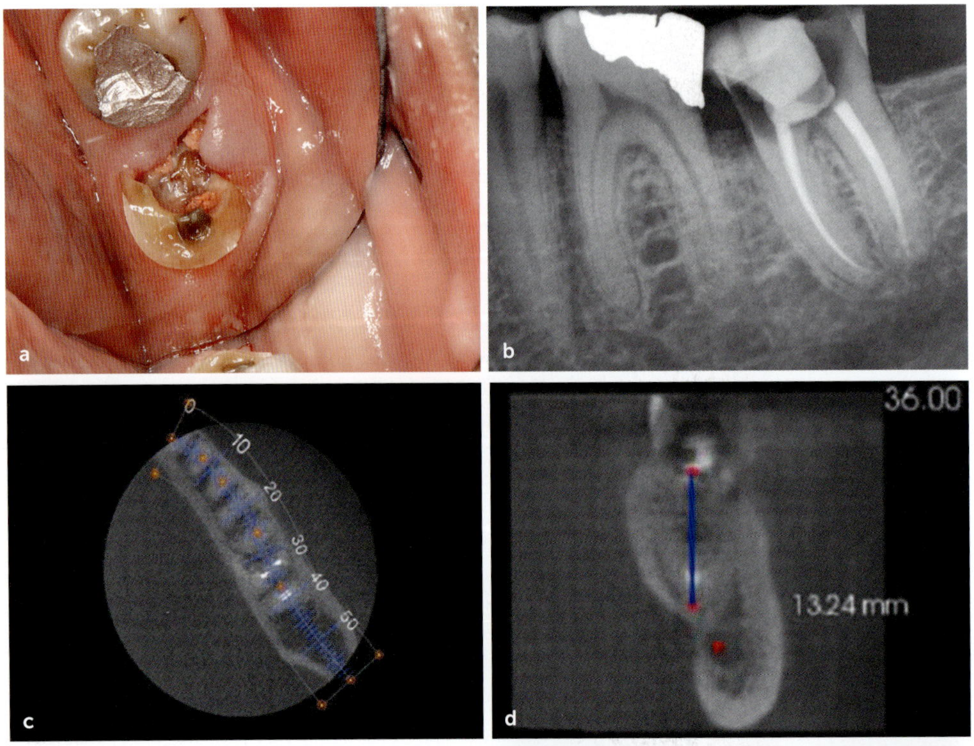

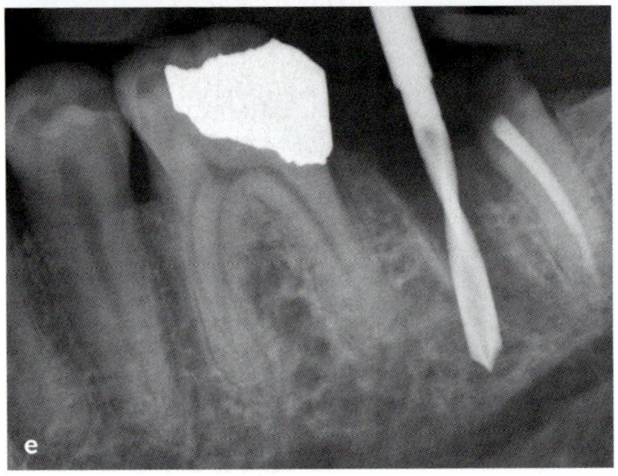

FIG 3-18 *(a)* The left second molar had lost its restoration and was deemed to be nonrestorable. *(b)* The preoperative radiograph showed the tooth to be typical of many mandibular second molars with its type C IRS. *(c)* The axial CBCT scans of the left second molar indicated thick buccal and lingual bone cortices and good buccolingual ridge width for an IMI. *(d)* The coronal CBCT slices showed a reasonable bone height (> 13 mm) in the furcation area but uncovered a deep lingual undercut. *(e)* After removing the mesial root, the pilot bur was positioned in contact with the mesial aspect of the IRS and positioned to engage bone mesial to the mesial root. This radiograph verifies that the osteotomy apex is a safe distance from the IAN.

The same patient had a hopeless left mandibular second molar with a type C IRS (Figs 3-18a and 3-18b; see also Fig 3-17c). The axial slices of the CBCT scan showed the buccal and lingual cortical bone plates to be thick and the buccolingual ridge width favorable for an IMI (Fig 3-18c). However, there was one caution raised, as there was a deep lingual undercut of the body of the mandible approximately 13 mm apical to the tooth furcation (Fig 3-18d). Based on these radiographic findings, the decision was made to place a 10-mm-long × 5-mm-diameter implant with aggressive cutting threads (NobelActive TiUltra, Nobel Biocare) to stabilize the implant apically in bone mesial to the apex of the mesial root socket. The surgical approach was largely flapless, although a midcrestal incision was made distally to improve visibility. After separating the tooth roots using a high-speed handpiece and bur, the mesial root was removed atraumatically with the aid of periotomes. The mesial aspect of the IRS and the distal root were then used to help stabilize the pilot bur for creation of the initial osteotomy and a radiograph taken to check (Fig 3-18e). Osteotomy preparation was then continued using the 2.4/2.8-mm- and 3.2/3.6-mm-diameter implant burs (here the smaller number refers to the diameter at the tip of the bur and the larger the diameter of the drill bit body) to the same depth as the pilot drill preparation, and the 10 × 5-mm

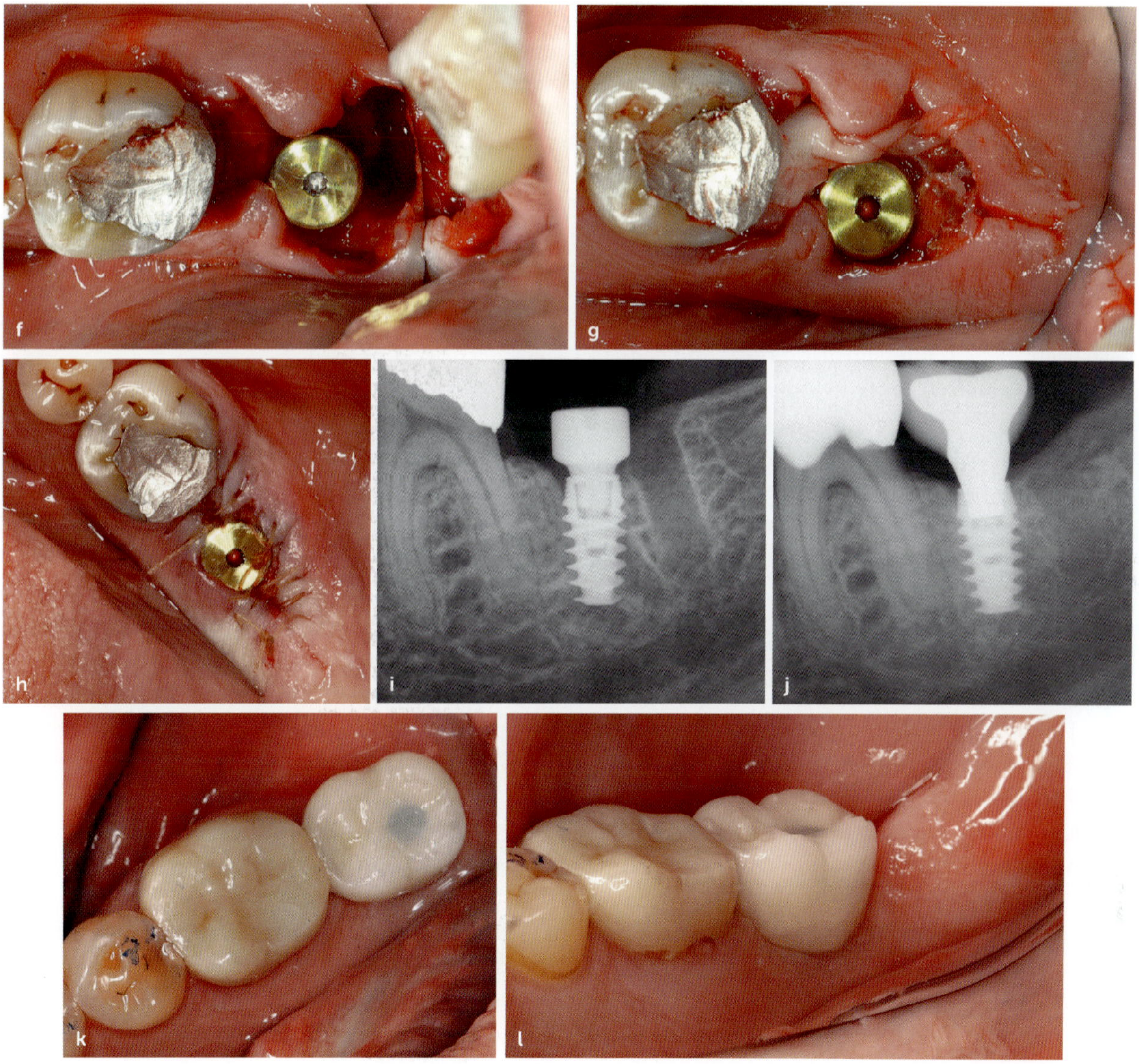

FIG 3-18 *(cont) (f)* Following implant insertion, a wide-diameter healing abutment was added to the implant. *(g)* Three large CGF-containing fibrin clots were condensed into the peri-implant gaps and the distal root socket. *(h)* The soft tissues were repositioned and sutured with chromic gut sutures, leaving the top of the healing abutment exposed. *(i)* The immediate postoperative radiograph showing the implant apex to be a safe distance from the IAN. A 10-mm-long × 5-mm-diameter implant with aggressive cutting threads (Nobel-Active TiUltra) was selected to ensure good initial stability. *(j)* A periapical radiograph of the restored implant. *(k)* A clinical photograph of the occlusal of the restoration. *(l)* A mirror view of the implant restoration. (Surgery performed by Dr Quang Nguyen, University of Toronto.)

implant placed. The combination of the aggressive implant cutting threads and the slightly undersized osteotomy resulted in the handpiece torquing out at 35 Ncm during implant insertion but with 2 mm of implant length still needing submergence. Therefore, final seating of the implant was accomplished with a hand torque wrench. Stability was felt to be adequate to allow the addition of a 6-mm-diameter healing abutment, after which three CGF clots were packed into the remaining gaps (Figs 3-18f and 3-18g) before suturing (Fig 3-18h). Figure 3-18i shows the immediate postoperative radiograph of the implants in place, while the clinical and radiographic images of the restored implant are seen in Figs 3-18j to 3-18l.

Gap management with mandibular IMIs

Following placement of most mandibular IMIs, there will be peri-implant gaps remaining between the implant perimeter and internal walls of the socket, and indeed efforts should be made to ensure that adequate (≥ 2 mm) gaps remain buccally at both root sockets to minimize risk of buccal bone loss and buccolingual alveolar ridge shrinkage.[56] These gaps have been termed "jumping distances"[57] and need to fill with new bone in order to integrate the implant. However, whether gap grafting is needed to ensure this bone fill has become controversial. Historically, the decision whether or not to graft was based on gap widths, with some clinicians suggesting grafting with gap widths of 2 mm or more.[58,59] Others suggested grafting if a midbuccal gap of ≥ 1.25 mm and/or a mesial, distal, or midlingual/palatal gap width of ≥ 2.25 mm remained.[60] However, growing evidence suggests that grafting may be unnecessary regardless of gap size, at least in supporting bone fill of any gaps. For example, Smith et al[61] recently reported on a successful case series of 300 IMIs placed using flapless surgery and no gap grafting. Instead, large-diameter healing abutments were placed to shelter the gaps during normal socket healing by secondary intention as would happen if an IMI had not been placed into the extraction socket.[62] Others have made similar observations.

Deporter et al[63] recently presented a classification of gaps based on location about the implant periphery. Seven gap types were proposed, and all but one type were suggested to heal without gap grafting, provided that flapless surgery and atraumatic extraction had been achieved. The exception was their type II gap, which they reported happening when an implant is placed too far buccally with little to no gap remaining and/or contact with a thin buccal plate of bone. The remaining thickness of the buccal bone wall is crucial,[28,64] although a thin buccal plate may be less likely to be present at molar than anterior sites, for example. Nevertheless, if after implant placement, the buccal bone thickness crestally is less than 1.5 mm and if the implant could not be placed sufficiently subcrestally to compensate, it may be helpful to augment buccally with a slow-resorbing material.[65] This can easily be done by inserting graft particles under the periosteum after creating a small full-thickness submucosal pouch.[66–68] This grafting also will reduce the degree of alveolar ridge shrinkage and the risk of having buccal ridge anatomical depressions that later trap food debris.[68]

Submerged or nonsubmerged protocol for initial stability

IMIs must have good initial stability to integrate. Stability should be verified with a torque wrench or resonance frequency device. Submerged healing is often recommended for IMIs with an insertion torque of less than 15 Ncm. If resonance frequency is being used to test stability, implant stability quotient values of greater than 65 are recommended if a long-profile (eg, ≥ 3 mm) stock or custom healing abutment is to be used straightaway.[69] If the implant stability quotient value is less than 65, placing a cover screw rather than a healing abutment may be advisable.

Conclusion

It is possible to obtain good outcomes following mandibular IMI placement, particularly at first molar sites. Considerations with second molars include whether its replacement is truly necessary, proximity of the mandibular canal, presence of lingual concavities, and limited patient opening. Placing a mandibular IMI is a difficult procedure meant for skilled and experienced surgeons (Fig 3-19). Complete intraoral examination and careful pretreatment CBCT analysis are both highly recommended. Proper case selection includes considering the reason for tooth extraction; the socket anatomy remaining after extraction; planning for a flap or flapless approach; the dimensions of the IRS bone; the appropriate implant shape, length, and diameter; the depth and 3D positioning of the implant; the size of peri-implant gaps; and the appropriateness of including soft tissue grafting at sites with a thin and/or narrow gingival biotype.

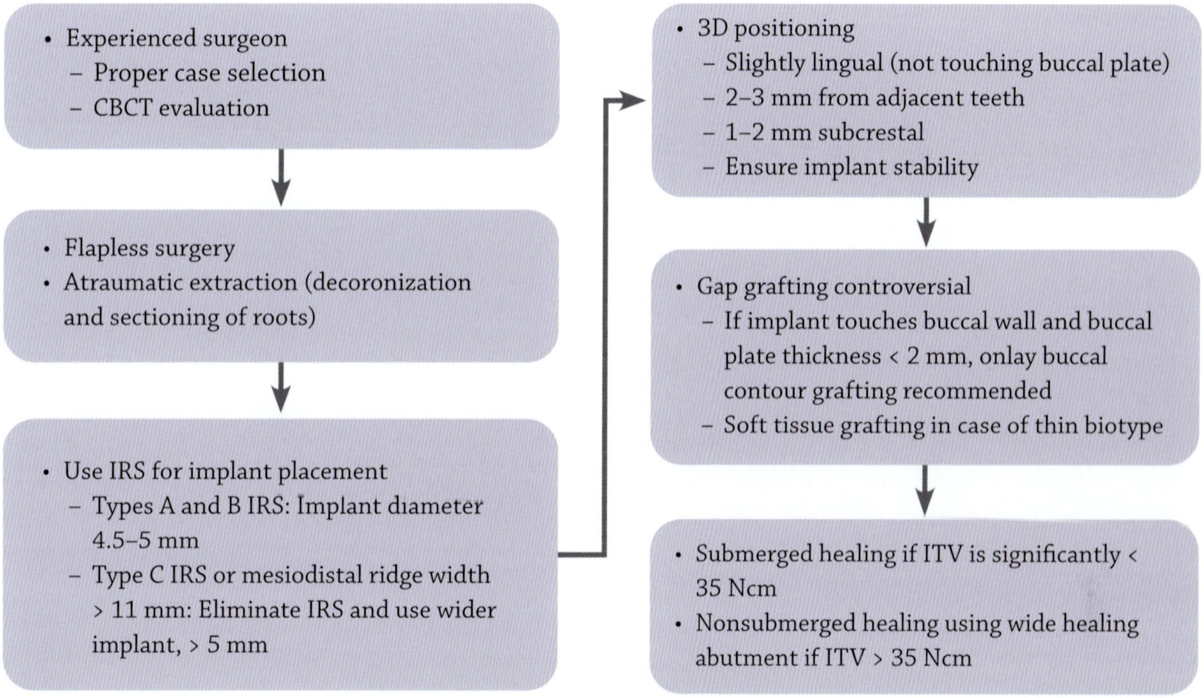

FIG 3-19 Summary flowchart for mandibular IMIs. ITV = insertion torque value.

KEY POINTS

- Sites with a thick, wide gingival biotype are preferred.
- Flapless surgery is recommended, provided there is intact buccal bone.
- Atraumatic tooth removal is crucial, meaning that the crown should first be removed with a high-speed handpiece, exposing the root furcation.
- Osteotomy preparation should be initiated in the IRS bone if this exists in sufficient volume.
- Given that a mandibular first molar tooth socket will likely have a type B IRS, beginning osteotomy preparation through the furcation of the tooth and slightly to the lingual before removal of the tooth roots will assist in minimizing bur drift and optimizing location.
- Tooth roots can be removed individually before or more likely after partial or complete osteotomy preparation.
- IMIs ideally will be submerged to the point where the buccal bone thickness is 1.5 mm or greater.
- Leaving a buccal gap that can be grafted will guard against unwanted buccal bone loss, but buccal onlay grafting also may be used to retain the alveolar ridge anatomy.
- Placing IMIs in mandibular second molar sockets is generally more difficult for various reasons, including the likelihood of having a type C IRS, the increased incidence of lingual undercuts, closer proximity to the mandibular canal, and limited operator access.
- Crucial to success is good initial implant stability, ideally 35-Ncm torque or greater.

References

1. Atieh MA, Payne AG, Duncan WJ, de Silva RK, Cullinan MP. Immediate placement or immediate restoration/loading of single implants for molar tooth replacement: A systematic review and meta-analysis. Int J Oral Maxillofac Implants 2010;25:401–415.
2. Ketabi M, Deporter D, Atenafu EG. A systematic review of outcomes following immediate molar implant placement based on recently published studies. Clin Implant Dent Relat Res 2016; 18:1084–1094.
3. Moy PK, Nishimura GH, Pozzi A, Danda AK. Single implants in dorsal areas: A systematic review. Eur J Oral Implantol 2016; 9(suppl 1):S163–S172.
4. Becker W, Becker BE. Replacement of maxillary and mandibular molars with single endosseous implant restorations: A retrospective study. J Prosthet Dent 1995;74:51–55.
5. Albrektsson T, Wennerberg A. Oral implant surfaces: Part 1—Review focusing on topographic and chemical properties of different surfaces and in vivo responses to them. Int J Prosthodont 2004;17:536–543.
6. Dawson A, Chen S (eds). The SAC Classification in Implant Dentistry. Berlin: Quintessence, 2009.
7. Sgolastra F, Petrucci A, Severino M, Gatto R, Monaco A. Periodontitis, implant loss and peri-implantitis. A meta-analysis. Clin Oral Implants Res 2015;26:e8–e16.
8. Aoki M, Takanashi K, Matsukubo T, et al. Transmission of periodontopathic bacteria from natural teeth to implants. Clin Implant Dent Relat Res 2012;14:406–411.
9. Wen X, Liu R, Li G, et al. History of periodontitis as a risk factor for long-term survival of dental implants: A meta-analysis. Int J Oral Maxillofac Implants 2014;29:1271–1280.
10. Roccuzzo M, De Angelis N, Bonino L, Aglietta M. Ten-year results of a three-arm prospective cohort study on implants in periodontally compromised patients. Part 1: Implant loss and radiographic bone loss. Clin Oral Implants Res 2010;21:490–496.
11. Matarasso S, Rasperini G, Iorio Siciliano V, Salvi GE, Lang NP, Aglietta M. A 10-year retrospective analysis of radiographic bone-level changes of implants supporting single-unit crowns in periodontally compromised vs. periodontally healthy patients. Clin Oral Implants Res 2010;21:898–903.
12. Bain CA, Moy PK. The association between the failure of dental implants and cigarette smoking. Int J Oral Maxillofac Implants 1993;8:609–615.
13. Chrcanovic BR, Albrektsson T, Wennerberg A. Bruxism and dental implants: A meta-analysis. Implant Dent 2015;24:505–516.
14. El Haddad E, Lauritano D, Carinci F. Interradicular septum as guide for pilot drill in postextractive implantology: A technical note. J Contemp Dent Pract 2015;16:81–84.
15. Froum S, Casanova L, Byrne S, Cho SC. Risk assessment before extraction for immediate implant placement in the posterior mandible: A computerized tomographic scan study. J Periodontol 2011;82:395–402.
16. Agostinelli C, Agostinelli A, Berardini M, Trisi P. Radiological evaluation of the dimensions of lower molar alveoli. Implant Dent 2018;27:271–275.
17. Smith RB, Tarnow DP. Classification of molar extraction sites for immediate dental implant placement: Technical note. Int J Oral Maxillofac Implants 2013;28:911–916.
18. Padhye NM, Shirsekar VU, Bhatavadekar NB. Three-dimensional alveolar bone assessment of mandibular first molars with implications for immediate implant placement. Int J Periodontics Restorative Dent 2020;40:e163–e167.
19. Hattingh AC, De Bruyn H, Ackermann A, Vandeweghe S. Immediate placement of ultrawide-diameter implants in molar sockets: Description of a recommended technique. Int J Periodontics Restorative Dent 2018;38:17–23.
20. Juodzbalys G, Wang HL, Sabalys G, Sidlauskas A, Galindo-Moreno P. Inferior alveolar nerve injury associated with implant surgery. Clin Oral Implants Res 2013;24:183–190.
21. Chan HL, Benavides E, Yeh CY, Fu JH, Rudek IE, Wang HL. Risk assessment of lingual plate perforation in posterior mandibular region: A virtual implant placement study using cone-beam computed tomography. J Periodontol 2011;82:129–135.
22. Chan HL, Brooks SL, Fu JH, Yeh CY, Rudek I, Wang HL. Cross-sectional analysis of the mandibular lingual concavity using cone beam computed tomography. Clin Oral Implants Res 2011;22: 201–206.
23. Huang RY, Cochran DL, Cheng WC, et al. Risk of lingual plate perforation for virtual immediate implant placement in the posterior mandible: A computer simulation study. J Am Dent Assoc 2015;146:735–742.
24. Lin MH, Mau LP, Cochran DL, Shieh YS, Huang PH, Huang RY. Risk assessment of inferior alveolar nerve injury for immediate implant placement in the posterior mandible: A virtual implant placement study. J Dent 2014;42:263–270.
25. Yu DC, Friedland BD, Karimbux NY, Guze KA. Supramandibular canal portion superior to the fossa of the submaxillary gland: A tomographic evaluation of the cross-sectional dimension in the molar region. Clin Implant Dent Relat Res 2013;15:750–758.
26. Chrcanovic BR, de Carvalho Machado V, Gjelvold B. Immediate implant placement in the posterior mandible: A cone beam computed tomography study. Quintessence Int 2016;47:505–514.
27. Theye CEG, Hattingh A, Cracknell TJ, Oettlé AC, Steyn M, Vandeweghe S. Dento-alveolar measurements and histomorphometric parameters of maxillary and mandibular first molars, using micro-CT. Clin Implant Dent Relat Res 2018;20:550–561.
28. Monje A, Chappuis V, Monje F, et al. The critical peri-implant buccal bone wall thickness revisited: An experimental study in the beagle dog. Int J Oral Maxillofac Implants 2019;34:1328–1336.
29. Domic D, Bertl K, Ahmad S, Schropp L, Hellén-Halme K, Stavropoulos A. Accuracy of cone-beam computed tomography is limited at implant sites with a thin buccal bone: A laboratory study. J Periodontol 2021;92:592–601.
30. Welander M, Abrahamsson I, Berglundh T. Subcrestal placement of two-part implants. Clin Oral Implants Res 2009;20:226–231.
31. Koutouzis T, Fetner M, Fetner A, Lundgren T. Retrospective evaluation of crestal bone changes around implants with reduced abutment diameter placed non-submerged and at subcrestal positions: The effect of bone grafting at implant placement. J Periodontol 2011;82:234–242.
32. Urdaneta RA, Seemann R, Dragan IF, Lubelski W, Leary J, Chuang SK. A retrospective radiographic study on the effect of natural tooth-implant proximity and an introduction to the concept of a bone-loading platform switch. Int J Oral Maxillofac Implants 2014;29:1412–1424.
33. Madani E, Smeets R, Freiwald E, et al. Impact of different placement depths on the crestal bone level of immediate versus delayed placed platform-switched implants. J Craniomaxillofac Surg 2018;46:1139–1146.
34. Blanco J, Alves CC, Nuñez V, Aracil L, Muñoz F, Ramos I. Biological width following immediate implant placement in the dog: Flap vs. flapless surgery. Clin Oral Implants Res 2010;21:624–631.
35. Fickl S, Zuhr O, Wachtel H, Bolz W, Huerzeler M. Tissue alterations after tooth extraction with and without surgical trauma: A volumetric study in the beagle dog. J Clin Periodontol 2008; 35:356–363.

36. Koh RU, Rudek I, Wang HL. Immediate implant placement: Positives and negatives. Implant Dent 2010;19:98–108.
37. Sharma SD, Vidya B, Alexander M, Deshmukh S. Periotome as an aid to atraumatic extraction: A comparative double blind randomized controlled trial. J Maxillofac Oral Surg 2015;14:611–615.
38. Blus C, Szmukler-Moncler S. Atraumatic tooth extraction and immediate implant placement with Piezosurgery: Evaluation of 40 sites after at least 1 year of loading. Int J Periodontics Restorative Dent 2010;30:355–363.
39. Pei X, Wang L, Chen C, Yuan X, Wan Q, Helms JA. Contribution of the PDL to osteotomy repair and implant osseointegration. J Dent Res 2017;96:909–916.
40. Nelson S, Thomas G. Bacterial persistence in dentoalveolar bone following extraction: A microbiological study and implications for dental implant treatment. Clin Implant Dent Relat Res 2010;12:306–314.
41. Hayacibara RM, Gonçalves CS, Garcez-Filho J, Magro-Filho O, Esper H, Hayacibara MF. The success rate of immediate implant placement of mandibular molars: A clinical and radiographic retrospective evaluation between 2 and 8 years. Clin Oral Implants Res 2013;24:806–811.
42. Lahens B, Neiva R, Tovar N, et al. Biomechanical and histologic basis of osseodensification drilling for endosteal implant placement in low density bone. An experimental study in sheep. J Mech Behav Biomed Mater 2016;63:56–65.
43. Fugazzotto PA. Implant placement at the time of mandibular molar extraction: Description of technique and preliminary results of 341 cases. J Periodontol 2008;79:737–747.
44. Atieh MA, Alsabeeha NH, Duncan WJ, et al. Immediate single implant restorations in mandibular molar extraction sockets: A controlled clinical trial. Clin Oral Implants Res 2013;24:484–496.
45. Prosper L, Crespi R, Valenti E, Capparé P, Gherlone E. Five-year follow-up of wide-diameter implants placed in fresh molar extraction sockets in the mandible: Immediate versus delayed loading. Int J Oral Maxillofac Implants 2010;25:607–612.
46. Lazzara RJ, Porter SS. Platform switching: A new concept in implant dentistry for controlling postrestorative crestal bone levels. Int J Periodontics Restorative Dent 2006;26:9–17.
47. Botticelli D, Persson LG, Lindhe J, Berglundh T. Bone tissue formation adjacent to implants placed in fresh extraction sockets: An experimental study in dogs. Clin Oral Implants Res 2006;17:351–358.
48. Araújo MG, Sukekava F, Wennström JL, Lindhe J. Ridge alterations following implant placement in fresh extraction sockets: An experimental study in the dog. J Clin Periodontol 2005;32:645–652.
49. Malkoç S, Basçiftçi FA, Nur M, Catalbas B. Maxillary and mandibular mesiodistal tooth sizes among different malocclusions in a sample of the Turkish population. Eur J Orthod 2011;33:592–596.
50. Rodriguez-Tizcareño MH, Bravo-Flores C. Anatomically guided implant site preparation technique at molar sites. Implant Dent 2009;18:393–401.
51. Scarano A. Traditional postextractive implant site preparation compared with pre-extractive interradicular implant bed preparation in the mandibular molar region, using an ultrasonic device: A randomized pilot study. Int J Oral Maxillofac Implants 2017;32:655–660.
52. Rebele SF, Zuhr O, Hürzeler MB. Pre-extractive interradicular implant bed preparation: Case presentations of a novel approach to immediate implant placement at multirooted molar sites. Int J Periodontics Restorative Dent 2013;33:89–96.
53. Sohn DS, Huang B, Kim J, Park I, Park CC. Utilization of autologous concentrated growth factors (CGF) enriched bone graft matrix (sticky bone) and CGF-enriched fibrin membrane in implant dentistry. J Implant Adv Clin Dent 2015;7(10):11–29.
54. Zheng RC, Park YK, Kim SK, et al. Bone regeneration of blood-derived stem cells within dental implants. J Dent Res 2015;94:1318–1325.
55. Zhou J, Li X, Sun X, et al. Bone regeneration around immediate placed implant of molar teeth with autologous platelet-rich fibrin: Two case reports. Medicine (Baltimore) 2018;97(44):e13058.
56. Noelken R, Pausch T, Wagner W, Al-Nawas B. Peri-implant defect grafting with autogenous bone or bone graft material in immediate implant placement in molar extraction sites: 1- to 3-year results of a prospective randomized study. Clin Oral Implants Res 2020;31:1138–1148.
57. Botticelli D, Berglundh T, Lindhe J. Resolution of bone defects of varying dimension and configuration in the marginal portion of the peri-implant bone. An experimental study in the dog. J Clin Periodontol 2004;31:309–317.
58. Araújo MG, Linder E, Lindhe J. Bio-Oss collagen in the buccal gap at immediate implants: A 6-month study in the dog. Clin Oral Implants Res 2011;22:1–8.
59. Pluemsakunthai W, Le B, Kasugai S. Effect of buccal gap distance on alveolar ridge alteration after immediate implant placement: A microcomputed tomographic and morphometric analysis in dogs. Implant Dent 2015;24:70–76.
60. Botticelli D, Berglundh T, Lindhe J. Hard-tissue alterations following immediate implant placement in extraction sites. J Clin Periodontol 2004;31:820–828.
61. Smith RB, Tarnow DP, Sarnachiaro G. Immediate placement of dental implants in molar extraction sockets: An 11-year retrospective analysis. Compend Contin Educ Dent 2019;40:166–170.
62. Gober DD, Fien MJ. Flapless extraction socket healing around an immediate implant placed into a mandibular molar site without the use of regenerative materials: A case report. Int J Periodontics Restorative Dent 2016;36:e26–e32.
63. Deporter D, Khoshkhounejad AA, Khoshkhounejad N, Ketabi M. A new classification of peri implant gaps based on gap location (A case series of 210 immediate implants). Dent Res J (Isfahan) 2021;18:29–39.
64. Tomasi C, Sanz M, Cecchinato D, et al. Bone dimensional variations at implants placed in fresh extraction sockets: A multilevel multivariate analysis. Clin Oral Implants Res 2010;21:30–36.
65. Poulias E, Greenwell H, Hill M, et al. Ridge preservation comparing socket allograft alone to socket allograft plus facial overlay xenograft: A clinical and histologic study in humans. J Periodontol 2013;84:1567–1575.
66. Brugnami F, Caiazzo A. Efficacy evaluation of a new buccal bone plate preservation technique: A pilot study. Int J Periodontics Restorative Dent 2011;31:67–73.
67. Birang E, Deporter D, Birang R, Mahabadi M, Atenafu E, Ketabi M. Effectiveness of buccal pouch grafting in minimizing loss of alveolar dimension: A canine investigation. Dent Res J (Isfahan) 2019;16:338–345.
68. Caiazzo A, Brugnami F, Galletti F, Mehra P. Buccal plate preservation with immediate implant placement and provisionalization: 5-year follow-up outcomes. J Maxillofac Oral Surg 2018;17:356–361.
69. Block MS. Placement of implants into fresh molar sites: Results of 35 cases. J Oral Maxillofac Surg 2011;69:170–174.

4

IMMEDIATE MAXILLARY MOLAR IMPLANT PLACEMENT

Douglas Deporter
Ali Akbar Khoshkhounejad
Mohammad Ketabi
Azadeh Rahmati

Literature Review

Lost maxillary molars have been reported to account for 17% to 26% of all missing teeth in some adult populations.[1,2] Within the first 3 to 6 months postextraction, substantial loss in vertical and buccopalatal alveolar ridge width is expected to occur at molar sites,[3,4] and teeth distal to the extracted molar can sometimes be expected to develop drifting and mesial inclinations.[5] In one recent study, Chen et al[6] reported CBCT data before and at least 6 months after maxillary molar extraction. Excluded were teeth with large periapical lesions or substantial periodontal bone loss (> 3 mm), those with significant root resorption, and those that were traumatic to extract. Their results indicated an average reduction in vertical bone height of 2.61 ± 1.76 mm (35.2%), reduction in buccopalatal ridge width of 8.33 ± 4.51 mm (65.1%), and a reduction in area of the remodeled alveolus of 56.08 ± 44.23 mm (18.89%). After more than one molar is lost in the same maxillary quadrant, further reductions in subantral bone height of 2.0 to 5.27 mm can occur.[7] In addition, subsequent sinus pneumatization may further limit the bone available for placement of implants to replace the lost molars[8] (Fig 4-1a). Such sinus expansion can be considerably greater following extraction of maxillary posterior teeth previously enveloped by an inferiorly curving sinus floor (Fig 4-1b). Also, sinus expansion can be larger in cases of second molar extractions (in comparison to first molars) and in instances of extraction of two or more adjacent posterior teeth.[8] Once all of these changes have occurred, it often becomes challenging and laborious to place dental implants to replace the lost molars. As a result, a keen interest has developed in employing immediate maxillary molar implant treatment if certain prerequisites can be met.

One of the earliest reports on immediate maxillary molar placement was that of Schwartz-Arad et al.[9] From 1989 to 1996, these clinicians placed 56 immediate molar implants (IMIs) in 43 patients. As expected for the era, the

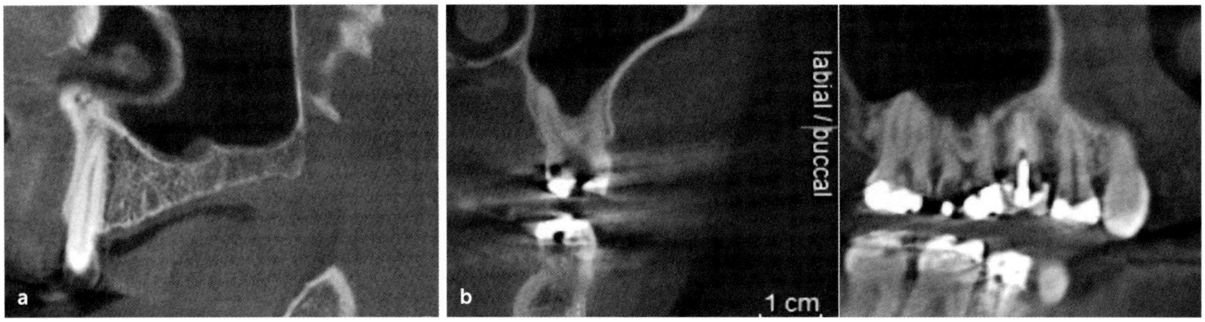

FIG 4-1 *(a)* A site where all posterior teeth have been removed. Both crestal bone resorption and sinus pneumatization will make molar implant placement challenging. *(b)* The sinus floor curves inferiorly, creating intimate contact with the tooth roots with little bone height in the first molar furcal region, making the site not amenable to immediate implant placement in the interradicular septum (IRS) bone.

majority (47/56) of the implants were machine-turned titanium screw-type, and every attempt was made to create the implant osteotomies in the furcal bone to position the implants optimally for later restoration. Mean implant length used was 12.8 mm (range: 10–16 mm) with a mean implant diameter of 4.28 mm (range: 3.25–5.0 mm). Otherwise, technical details were scant. Mean healing time before restoration was 6.8 months, following which some implants were restored using single crowns, but most were used as part of 52 splinted fixed prostheses. The 5-year cumulative survival rate was estimated to be an amazing 89%. However, there was a sex difference, with males having 5-year survival of 84% compared to 93.5% in females. Smoking cigarettes also had an impact, with nonsmokers showing 90% implant survival versus 83% among smokers.

In an earlier literature review of the topic,[10] the same authors reached the following conclusions:

- IMIs can help to reduce vertical and horizontal alveolar bone loss that would otherwise occur.
- Ideal implant placement could be achieved, assuming that the extracted tooth had been normally positioned.
- Crown length in harmony with adjacent teeth along with favorable gingival architecture was more likely to be achieved with IMIs than with delayed molar implant placement.

However, they also cited the following situations as causing possible difficulties:

- If the tooth to be replaced originally had been abnormally positioned
- If there remained insufficient native bone apically to stabilize the implant
- If the condition of surrounding soft tissues was unfavorable (eg, inadequate thickness, width, or health)

The authors also stressed that immediate replacement was not suitable if there was local acute infection, or if the tooth had been condemned due to advanced periodontal disease, having lost one or more of its bony socket walls. They also concluded that atraumatic tooth extraction with preparatory sectioning of molar roots for their individual removal was crucial to minimize damage to socket walls, and that if the implant was to have adequate primary stability, it was recommended that its apex engage 3 to 5 mm of native bone.

Some years later, Fugazzotto defined a recommended protocol for replacing maxillary molar teeth with immediate implants.[11] By this stage in implant development (2006), it had become evident that threaded implants modified with rough (eg, titanium plasma-sprayed) and eventually with moderately roughened surface treatments such as acid-etching and particle-blasting[12] generally performed better in the average clinician's hands than did machine-turned implants. At the time of publication of his results, Fugazzotto was able to report early outcomes with 83 Straumann tapered-end, tissue-level implants with an apical diameter of 4.1 mm and a neck diameter of 6.5 mm, the majority having been placed in first molar sites. Prior to tooth removal, buccal full-thickness mucoperiosteal flaps were raised, along with vertical releasing incisions that extended well beyond the mucogingival junction so as to later be able to achieve primary soft tissue closure. As well, horizon-

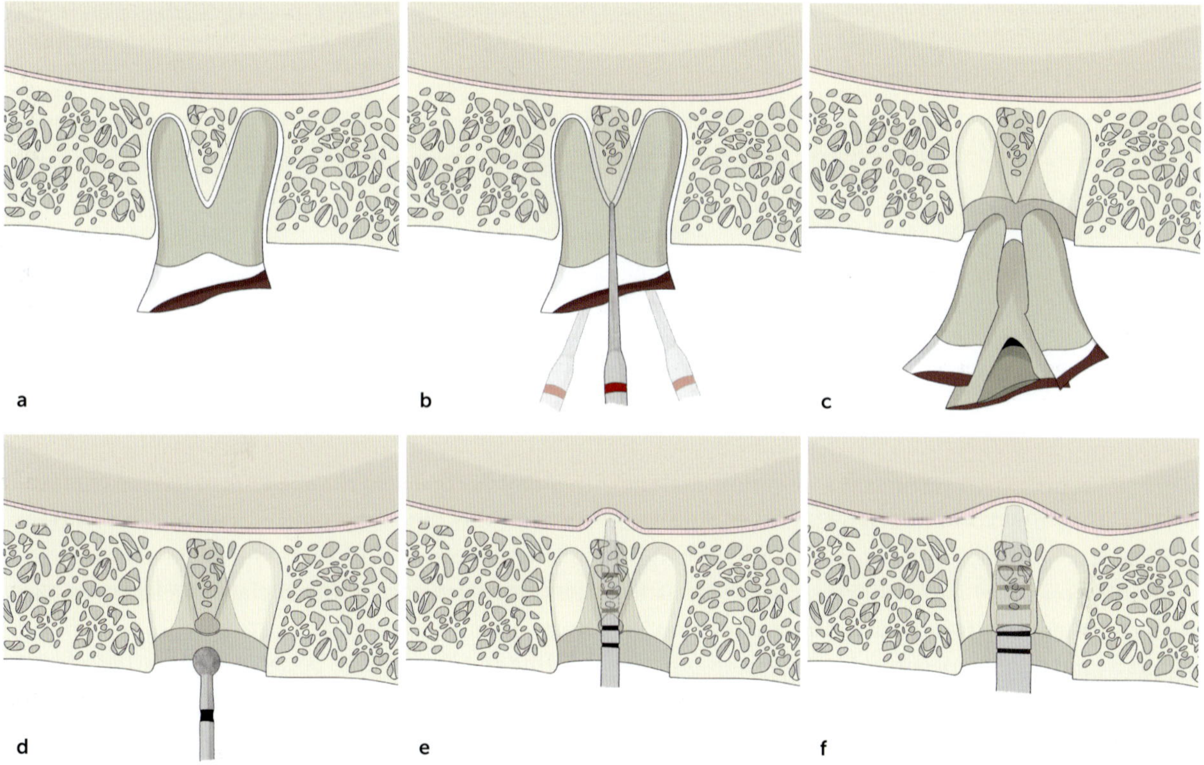

FIG 4-2 *(a)* The condemned tooth is decoronated if need be. *(b)* It is separated into three separate roots with a high-speed handpiece and bur. *(c)* This allows removal of each root separately and atraumatically. *(d)* A round bur creates the entry point into the IRS. *(e)* A tapered, blunt-ended osteotome of maximum diameter 2.2 mm is used with a surgical mallet to initiate the osteotomy. *(f)* This is followed by enlargement of the osteotomy and upfracture of the sinus floor with a series of osteotomes of increasing diameter. →

tal releasing incisions were placed at the most apical extents of the buccal vertical releasing incisions and extended 6 to 7 mm horizontally.[13] A palatal sulcular incision was made on the tooth to be removed and extended to the adjacent teeth. As well, palatal vertical releasing incisions were used at the mesial and distal aspects of the condemned tooth to allow elevation of a full-thickness palatal flap. Presence of chronic periodontal and/or periapical pathology was not taken as a contraindication (see also chapter 5). Eight treated teeth presented originally with periapical infection, while 11 demonstrated evidence of exudate. In each instance, the tooth to be removed was trisected and each root removed individually (Figs 4-2a to 4-2c), unless three distinct roots did not exist, as may occur with some type C sockets as classified by Smith and Tarnow.[14] Sockets were carefully debrided to remove all granulation tissue and, if present, any periapical lesions. The plan was to use 11.8-mm-long tissue-level implants (10 mm of roughened surface and 1.8 mm of polished collar), and in order to do this, osteotomies were started in the center of the remaining interradicular septum (IRS) bone using a round bur at 550 rpm (Fig 4-2d). Thereafter, a tapered, blunt-ended, handheld osteotome of maximum diameter 2.2 mm was used with a surgical mallet to initiate the osteotomy (Fig 4-2e) by compressing the IRS bone and widening the osteotomy without any bone removal, as recommended by Summers.[15,16] If there was insufficient native bone height to fully house the 10-mm length of roughened implant surface, the osteotome was simply malleted to the required depth with localized lifting of the sinus floor[15] (Fig 4-2f). Care was taken to never elevate the sinus floor more than two times the height of the original residual IRS bone. At this point, osteotome tips of 2.8- and 3.5-mm diameter were used in sequence to further widen the osteotomy. Next, the tapered implant was placed (Fig 4-2g) using a hand-

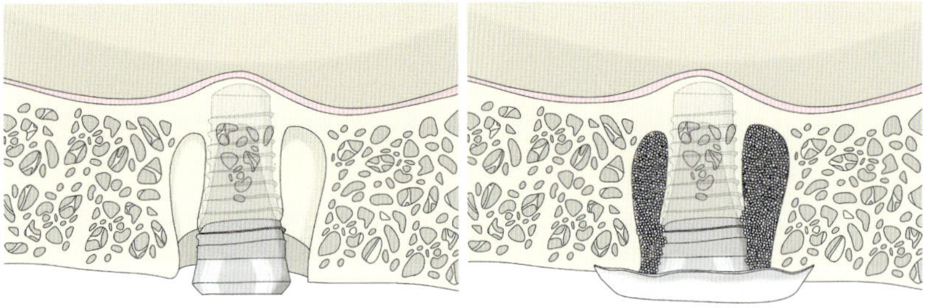

g h

FIG 4-2 *(cont) (g)* Seating of the implant was such as to submerge the roughened implant surface below the crestal bone. *(h)* After grafting the peri-implant gaps, an ePTFE barrier membrane covered the site before primary soft tissue closure.

piece at 30 rpm with copious saline irrigation, making certain that the 10-mm-long roughened implant surface was at or below the anticipated final height of crestal bone. Any peri-implant gaps were grafted with collected particulate autogenous bone and/or allograft, and the site covered using either a resorbable collagen barrier membrane or a titanium-reinforced expanded polytetrafluoroethylene (ePTFE; ie, GORE-TEX, W. L. Gore) membrane (Fig 4-2h) secured with titanium tacks apically. That he was able to use the latter membrane successfully was a testament to how skilled the operator was. Unwanted early exposure of this nonresorbable membrane during site healing would most likely have led to infection and early implant failures. Finally, the soft tissue flaps were manipulated to achieve primary, tension-free wound closure. Worth noting is the fact that patients were not allowed to use any removable prostheses throughout the entire 6-month healing interval. To summarize, 83 maxillary first molar implants were placed in 83 patients, and all but 2 implants remained totally submerged during the 6-month healing interval. All implants became successfully integrated and subsequently were restored using single porcelain-fused-to-metal crowns. The author reported 100% survival at the 12- to 18-month follow-up.

This same clinician again reported on his experiences with maxillary IMIs in 2008.[17] By this time, he had used 391 IMIs in 386 patients. At the time of the report, 389 of 391 implants had been functioning successfully for up to 75 months with a cumulative survival rate of 99.5%. All patients had been treated between 2003 and 2006. While his earlier patients had all been nonsmokers, more recent candidates had been accepted if they smoked not more than 10 cigarettes per day. He had also changed his preferred choices of implant size, choosing a tapered implant with a 4.8-mm diameter apically and a 6.5-mm-diameter prosthetic platform. However, if this implant size had been likely to result in significant damage to and/or loss of the IRS during site preparation because of the latter's limited width, a cylindrical (ie, nontapered) 4.8-mm-diameter implant with a 6.5-mm-diameter restorative platform was used. His preference was still to use particulate graft material to fill any peri-implant extraction socket defects, but only if these defects or gaps exceeded 3 mm in width. Membranes and primary wound closure were still used routinely.

In this more recent paper, Fugazzotto also revealed that he did modify the procedure according to the different widths of IRS encountered.[17] For example, if this bone was not sufficiently wide to achieve complete housing of the roughened implant surface, he elected to place a tapered implant with an apical diameter of only 4.0 mm. With more recent experiences, others have reported successful outcomes using maxillary IMIs using smaller flaps or a flapless approach and nonsubmerged healing, thus eliminating the tedious and often risky use of barrier materials. For example, Jiansheng et al[18] presented 2-year retrospective data for 162 maxillary IMIs used to treat 145 primarily nonsmoking patients without complete soft tissue closure at sites with a 2-mm minimal width of keratinized gingiva. They also pushed the limit by using short, wider-diameter single-tooth implants to avoid the need for dedicated sinus floor manipulation. Sites selected required a minimal 7-mm residual bone height and 9-mm ridge width, which is often found at maxillary molar extraction sites[19,20] (Fig 4-3). Implants were threaded with a moderately rough surface and used in lengths of 5.7 to 8.0 mm and widths of 5.0 to 7.0 mm. After a mean time of 2 years, the implant survival rate was reported as 99.4%. As a result of their work and that of many others, assuming good initial stability, maxillary IMIs are now generally placed using a nonsubmerged, one-stage technique.

There have been a number of systematic literature reviews on the topic of maxillary IMI usage. Lang et al[21] identified and examined a total of 46 prospective maxillary IMI studies, with a mean follow-up time of 2.08 years. The 2-year mean survival rate calculated from the available data was 98.4% (range: 97.3%–99%). Among the factors analyzed as possible contributors to failure were the reason for extraction and the use of antibiotics. The latter factor was notable in that patients who had been prescribed an antibiotic for use postoperatively for 5 to 7 days did better than those given only a single preoperative loading dose. A more recent systematic literature review[22] with meta-analysis of the findings in 15 IMI studies published between November 2008 and May 2015 reported survival of 98% after 1 or more years for 768 IMIs placed in 757 patients. No differences in survival were found between maxillary and mandibular molar sites. As well, five of the reviewed studies had included within-study delayed molar implant placement as controls, and the authors had reported no significant difference compared with IMIs.

With the above information as background, this chapter is meant to provide key information on the use of maxillary IMIs, including case selection, anatomical considerations, and suggested surgical procedures.

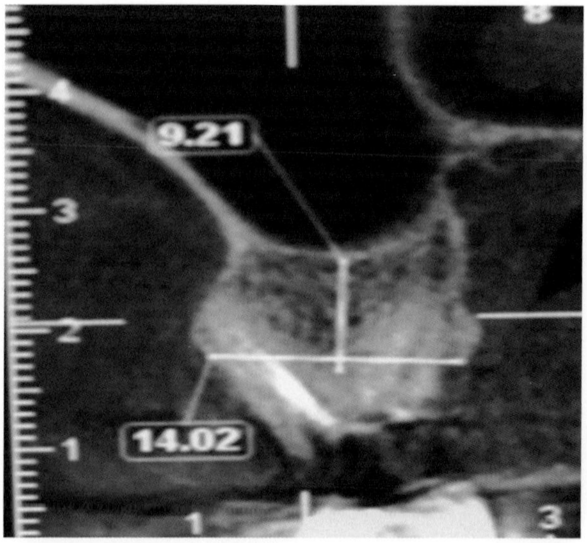

FIG 4-3 If a short implant (≤ 8 mm) is chosen for this site, since the IRS is wide buccopalatally, the implant could be ≥ 6 mm in diameter, helping to compensate for the shorter length.[20]

Case Selection

Recognizing that placing maxillary IMIs can be challenging, treatment planning is best undertaken with the assistance of CBCT scans to allow assessment of the thicknesses of buccal and palatal cortical plates, the thickness and type of IRS bone, the distance from alveolar crest to maxillary sinus, the distance from the molar tooth furcation to sinus floor, the relationships of the sinus floor to the molar roots in both the coronal and sagittal planes, any intrusions of maxillary molar roots into the sinus domain, and any possible thickening of sinus membrane or pathologies such as chronic sinusitis, retention cysts, mucoceles, or sinus opacities (Fig 4-4). As with mandibular IMIs, any patient with a history of severe periodontitis, even if successfully treated, should be approached with caution because they may continue to harbor pathogenic microbiota,[23] increasing risk of late implant failure due to peri-implantitis.

Nonsmokers are more likely to have successful outcomes with maxillary IMI treatment because the posterior maxilla has long been known to be the jaw site at highest risk to implant failure in patients with the habit.[24] Cigarette smoking also is a recognized risk factor for sinus grafting, which is often a key ancillary measure with maxillary IMI treatment. Lin et al[25] investigated the effect of cigarette smoking and residual native bone height on the survival of dental implants placed immediately in transcrestally elevated and grafted sinuses. In this retrospective study, 75 patients received 155 implants. The implant survival rates for nonsmokers and smokers at stage-two surgery were 93% and 84%, respectively. Further data analysis revealed that the effect of smoking on implant survival also was related to the pretreatment residual subantral bone height. Where this bone height had been less than 4 mm before treatment, the survival rate in nonsmokers was 82.4%, compared with 60% in smokers ($P < .05$). It was concluded that smoking presents a high risk factor when implants are placed simultaneously with sinus grafting.

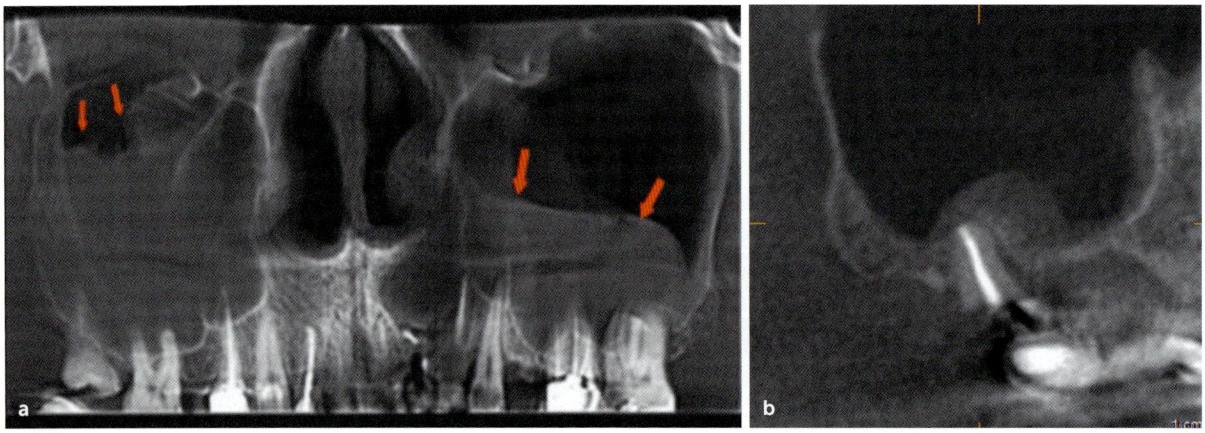

FIG 4-4 *(a)* This panoramic radiograph shows a patient with marked opacities of both maxillary sinuses indicative of pathology. IMI treatment should not be considered before referral for sinus diagnosis and resolution. *(b)* This molar planned for IMI replacement was found to have a cystic lesion that had penetrated the sinus floor, which altered the treatment plan.

Anatomical Factors to Consider

Socket anatomy and proximity to the maxillary sinus

Socket anatomy is central for successful maxillary IMI outcomes. Firstly, intact socket walls are preferred to avoid the concomitant need and challenges/complications of simultaneous guided bone augmentation grafting. Where one or more socket walls are missing or have a significant dehiscence, socket preservation grafting[26,27] and delayed implant placement are often more appropriate, although recent innovations may alter this approach in the future. A key factor in success with maxillary IMIs is choosing the implant size that will most suitably fit the socket of the extracted molar but without contact with the buccal bone plate. In a recent study,[19] CBCT images were used to assess socket dimensions of 150 healthy maxillary first molar sites in 95 patients. Mean overall socket widths crestally were determined to be 10.5 mm (SD [standard deviation]: 0.90 mm) buccopalatally (Fig 4-5) and 7.3 mm (SD: 0.84 mm) mesiodistally, although these dimensions are generally smaller in females than in males.[28] The corresponding figures for maxillary second molars are 9.9 mm and 9.8 mm, respectively.[29] For both type A and B sockets and subantral bone height greater than 8 mm, appropriate IMI implant diameters will likely be 4.5 to 5 mm. If subantral bone height is less than 8 mm and the clinician prefers to avoid the sinus, a short implant with diameter greater than 5 mm may be considered. Larger-diameter implants can also be an option in maxillary type C septa and where the mesiodistal ridge length is greater than 11 mm, again if width permits.

Mean thicknesses of buccal and palatal bony walls at 2 mm from the bone crest have been reported to be 1.58 (SD: 0.6 mm) buccally and 1.34 mm (SD: 0.54 mm) palatally at maxillary first molar sites,[19] although they do tend to thicken further apically (Fig 4-6). At 8% of sites, the buccal plate was less than 1 mm in thickness compared with 25% of palatal plates. It should be noted, however, that CBCT measurements of buccal bone 1 mm or less in thickness can be highly inaccurate, leading to dehiscences being misdiagnosed.[30] Generally, buccal bone 2 mm or less in crestal thickness is likely to experience significant resorption.[31,32] This being the case, it is best to do maxillary IMI placement without raising flaps, to avoid direct contact between buccal crestal bone and the implant periphery, leaving a gap to fill with a blood clot or for grafting,[33] and to submerge the implant subcrestally by at least 1 mm (Fig 4-7).

It has also been reported that the mean distance from sinus floor to molar furcation, ie, the height of the IRS, is about 6.51 mm (SD: 2.94 mm) with a range of 0 to 16 mm (Fig 4-8). In order to position a maxillary first molar IMI optimally, it most likely needs to be placed into this IRS bone, and it may require some indirect sinus floor elevation if the clinician is

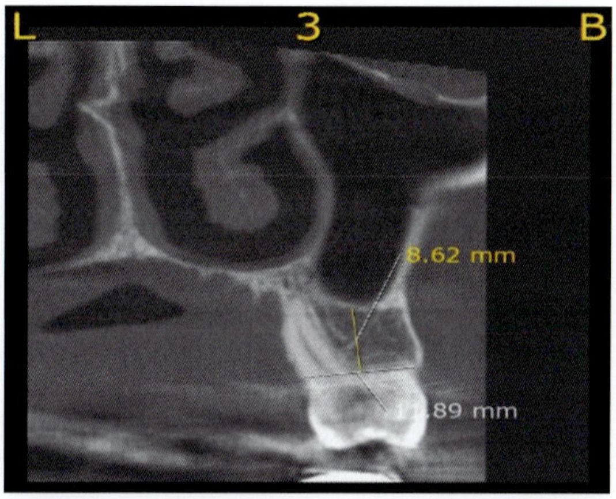

FIG 4-5 This CBCT slice shows a maxillary first molar with 11.89-mm buccopalatal width and 8.62-mm height of bone from the furcation to the sinus floor.

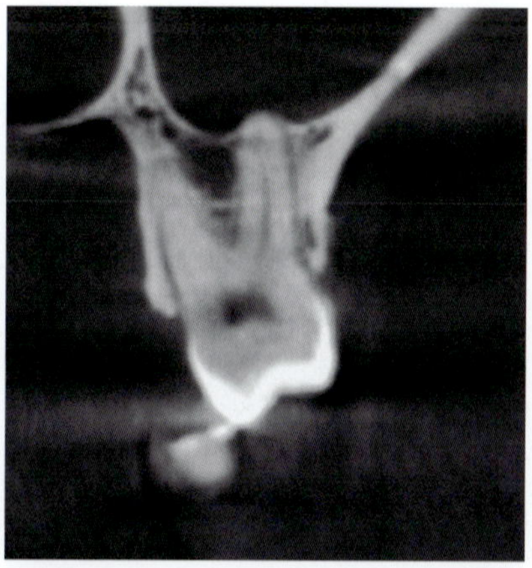

FIG 4-6 Buccal and palatal bone of maxillary first molar sockets generally thicken toward the root apices.

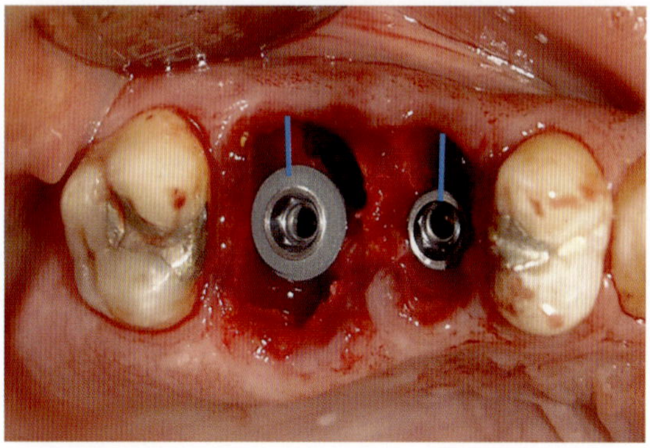

FIG 4-7 Leaving gaps between the buccal cortical bone plates and the implant periphery will allow blood clots to fill the spaces, leading to subsequent bone fill. Ideally, the implants will be submerged subcrestally by at least 1 mm.

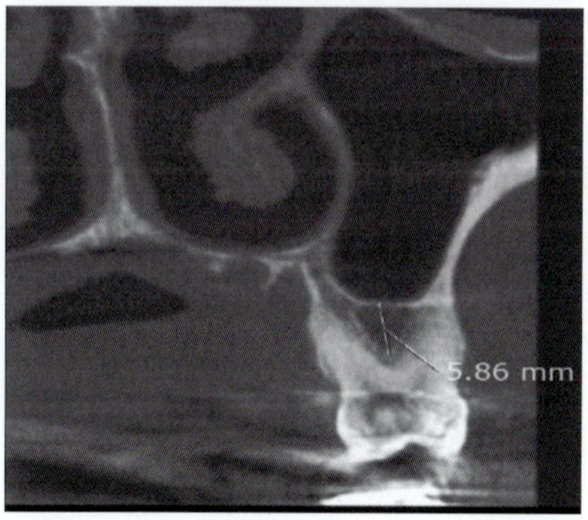

FIG 4-8 The example shown has only 5.86 mm of bone height available from the furcation to the sinus floor and will require some minor indirect sinus floor elevation during osteotomy site preparation.

not prepared to place a short implant. Keeping to the IRS also helps to minimize the risk of sinus damage given the usual small distances between sinus floor and molar root apices. For example, in Matsuda et al's survey of 150 healthy maxillary first molars,[19] mean distances between sinus floor and the apices of the mesiobuccal, distobuccal, and palatal roots were –0.36 mm, 0.32 mm, and –2.2 mm, with the negative numbers indicating root apex intrusion into the sinus domain. Demircan and Çankaya[28] reported that while 69.1% of their patients had no root intrusions into the sinus at first molar sites, 5.9% had buccal root intrusions, and 19.1% had both buccal and palatal root intrusions. Such intrusions would of course increase the risk of sinus membrane perforation if the clinician opted to use a root socket to develop the osteotomy (Fig 4-9).

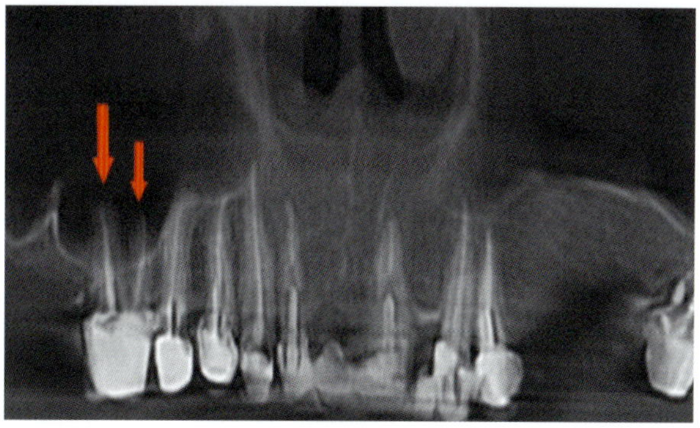

FIG 4-9 The roots of the maxillary right first molar can clearly be seen to be protruding into the maxillary sinus, making this tooth a poor choice for IMI placement.

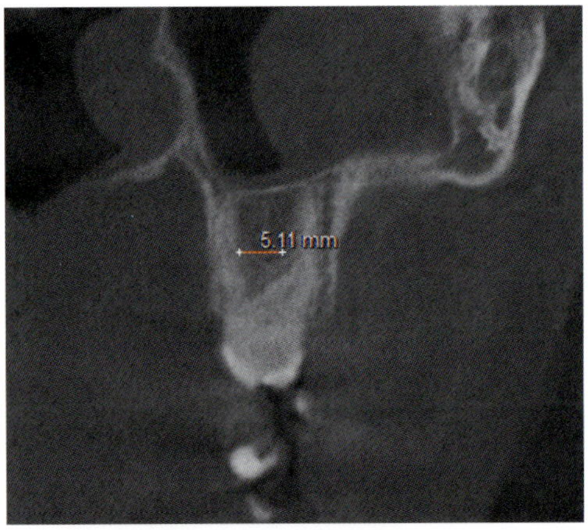

FIG 4-10 An example of a type A IRS. The IRS bone is sufficient to house the entire implant buccopalatally, although some minor indirect sinus floor elevation may be needed unless a short implant can be used.

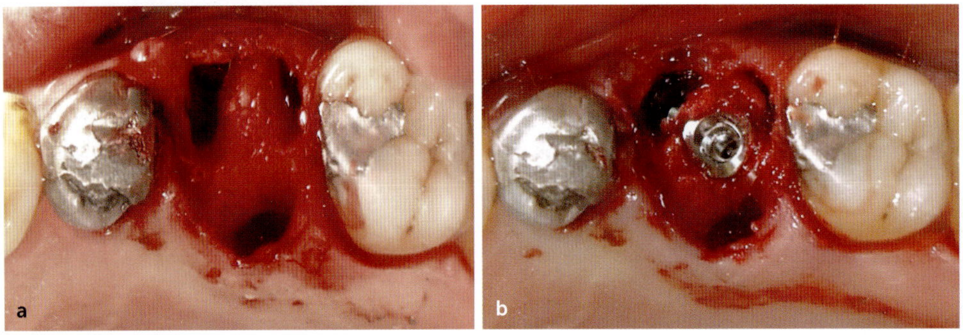

FIG 4-11 *(a)* This maxillary first molar extraction socket showed typical type A interseptal bone anatomy. *(b)* The implant placed was completely housed in the IRS without a need for gap grafting.

IRS bone anatomy

Demircan and Çankaya[28] estimated that 89.5% of maxillary first molars have some IRS, the mean mesiodistal width of which was reported to be 3.3 mm. Smith and Tarnow[14] classified molar IRS into three types, stressing that they varied in difficulty to manipulate successfully. Type A sockets (Fig 4-10) are those with sufficient IRS bulk to contain the implant osteotomy in its entirety and can be the most straightforward type to manage[14] (Fig 4-11). While this type of IRS is infrequent at second molar sites, recent data has shown that it exists at 61.7% of maxillary first molar sites.[34] If the implant can be fully seated in the IRS, any remaining root socket defects or gaps like those shown in Fig 4-7 should not need grafting.[14] This would, however, assume that the defects can be fully sheltered by repositioned thick keratinized gingiva adequately supported by wide-diameter healing abutments.

Type B sockets are those with sufficient IRS volume to stabilize an IMI, but not completely house it, at least crestally[14,35] (Figs 4-12 and 4-13). In this case, the buccal and palatal buttresses of the IRS can be used to assist with initial implant stabilization. Then, once the implant has been placed, any implant surface not housed in IRS and associated socket spaces may need socket grafting. Managing type B sockets by placing the implant into the palatal root socket of the molar[36] also has been advocated (Fig 4-14), but it may result in a less than ideal restorative emergence profile and compromised home care if placed too far palatally. However, with the advent of angulated abutments, the practice is still used by some clinicians, allowing them to eliminate the need for sinus floor manipulation[37] (Fig 4-15).

Type C sockets are those with insufficient septal bone to stabilize an IMI (Fig 4-16). This IRS situation is the most difficult to manage with IMIs and often is best managed by utilizing the palatal root socket or with socket preservation grafting and delayed implant placement (see chapter 1). Another option for the experienced clinician might be placing an ultra-wide-diameter implant (see chapter 8).

FIG 4-12 While this type B IRS has minimal width crestally, it widens significantly, making it a good candidate for an IMI.

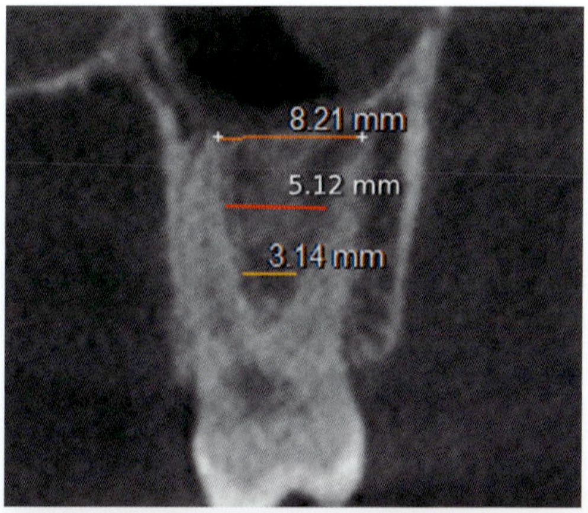

FIG 4-13 *(a)* The figure shows an example of a type B IRS at a maxillary first molar extraction socket. *(b)* The implant placed in this type B IRS was adequately stabilized but showed dehiscences at the mesiobuccal, distobuccal, and palatal aspects. The remaining gaps seen here would be considered for grafting with allograft by most clinicians, although others prefer to avoid grafting.[35]

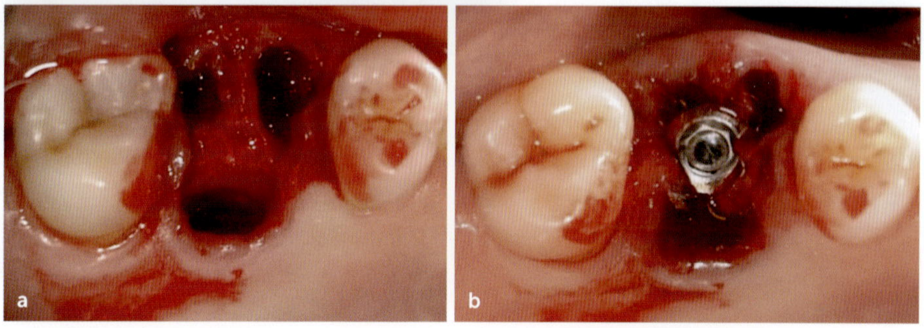

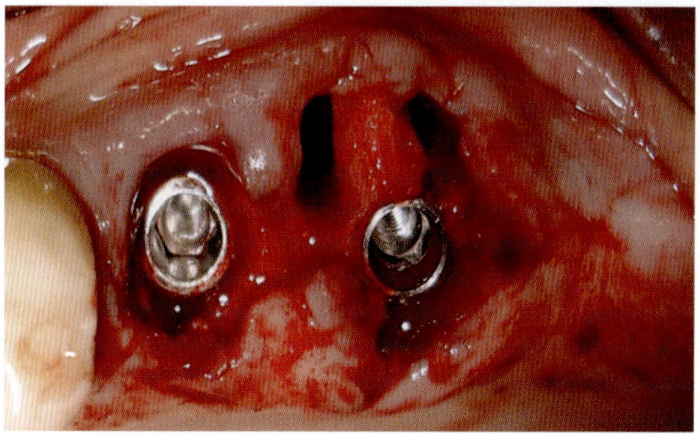

FIG 4-14 In this patient, the operator opted to place an IMI into the palatal root socket.

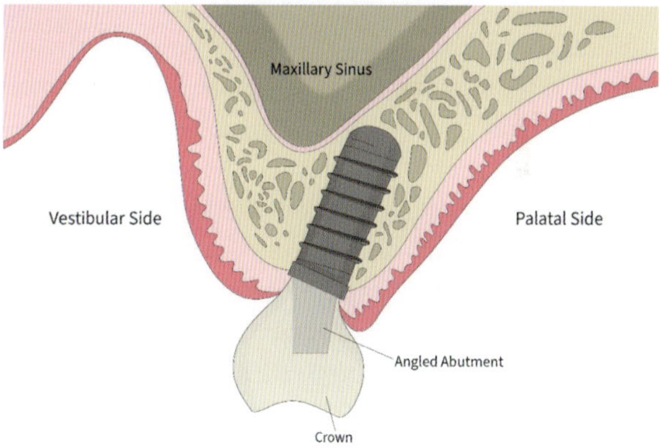

FIG 4-15 This illustration depicts the placement of an IMI into the palatal root socket of a maxillary molar.

FIG 4-16 *(a)* An example of a maxillary type C IRS. The simplest approach would be to place an IMI into the palatal root socket or to do socket preservation grafting and delayed implant surgery. *(b)* A typical type C IRS with insufficient septal bone to receive an IMI.

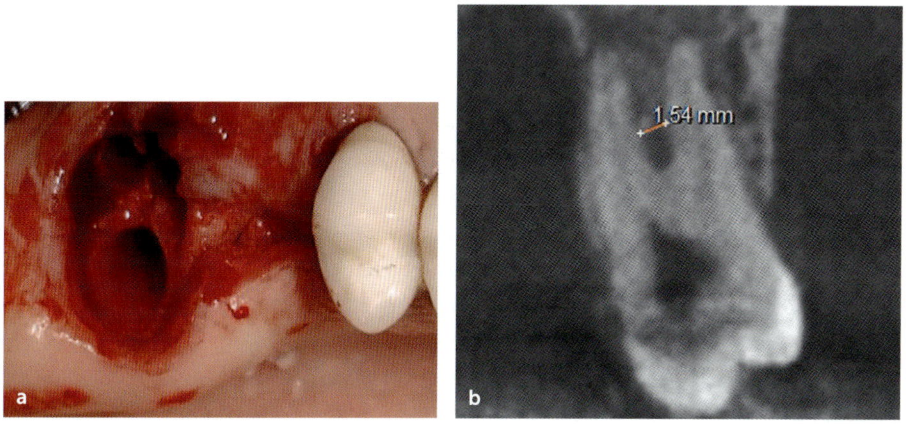

Suggested Surgical Protocols

Prior to treatment, patients must receive a thorough oral examination, including assessment of maximal jaw opening, intra-arch relationships, site-specific buccopalatal alveolar ridge width, and specific as well as general intermaxillary relationships. Panoramic radiographs and CBCT records are recommended to evaluate the overall 3D anatomy of the site. Impressions should be taken and, if appropriate, study casts mounted on an articulator. Based on the information obtained, diagnostic wax-ups are made and surgical templates fabricated. Ideally, during the week before surgery, a full-mouth professional scaling and prophylaxis will be carried out. Use of a systemic antibiotic is also common practice, as is having the patient rinse with a chlorhexidine solution several times daily for 2 to 3 days preoperatively.

Flap design and atraumatic extraction

As with all IMIs, a flapless approach is preferred with maxillary IMI placement in order to minimize post-surgical crestal bone loss,[38,39] but this generally should only be done if an intact buccal plate of bone exists. Flapless surgery also will reduce postoperative discomfort for the patient.[40] If, on the other hand, a dehiscence or fenestration is present or the buccal plate is thin, most clinicians likely would opt to raise a flap in order to perform a regenerative grafting procedure to help to limit unfavorable dimensional changes during and following healing.[41] Interestingly, however, recent data suggests that a flapless approach for IMI sites with buccal dehiscences can give successful outcomes simply by densely packing xenograft particles without a barrier membrane under the periosteum.[42] This approach is appealing because it reduces cost and simplifies the implant surgery, but it may require longer healing intervals (ie, up to 6 months) before delivering the definitive restorations.

The need for thorough socket debridement after all tooth fragments have been removed will depend on the health of the surrounding bone tissue and, by extension, the reason for tooth extraction. If no periapical pathology exists, there is likely little to no need to perform aggressive socket debridement, particularly because remnants of healthy periodontal ligament with its vascularity may be beneficial in achieving osseointegration of immediate implants.[43] However, if the condemned tooth has granulation or cystic tissue related to pulpal or periodontal disease, most clinicians prefer meticulous removal of this tissue using sharp curettes and even rotary or piezoelectric surgical instruments because pathogenic organisms can persist in dormancy in periapical bone, possibly leading to delayed implant failure.[44,45]

Osteotomy preparation

Because the mean bone height of the IRS of maxillary first molars is approximately 6.5 mm, unless a short (ie, ≤ 8 mm) implant can be successfully employed, it can be anticipated that some localized indirect sinus floor elevation will be needed to place an IMI of sufficient dimensions to ensure a successful outcome.[46] As already stated, this can be accomplished using hand osteotomes and a surgical mallet[15] or other specialized instrument kits to upfracture the sinus floor. If a short implant is selected, one with a wider than standard diameter should be considered.[18] In addition to providing added bone-to-implant surface contact, the wider prosthetic platform will enable a more favorable emergence profile for a molar crown. If the clinician wishes to use a longer implant, combining it with indirect sinus floor elevation will also allow for the IMI to be placed up to 2 mm subcrestally in order to reduce the risk of early micromovements, help with minimizing the impact of postoperative crestal bone loss,[47,48] and provide adequate running room (ie, apicocoronal distance between the implant platform and the gingival margin) to ensure a favorable and stable emergence profile for the final molar prosthesis.[14,49]

The heavily restored first molar seen in Fig 4-17a was condemned due to a failed endodontic treatment with apical pathosis at its mesiobuccal root. The tooth was first decoronated to allow removal of its three roots separately (Fig 4-17b), revealing a type A septum. Osteotomy preparation was begun and completed at the central point of the IRS (Fig 4-17c), after which a 12 × 4.9–mm Dentium implant was placed with complete housing in the IRS. No gap grafting or sutures were employed (Fig 4-17d). At the 8-week postoperative visit, the large palatal defect shows ongoing healing by secondary intention (Fig 4-17e). Figs 4-17f and 4-17g show radiographic and clinical images of the restored implant after 1 year in function.

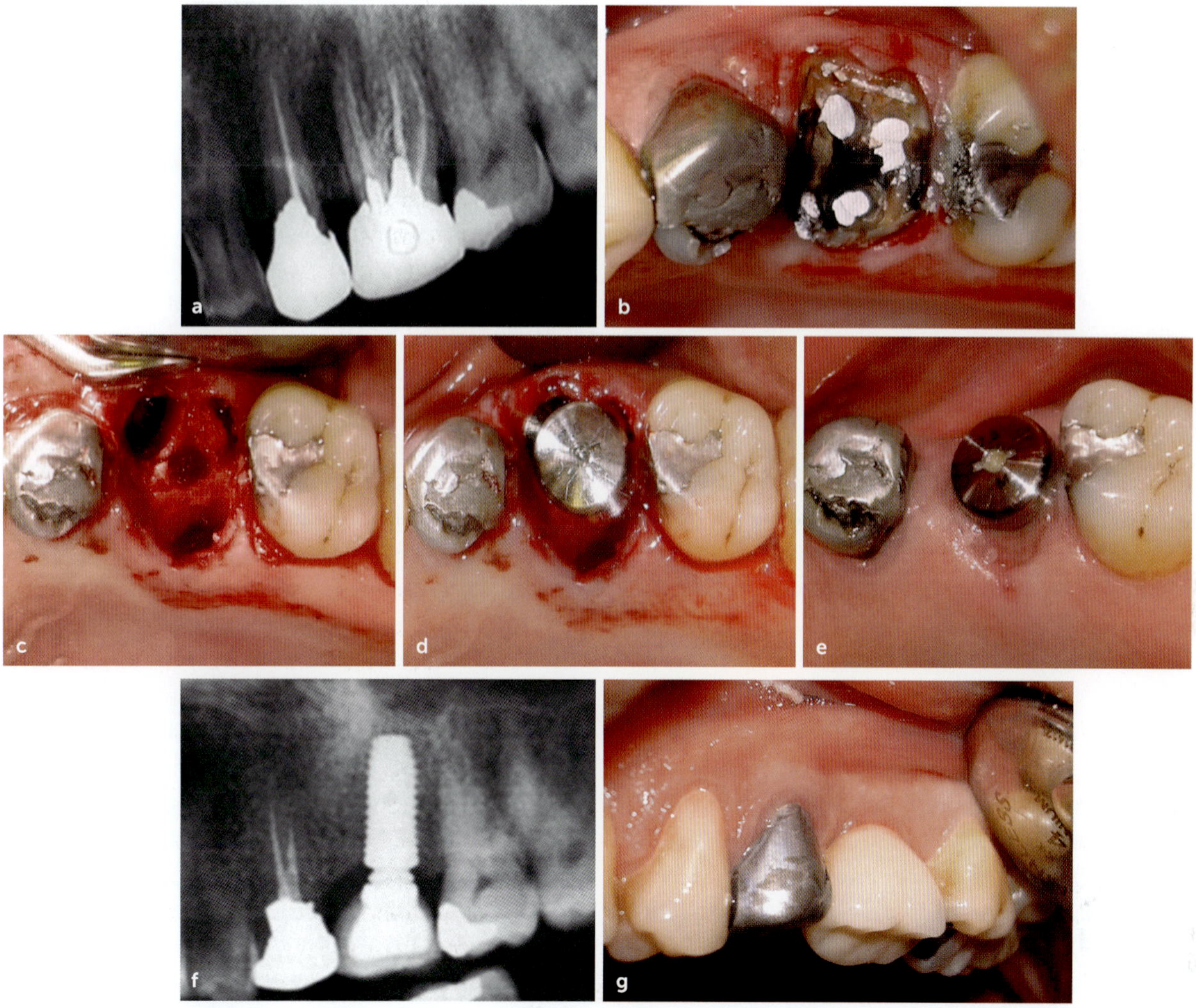

FIG 4-17 *(a)* This maxillary left first molar was deemed hopeless. *(b)* The tooth was decoronated in preparation for removal of the three roots separately. A flapless approach was used. *(c)* Osteotomy preparation was begun in the exposed type A IRS. *(d)* A 12 × 4.9-mm Dentium implant was placed successfully and fully encased by the IRS. A large (6-mm-diameter) healing abutment was added to shelter the remaining buccal and interproximal peri-implant gaps, which were not grafted. The large palatal gap was left untreated, and no sutures were used as the procedure had been flapless. *(e)* This clinical photograph taken at the 8-week postoperative visit shows closure of the large palatal gap by secondary intention healing. *(f)* A periapical radiograph of the restored implant after 1 year in function. *(g)* A clinical photograph of the implant restoration.

As already mentioned, a common scenario with maxillary molars is insufficient remaining bone height to place an appropriate IMI without simultaneous sinus floor elevation. The combination of IMI placement into the IRS of fresh sockets and simultaneous transcrestal sinus floor elevation has been shown to be a viable approach.[50,51] Indeed, it is generally held that up to 5 mm of transcrestal sinus floor elevation can safely be done without sinus membrane damage,[52,53] and because maxillary molar IRS commonly widens with increasing distance from the furcation (see Fig 4-12), good implant stability can be achieved. Most clinicians who have published maxillary IMI results following transcrestal sinus floor elevation have used hand osteotomes advanced using a surgical mallet to elevate the sinus floor apical to the IRS.[17,54] Using osteotomes has the added advantage that none of the septal bone will be removed, but rather simply expanded laterally and compressed apically (see Fig 4-2). The minimal coronal width of IRS generally considered to be acceptable for this procedure is 2.5 mm, provided that it does widen more apically.

Liu et al[55] recently published results of a prospective clinical study in which patients were randomized into two groups: a test group that received IMIs with simultaneous indirect sinus grafting and a control group for whom delayed implant placement with indirect sinus elevation using osteotomes was performed. Potential IMI sites needed to have a minimum of 4 mm IRS height below the sinus floor, and as a result, the mean sinus floor elevation needed was 3.6 ± 0.41 mm. The implants used (TS-III, Osstem Implant) were 6 mm in diameter and were submerged subcrestally by 1 mm. While the actual implant lengths were not provided in the paper, given the IRS heights and minimal sinus floor elevation data, the implants were likely short in length (ie, ≤ 8 mm). It appeared that no grafting materials were used either for the sinus elevation or for the peri-implant gaps. Twenty-seven of the 33 IMI sites were type A, and all implants were left nonsubmerged during healing. The survival rate at 1 year was 100% for both groups. Most interesting, however, was the finding that at the time of permanent restoration, the horizontal alveolar shrinkage on the buccal aspect was significantly less with the IMIs than with the control implants (0.65 ± 0.12 mm vs 1.23 ± 0.32 mm; $P < .0001$). Differences in vertical ridge resorption buccally also were significantly less at the IMI sites (0.60 ± 0.18 mm vs 1.53 ± 0.19 mm; $P < .0001$). If replicable in future prospective clinical trials, these findings offer more proof that IMI placement in the maxilla may offer distinct biologic advantages.

The osteotome technique for indirect (ie, transcrestal) sinus floor elevation can only be used if the bone is primarily cancellous, ie, type III or IV.[56] Otherwise, too much malleting force will be needed to advance the osteotomes, making the procedure unpleasant for the patient and with the risk of causing postoperative transient or even protracted vertigo.[57] In such cases, it is appropriate to begin site preparation with a pilot bur using drill stops[58] or piezoelectric tips so as to be able to closely develop the osteotomy's initial base at a depth of about 1 mm or less short of the sinus floor. At that point, osteotomes, specialized burs,[59] or specialized piezoelectric tips[60] can be used to upfracture the sinus floor. Another method could be to use densifying burs for osteotomy preparation and the transcrestal sinus elevation[61] (see chapters 7 and 11).

Most commonly in the past, particulate allograft or xenograft particles have been used with indirect sinus floor elevation procedures in order to maximize new bone formation around the implant apex. However, recent reports have indicated that autologous platelet-rich fibrin (PRF) clots also are appropriate as a graft,[62,63] and these have the added advantage of being an excellent means to seal any recognized or unrecognized small tears in the sinus membrane that may have occurred during upfracturing of the sinus floor.[64] This is particularly of interest since a recent cadaver study documented that with indirect sinus elevation of only 3 mm, sinus membrane perforations, often undetected clinically, may in fact be fairly common.[65] Autologous PRF clots are rich in growth factors, and as such have been shown to enhance the degree of osseointegration,[66,67] accelerate healing, and provide possible site-specific antibacterial[68] and anti-inflammatory properties, helping to reduce early postoperative discomfort.[69]

A sample case of a site requiring sinus elevation coincident to IMI placement is shown in Fig 4-18. A periapical radiograph taken immediately after the patient's first molar was removed showed favorable IRS but limited subantral bone height (Fig 4-18a). Osteotomy preparation was begun in the IRS using piezoelectric surgical tips.[60] Briefly, after developing the osteotomy to the sinus floor with a round piezoelectric tip, a hollow end-cutting specialized tip called the *hydrodynamic piezoelectric internal sinus elevation (HPISE)* tip (#S028I, BukBu Dental) was used to cut through the sinus floor and elevate the sinus membrane locally with hydraulic pressure via a stream of saline emitted from the HPISE tip[15,70] (Fig 4-18b). Next, autologous platelet-rich concentrated growth factor (CGF) clots prepared from the patient's venous blood were introduced into the elevated sinus space as the only graft material (Fig 4-18c). Following this, a 10-mm-long × 6-mm-diameter implant (Biotem) was inserted into the site (Fig 4-18d).

After the patient's tooth had been extracted, it was immediately prepared as a partially demineralized, osteoinductive particulate dentin autograft material using a dedicated processing machine (TOP Graft VacuaSonic System, CosmoBioMedicare), and subsequently mixed with autologous fibrin glue again prepared from the patient's blood. This resulted in a sticky mass of particulate dentin particles (Fig 4-18e), which was then used to fill all of the peri-implant gaps (Fig 4-18f). To complete the procedure, another

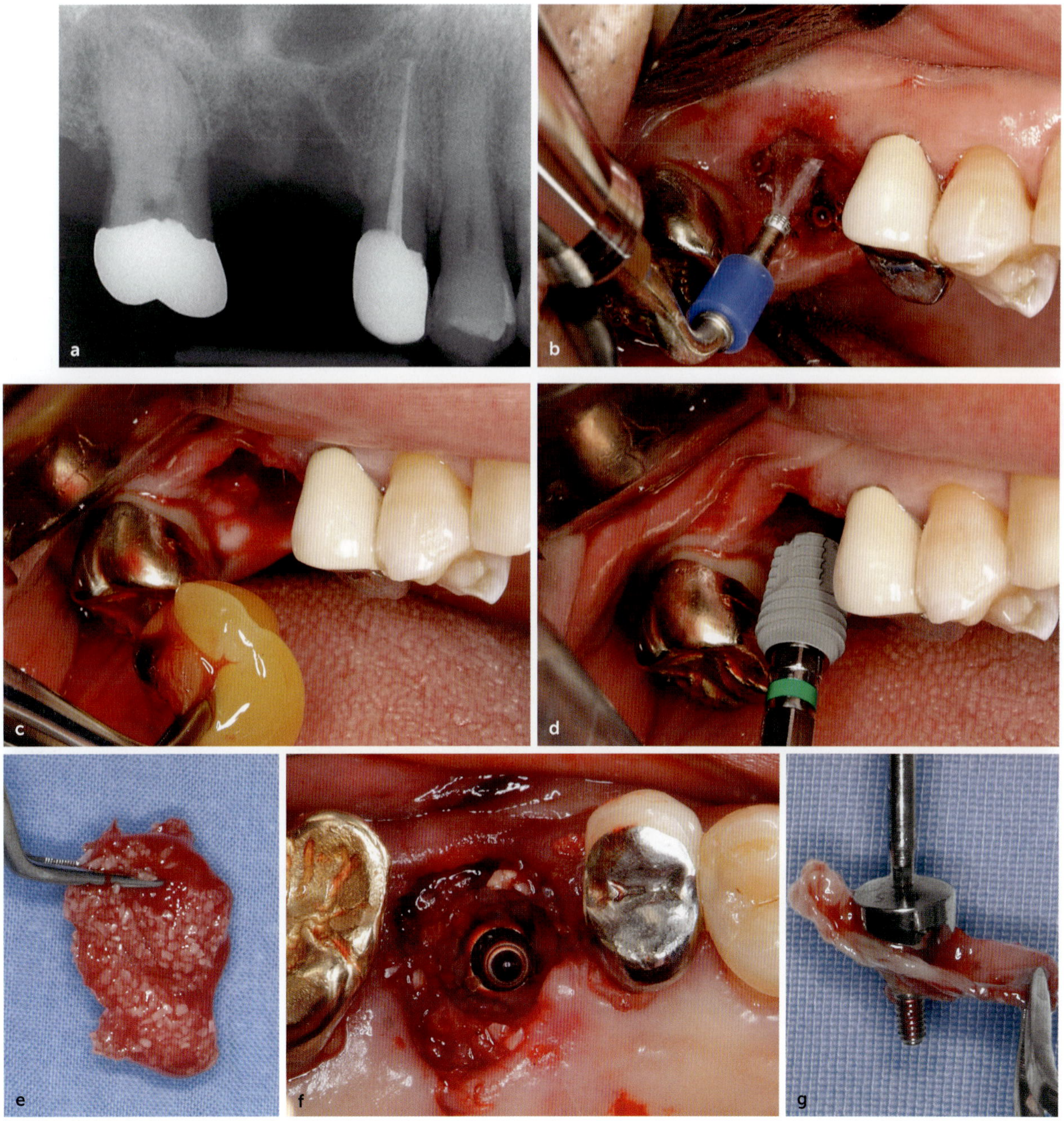

FIG 4-18 *(a)* The patient's maxillary right first molar required extraction because of advanced periodontal destruction. In the radiograph taken immediately after the extraction, while there is a favorable amount of IRS, there is limited bone remaining below the sinus floor. *(b)* Rather than using hand osteotomes and a surgical mallet to upfracture the sinus floor and elevate the sinus membrane,[15] a specialized piezoelectric tip that emitted saline under pressure was used.[69] *(c)* Autologous PRF clots prepared from the patient's venous blood were introduced in the localized sinus elevation space to act as the only graft material. *(d)* A moderately rough 10 × 6–mm implant was inserted into the osteotomy. *(e)* An autograft of partially demineralized dentin prepared from the extracted molar was prepared chairside and combined with autologous fibrin glue (see also chapter 6). *(f)* The sticky autograft was packed into the peri-implant gaps. *(g)* A platelet-rich autologous CGF clot was skewered onto the healing abutment before its connection to the implant. →

CGF clot was compressed into a membrane form and skewered like a poncho onto the threaded portion of a large-diameter healing abutment (Fig 4-18g), which was then connected to the implant (Fig 4-18h). This flattened clot acted as a membrane to help in protecting the sticky autograft material. A radiograph taken postoperatively is seen in Fig 4-18i. Healing was uneventful, as shown in the clinical photograph taken

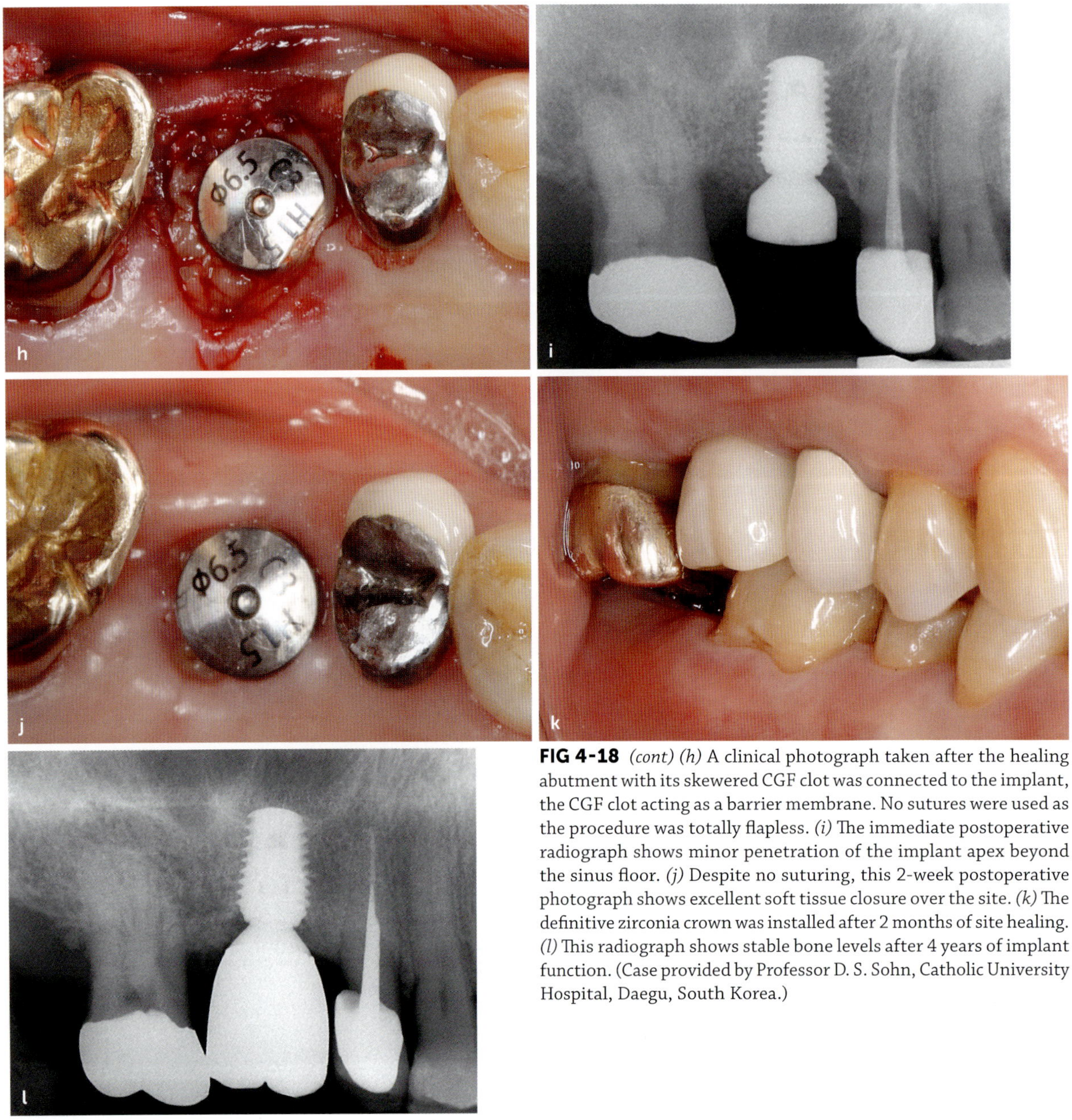

FIG 4-18 *(cont) (h)* A clinical photograph taken after the healing abutment with its skewered CGF clot was connected to the implant, the CGF clot acting as a barrier membrane. No sutures were used as the procedure was totally flapless. *(i)* The immediate postoperative radiograph shows minor penetration of the implant apex beyond the sinus floor. *(j)* Despite no suturing, this 2-week postoperative photograph shows excellent soft tissue closure over the site. *(k)* The definitive zirconia crown was installed after 2 months of site healing. *(l)* This radiograph shows stable bone levels after 4 years of implant function. (Case provided by Professor D. S. Sohn, Catholic University Hospital, Daegu, South Korea.)

at 2 weeks after surgery (Fig 4-18j). A definitive zirconia crown was inserted 2 months later (Fig 4-18k), while the radiographic appearance after 4 years in function is seen in Fig 4-18l.

Sometimes with type B IRS, it can be difficult to stabilize burs if the tooth roots are removed before osteotomy preparation is begun. The first molar shown in Fig 4-19a became symptomatic after suffering a vertical root fracture. Radiographic examination revealed a type B IRS and plenty of bone apically to receive an IMI without the need to manipulate the sinus floor. The CBCT scan confirmed adequate buccopalatal ridge width and favorable IRS (Fig 4-19b). The tooth crown was removed with a high-speed handpiece and fissure bur (Fig 4-19c), after which a long, narrow diamond pencil bur was used to create narrow channels in the periodontal ligament space to facilitate later removal of the molar roots (Fig 4-19d).

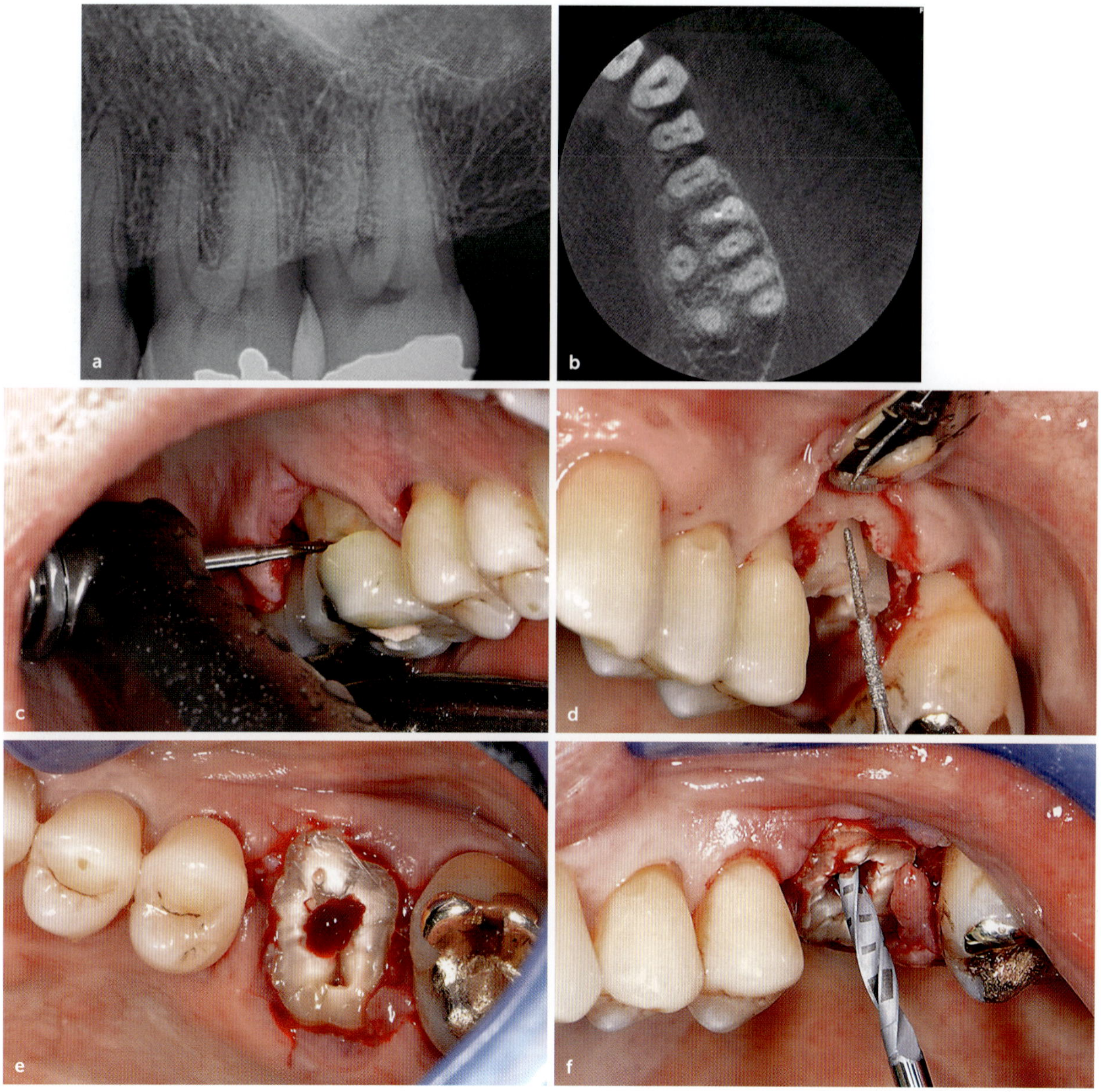

FIG 4-19 *(a)* The pretreatment periapical radiograph of a maxillary first molar that suffered a vertical root fracture. The site had plenty of native bone apically to place an implant without interfering with the maxillary sinus. *(b)* An occlusal horizontal CBCT slice of the tooth showing a favorable type B IRS. *(c)* After raising a flap sufficient to allow visualization for clinical photographs, a fissure bur and high-speed handpiece were used to remove the crown of the tooth. (Surgery performed by Dr Suzette Guo, University of Toronto.) *(d)* A long, small-diameter high-speed diamond bur was used to create narrow channels in the periodontal ligament spaces to facilitate removal of the molar roots. The penetration depth of this bur should be at least to two-thirds of the root length to reduce risk of root fracture during subsequent luxation/removal using small tipped elevators. For photographic purposes and because the buccal bone plate was thick, a small flap was raised to show the bur shaving tooth substance from the buccal aspect. More commonly, the bur would be used only at the proximal root surfaces and with a flapless protocol. *(e)* After coronectomy, a large round bur was used to localize the future osteotomy over the molar furcation. *(f)* After the round bur had created an adequate opening to avoid bur interference, a pilot bur was used to create the initial osteotomy to the predetermined depth.

Next, a large-diameter round bur was used to create an entry point for the pilot bur through the crown overlying the IRS (Figs 4-19e and 4-19f). The orientation of the initial osteotomy was checked after inserting a positioning pin (Figs 4-19g and 4-19h), and its depth was assessed with a radiograph (Fig 4-19i). The decision then was made to section and remove the three roots separately (Figs 4-19j and 4-19k). After

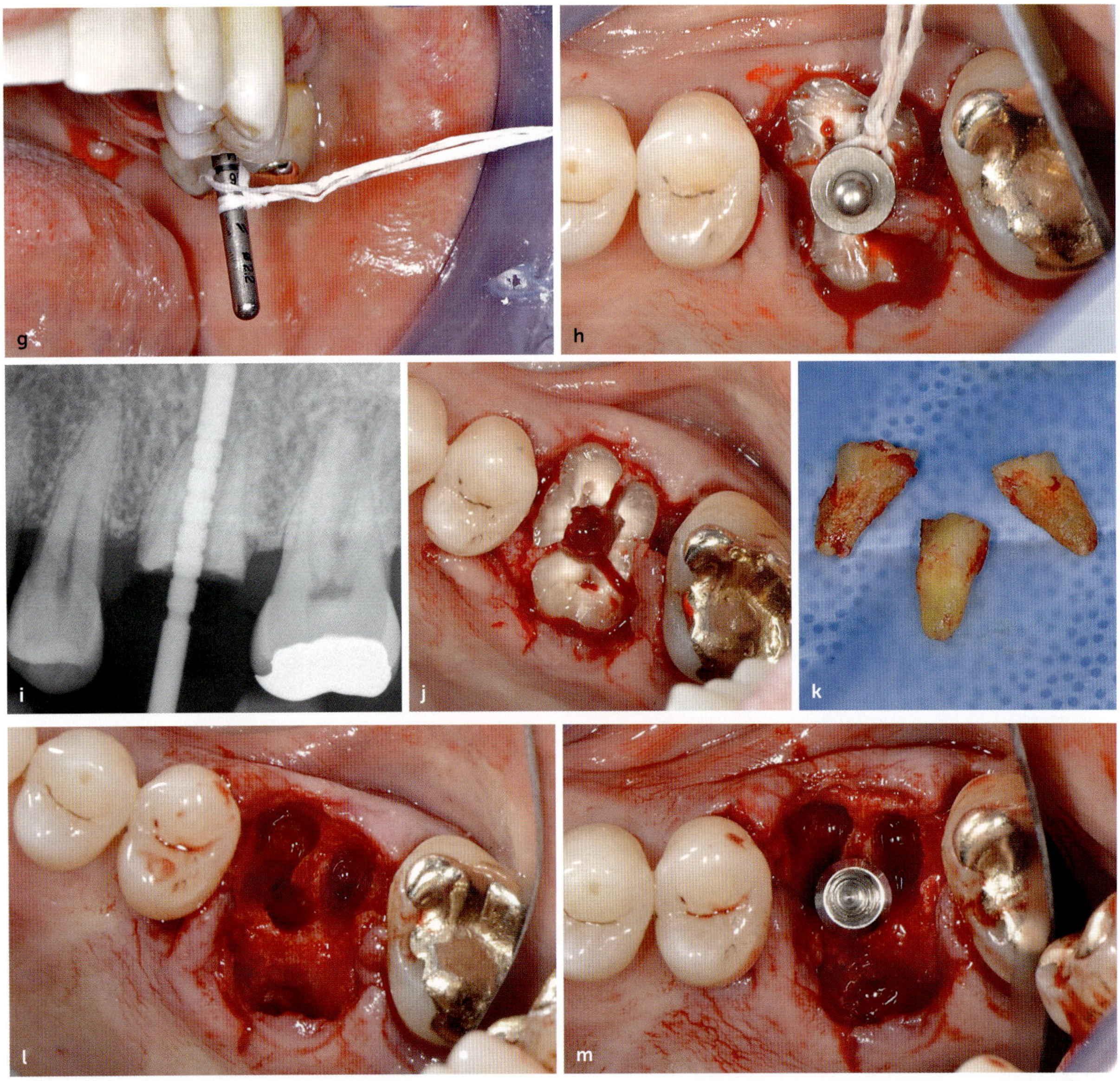

FIG 4-19 *(cont) (g)* A paralleling pin was used to verify the correct osteotomy orientation in 3D, and a radiograph was taken. *(h)* Optimal 3D implant positioning has been established before tooth root removal. *(i)* The radiograph verified that the osteotomy was adequate in depth to receive a 12-mm-long implant. *(j)* After completing the osteotomy preparation, the roots were separated for removal. *(k)* The roots were removed individually. *(l)* After root removal, the type B IRS was seen to have a dehiscence mesially. *(m)* A 4-mm-diameter implant was placed without further delay.

removing the roots atraumatically, the initial osteotomy was seen to have a major dehiscence mesially (Fig 4-19l), and the clinician elected to avoid additional drilling and placed the implant without further delay (Fig 4-19m). Due to the significant dehiscence, after adding a healing abutment to the implant, gap grafting was performed using sticky bone, ie, allograft particles mixed with autologous platelet-derived growth factors[71] (Fig 4-19n). The graft was covered like a poncho with a double layer of autologous growth factor–enriched fibrin membranes (Figs 4-19o and 4-19p), and the soft tissues were stabilized with sutures (Fig 4-19q). Figure 4-19r shows the immediate postoperative radiographic appearance, while Figs 4-19s and 4-19t show the clinical and radiographic appearances of the restored implant after 18 months in function.

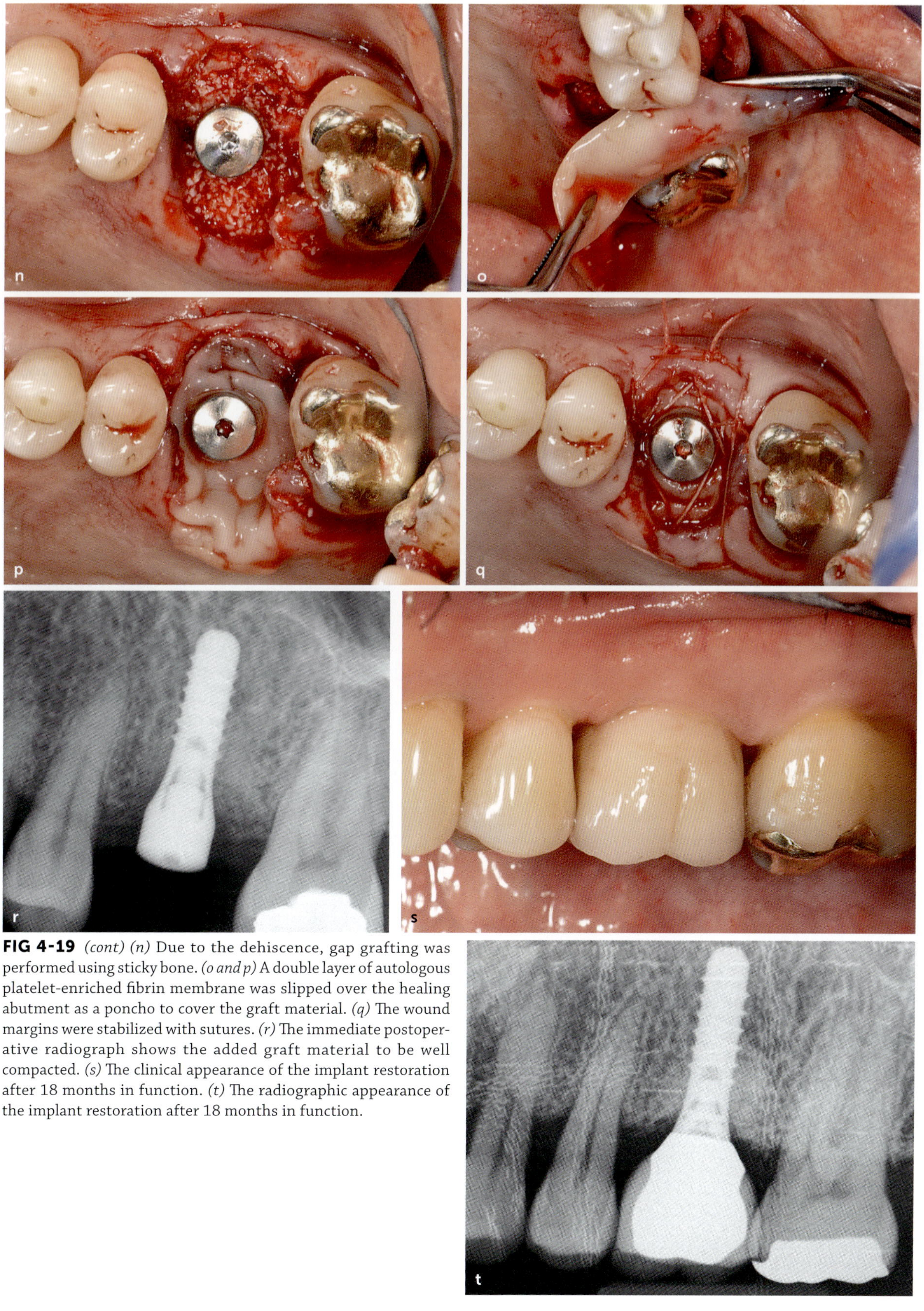

FIG 4-19 *(cont) (n)* Due to the dehiscence, gap grafting was performed using sticky bone. *(o and p)* A double layer of autologous platelet-enriched fibrin membrane was slipped over the healing abutment as a poncho to cover the graft material. *(q)* The wound margins were stabilized with sutures. *(r)* The immediate postoperative radiograph shows the added graft material to be well compacted. *(s)* The clinical appearance of the implant restoration after 18 months in function. *(t)* The radiographic appearance of the implant restoration after 18 months in function.

As mentioned previously, one way to avoid involving the sinus with maxillary IMIs can be to place the implant in the palatal root socket and later use an angulated prosthetic abutment to compensate for the awkward positioning of the implant. It needs to be stressed, however, that IMIs should never be placed in either of the buccal root sockets of a maxillary molar. Another option can be to use short, wide, or even ultra-wide-diameter implants. One group of investigators used 7- or 9-mm-long implants, mostly of 8-mm diameter, with the intention of avoiding specific sinus elevation steps[72] (see chapter 8). The mean preoperative bone height was 7.21 mm (SD: 1.78), but since the implants were generally submerged close to 2 mm subcrestally to minimize the impact of subsequent crestal bone loss, the majority of the implants appeared to have penetrated the sinus floor during insertion without untoward effects. Most likely in those instances, the implant apex simply became covered by sinus membrane without new bone formation. This conclusion can be based on work by others in animals and humans showing that small sinus perforations (up to 2 mm) resulting from implant seating can remain asymptomatic and of no consequence.[73,74] In fact, as the body of evidence grows, clinicians have observed that breaching the sinus floor during seating is far less of an issue than previously thought.[75]

Gap grafting and wound closure

As discussed in the introduction to this chapter, when IMIs were originally attempted, it was felt that any socket spaces or gaps that remained after implant insertion needed to be managed with some sort of mineralized particulate graft,[76] covered with a resorbable or nonresorbable barrier material, and submerged under a mucoperiosteal flap released sufficiently to allow tension-free complete wound closure. This added to the time involved for the procedure, its difficulty and cost, and the likelihood of postoperative complications. At present, most clinicians prefer to simplify the procedure by allowing nonsubmerged healing of IMIs, often with little or no gap grafting or suturing, provided that the procedure has been flapless (see chapter 11). Gap grafting at IMI sites may help to reduce horizontal bone loss, particularly on the crucial buccal aspect.[77] However, it is unlikely to reduce vertical bone loss, especially if a flap has been raised for the procedure, making it important to submerge the implant 1 to 2 mm subcrestally. While experts do vary in their choice of crucial gap size, most feel that, provided the IMI is adequately stabilized, gaps less than 3 mm and certainly less than 2 mm in width need not be grafted if they can be covered by the repositioned flap margins and sheltered by a stock wide-diameter or custom healing abutment (see chapter 12). Should the treating clinician choose to graft, a mineralized particulate allograft or xenograft is generally recommended. More experienced clinicians have suggested that gaps need no grafting regardless of their size.[78] Recent publication prescribed the use of wide-diameter or custom anatomical temporary immediate molar abutments to help in avoiding the need for gap grafting.[79,80] Additional advantages here would be the ability to add and subtract material for gingival support throughout the osseointegration phase and allowing for a precise customized socket seal over the immediately placed implant. One last issue with gap grafting is the situation where the buccal plate of bone is very thin even before extraction and therefore at great risk of resorption. In this situation, even if a large buccal gap can be left, it may be prudent to graft the gap with xenograft material.

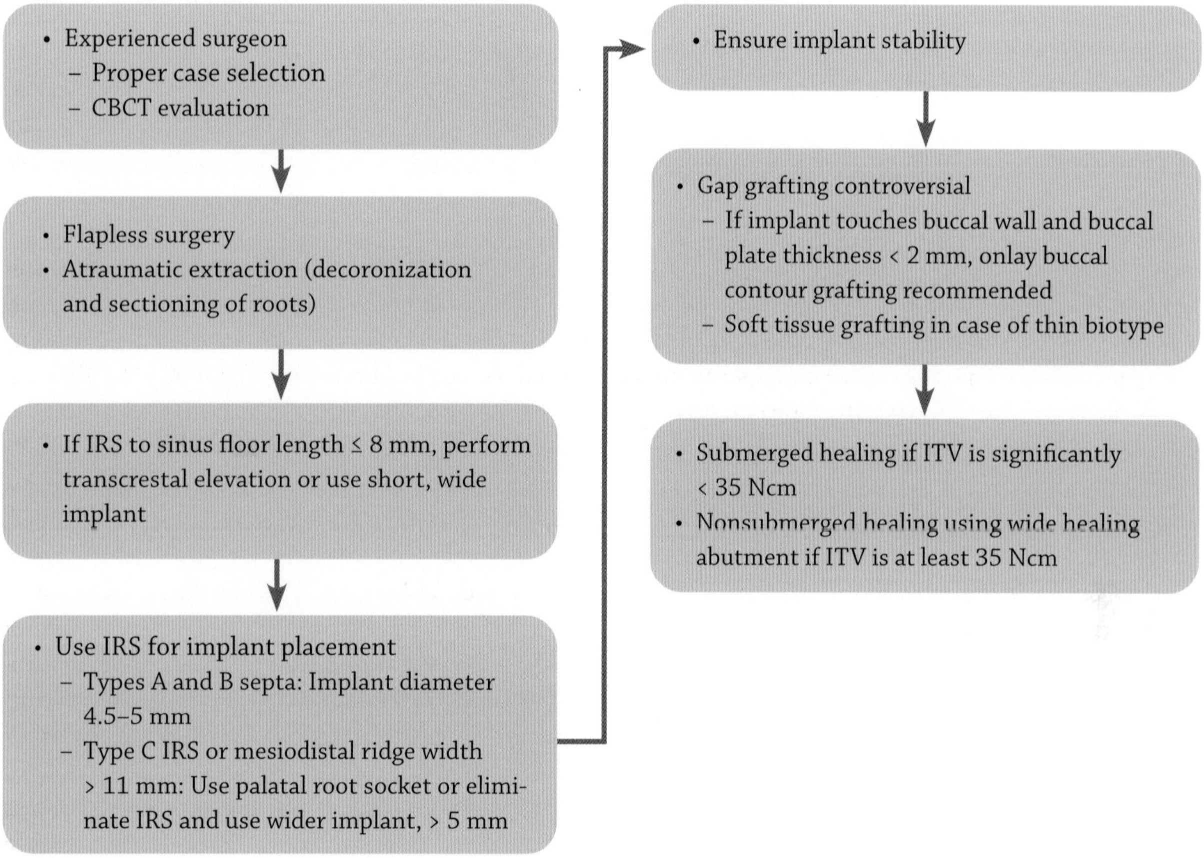

FIG 4-20 Flowchart for placing maxillary IMIs. ITV = insertion torque value.

Conclusion

IMI treatment in the maxilla is slowly becoming mainstream treatment (Fig 4-20). Adequate treatment planning must include CBCT scans to establish the condition of the remaining socket walls, the thickness of buccal and palatal cortical bone plates, the dimensions of the IRS, the distance from sinus floor to tooth furcation, and the condition of the sinus itself. In most instances, some indirect sinus floor elevation will be needed to allow the use of suitably long implants and achieve adequate initial implant stability. A flapless technique is preferred to minimize crestal bone loss. Unless the IRS has substantial volume (type A), after removing the molar crown and exposing the roots at the level of the trifurcation, osteotomy site preparation can be partially or completely finished before root removal and implant insertion. While IMIs placed in type B IRS will most likely be stabilized by contact with the remaining buccal and palatal IRS buttresses, no contact between implant periphery and the buccal bone of the two buccal root sockets should occur. Indeed, gaps of at least 1 mm should be left here to allow thickening of the buccal bone.

KEY POINTS

- Sites with a thick gingival biotype are preferred.
- Flapless surgery is recommended when there is intact buccal bone.
- Atraumatic tooth removal is crucial, meaning that the crown should first be removed with a high-speed handpiece and bur, exposing the root furcation.
- Tooth roots should be removed individually before, or if preferred, after osteotomy preparation.
- Osteotomy preparation should be centrally located in the IRS bone, if this exists.
- Good initial implant stability is crucial to success.
- Some transcrestal sinus floor elevation often will be needed, and this can be achieved using a variety of instruments.
- Ideally, at least 4 to 5 mm of native subantral bone will be present to help to stabilize the implant.
- Subcrestal implant placement of up to 2 mm will help to reduce the impact of any crestal bone resorption postoperatively.
- The decision whether or not to graft peri-implant gaps should be made by the treating clinician, recognizing that its necessity is presently controversial.
- Use of stock wide-diameter or custom healing abutments will reduce the need for gap grafting and help to guide soft tissue healing.

References

1. Yoshino K, Ishizuka Y, Watanabe H, Fukai K, Sugihara N, Matsukubo T. Sex- and age-based differences in single tooth loss in adults. Bull Tokyo Dent Coll 2015;56:63–67.
2. Müller F, Naharro M, Carlsson GE. What are the prevalence and incidence of tooth loss in the adult and elderly population in Europe? [published correction appears in Clin Oral Implants Res 2008;19:326–8]. Clin Oral Implants Res 2007;18(suppl 3): 2–14.
3. Covani U, Ricci M, Bozzolo G, Mangano F, Zini A, Barone A. Analysis of the pattern of the alveolar ridge remodelling following single tooth extraction. Clin Oral Implants Res 2011;22:820–825.
4. Tan WL, Wong TL, Wong MC, Lang NP. A systematic review of post-extractional alveolar hard and soft tissue dimensional changes in humans. Clin Oral Implants Res 2012;23(suppl 5): 1–21.
5. Livas C, Halazonetis DJ, Booij JW, Pandis N, Tu YK, Katsaros C. Maxillary sinus floor extension and posterior tooth inclination in adolescent patients with Class II Division 1 malocclusion treated with maxillary first molar extractions. Am J Orthod Dentofacial Orthop 2013;143:479–485.
6. Chen YW, Finkelman M, Papaspirisdakos P, César-Neto JB, Weber HP, de Souza AB. Comparative analysis of dimensional alterations following extraction of maxillary molars using three-dimensional images' superimposition: A CBCT study. Odontology 2021;109:514–523.
7. Harorh A, Bocutoğlu O. The comparison of vertical height and width of maxillary sinus by means of Waters' view radiograms taken from dentate and edentulous cases. Ann Dent 1995;54:47–49.
8. Sharan A, Madjar D. Maxillary sinus pneumatization following extractions: A radiographic study. Int J Oral Maxillofac Implants 2008;23:48–56.
9. Schwartz-Arad D, Grossman Y, Chaushu G. The clinical effectiveness of implants placed immediately into fresh extraction sites of molar teeth. J Periodontol 2000;71:839–844.
10. Schwartz-Arad D, Chaushu G. The ways and wherefores of immediate placement of implants into fresh extraction sites: A literature review. J Periodontol 1997;68:915–923.
11. Fugazzotto PA. Implant placement at the time of maxillary molar extraction: Technique and report of preliminary results of 83 sites. J Periodontol 2006;77:302–309.
12. Albrektsson T, Wennerberg A. Oral implant surfaces: Part 1—Review focusing on topographic and chemical properties of different surfaces and in vivo responses to them. Int J Prosthodont 2004;17:536–543.

13. Fugazzotto PA. Maintenance of soft tissue closure following guided bone regeneration: Technical considerations and report of 723 cases. J Periodontol 1999;70:1085–1097.
14. Smith RB, Tarnow DP. Classification of molar extraction sites for immediate dental implant placement: Technical note. Int J Oral Maxillofac Implants 2013;28:911–916.
15. Summers RB. The osteotome technique: Part 3—Less invasive methods of elevating the sinus floor. Compendium 1994;15:698–710.
16. Summers RB. A new concept in maxillary implant surgery: The osteotome technique. Compendium 1994;15:152–162.
17. Fugazzotto PA. Implant placement at the time of maxillary molar extraction: Treatment protocols and report of results. J Periodontol 2008;79:216–223.
18. Jiansheng H, Dongying X, Xianfeng W, Baoyi X, Qiong L, Jincai Z. Clinical evaluation of short and wide-diameter implants immediately placed into extraction sockets of posterior areas: A 2-year retrospective study. J Oral Implantol 2012;38:729–737.
19. Matsuda H, Borzabadi-Farahani A, Le BT. Three-dimensional alveolar bone anatomy of the maxillary first molars: A cone-beam computed tomography study with implications for immediate implant placement. Implant Dent 2016;25:367–372.
20. Renouard F, Nisand D. Short implants in the severely resorbed maxilla: A 2-year retrospective clinical study. Clin Implant Dent Relat Res 2005;7(suppl 1):S104–S110.
21. Lang NP, Pun L, Lau KY, Li KY, Wong MC. A systematic review on survival and success rates of implants placed immediately into fresh extraction sockets after at least 1 year. Clin Oral Implants Res 2012;23(suppl 5):39–66.
22. Ketabi M, Deporter D, Atenafu EG. A systematic review of outcomes following immediate molar implant placement based on recently published studies. Clin Implant Dent Relat Res 2016; 18:1084–1094.
23. Lu H, He L, Xu J, et al. Well-maintained patients with a history of periodontitis still harbor a more dysbiotic microbiome than health. J Periodontol 2020;91:1584–1594.
24. Bain CA, Moy PK. The association between the failure of dental implants and cigarette smoking. Int J Oral Maxillofac Implants 1993;8:609–615.
25. Lin TH, Chen L, Cha J, et al. The effect of cigarette smoking and native bone height on dental implants placed immediately in sinuses grafted by hydraulic condensation. Int J Periodontics Restorative Dent 2012;32:255–261.
26. Tomlin EM, Nelson SJ, Rossmann JA. Ridge preservation for implant therapy: A review of the literature. Open Dent J 2014; 8:66–76.
27. Barber HD, Lignelli J, Smith BM, Bartee BK. Using a dense PTFE membrane without primary closure to achieve bone and tissue regeneration. J Oral Maxillofac Surg 2007;65:748–752.
28. Demircan S, Çankaya AB. Is immediate implant placement possible in the maxillary molar area? An anatomical study. Quintessence Int 2016;47:853–859.
29. Malkoç S, Basçiftçi FA, Nur M, Catalbas B. Maxillary and mandibular mesiodistal tooth sizes among different malocclusions in a sample of the Turkish population. Eur J Orthod 2011;33: 592–596.
30. Domic D, Bertl K, Ahmad S, Schropp L, Hellén-Halme K, Stavropoulos A. Accuracy of cone-beam computed tomography is limited at implant sites with a thin buccal bone: A laboratory study. J Periodontol 2021;92:592–601.
31. Spray JR, Black CG, Morris HF, Ochi S. The influence of bone thickness on facial marginal bone response: Stage 1 placement through stage 2 uncovering. Ann Periodontol 2000;5:119–128.
32. Qahash M, Susin C, Polimeni G, Hall J, Wikesjö UM. Bone healing dynamics at buccal peri-implant sites. Clin Oral Implants Res 2008;19:166–172.
33. Araújo MG, Linder E, Lindhe J. Bio-Oss collagen in the buccal gap at immediate implants: A 6-month study in the dog. Clin Oral Implants Res 2011;22:1–8.
34. Deporter D, Ebrahimi DM, Rahmati A, Atenafu E, Ketabi M. CBCT data relevant in treatment planning for immediate maxillary molar implant placement. J Adv Periodontol Implant Dent 2021;13:49–55.
35. Tarnow DP, Chu SJ. Human histologic verification of osseointegration of an immediate implant placed into a fresh extraction socket with excessive gap distance without primary flap closure, graft, or membrane: A case report. Int J Periodontics Restorative Dent 2011;31:515–521.
36. Peñarrocha-Oltra D, Demarchi CL, Maestre-Ferrín L, Peñarrocha-Diago M, Peñarrocha-Diago M. Comparison of immediate and delayed implants in the maxillary molar region: A retrospective study of 123 implants. Int J Oral Maxillofac Implants 2012; 27:604–610.
37. Wychowański P, Woliński J, Kacprzak M, et al. Immediate palatal molar implants: A simple, safe, minimally invasive technique. Int J Periodontics Restorative Dent 2017;37(37):e297–e301.
38. Araújo MG, Lindhe J. Dimensional ridge alterations following tooth extraction. An experimental study in the dog. J Clin Periodontol 2005;32:212–218.
39. Wood DL, Hoag PM, Donnenfeld OW, Rosenfeld LD. Alveolar crest reduction following full and partial thickness flaps. J Periodontol 1972;43:141–144.
40. Fortin T, Bosson JL, Isidori M, Blanchet E. Effect of flapless surgery on pain experienced in implant placement using an image-guided system. Int J Oral Maxillofac Implants 2006;21:298–304.
41. Kinaia BM, Kazerani S, Korkis S, Masabni OM, Shah M, Neely AL. Effect of guided bone regeneration on immediately placed implants: Meta-analyses with at least 12 months follow-up after functional loading. J Periodontol 2021;92:1749–1760.
42. Hu C, Gong T, Lin W, Yuan Q, Man Y. Immediate implant placement into posterior sockets with or without buccal bone dehiscence defects: A retrospective cohort study. J Dent 2017;65:95–100.
43. Pei X, Wang L, Chen C, Yuan X, Wan Q, Helms JA. Contribution of the PDL to osteotomy repair and implant osseointegration. J Dent Res 2017;96:909–916.
44. Nelson S, Thomas G. Bacterial persistence in dentoalveolar bone following extraction: A microbiological study and implications for dental implant treatment. Clin Implant Dent Relat Res 2010; 12:306–314.
45. Deporter DA. Complications after implant site ridge preservation and delayed implant placement: A case report. Clin Adv Periodontics 2014;4:14–18.
46. Renouard F, Nisand D. Impact of implant length and diameter on survival rates. Clin Oral Implants Res 2006;17(suppl 2):35–51.
47. Calvo-Guirado JL, Gomez Moreno G, Aguilar-Salvatierra A, Mate Sanchez de Val JE, Abboud M, Nemcovsky CE. Bone remodeling at implants with different configurations and placed immediately at different depth into extraction sockets. Experimental study in dogs. Clin Oral Implants Res 2015;26:507–515.
48. Vandeweghe S, Ackermann A, Bronner J, Hattingh A, Tschakaloff A, De Bruyn H. A retrospective, multicenter study on a novo wide-body implant for posterior regions. Clin Implant Dent Relat Res 2012;14:281–292.

49. Bishara M, Kurtzman GM, Krause ES. Implant restorations: Establishing a proper emergence profile. Compend Contin Educ Dent 2020;41:e16–e20.
50. Chen Y, Yuan S, Zhou N, Man Y. Transcrestal sinus floor augmentation with immediate implant placement applied in three types of fresh extraction sockets: A clinical prospective study with 1-year follow-up. Clin Implant Dent Relat Res 2017; 19:1034–1043.
51. Crespi R, Capparè P, Gherlone EF. Electrical mallet in implants placed in fresh extraction sockets with simultaneous osteotome sinus floor elevation. Int J Oral Maxillofac Implants 2013;28: 869–874.
52. Engelke W, Deckwer I. Endoscopically controlled sinus floor augmentation. A preliminary report. Clin Oral Implants Res 1997;8:527–531.
53. Artzi Z, Parson A, Nemcovsky CE. Wide-diameter implant placement and internal sinus membrane elevation in the immediate postextraction phase: Clinical and radiographic observations in 12 consecutive molar sites. Int J Oral Maxillofac Implants 2003;18:242–249.
54. Acocella A, Bertolai R, Sacco R. Modified insertion technique for immediate implant placement into fresh extraction socket in the first maxillary molar sites: A 3-year prospective study. Implant Dent 2010;19:220–228.
55. Liu H, Liu R, Wang M, Yang J. Immediate implant placement combined with maxillary sinus floor elevation utilizing the transalveolar approach and nonsubmerged healing for failing teeth in the maxillary molar area: A randomized controlled trial clinical study with one-year follow-up. Clin Implant Dent Relat Res 2019;21:462–472.
56. Lekholm U, Zarb G. Patient selection and preparation. In: Branemark P-I, Zarb G, Albrektsson T (eds). Tissue-Integrated Prostheses: Osseointegration in Clinical Dentistry. Chicago: Quintessence, 1985:199–209.
57. Peñarrocha M, Pérez H, Garciá A, Guarinos J. Benign paroxysmal positional vertigo as a complication of osteotome expansion of the maxillary alveolar ridge. J Oral Maxillofac Surg 2001;59:106–107.
58. Tilotta F, Lazaroo B, Gaudy JF. Gradual and safe technique for sinus floor elevation using trephines and osteotomes with stops: A cadaveric anatomic study. Oral Surg Oral Med Oral Pathol Oral Radiol Endod 2008;106:210–216.
59. Ahn SH, Park EJ, Kim ES. Reamer-mediated transalveolar sinus floor elevation without osteotome and simultaneous implant placement in the maxillary molar area: Clinical outcomes of 391 implants in 380 patients. Clin Oral Implants Res 2012;23:866–872.
60. Kim JM, Sohn DS, Heo JU, et al. Minimally invasive sinus augmentation using ultrasonic piezoelectric vibration and hydraulic pressure: A multicenter retrospective study. Implant Dent 2012;21:536–542.
61. Huwais S, Mazor Z, Ioannou AL, Gluckman H, Neiva R. A multicenter retrospective clinical study with up-to-5-year follow-up utilizing a method that enhances bone density and allows for transcrestal sinus augmentation through compaction grafting. Int J Oral Maxillofac Implants 2018;33:1305–1311.
62. Simonpieri A, Choukroun J, Del Corso M, Sammartino G, Dohan Ehrenfest DM. Simultaneous sinus-lift and implantation using microthreaded implants and leukocyte- and platelet-rich fibrin as sole grafting material: A six-year experience. Implant Dent 2011;20:2–12.
63. Kim JM, Sohn DS, Bae MS, Moon JW, Lee JH, Park IS. Flapless transcrestal sinus augmentation using hydrodynamic piezoelectric internal sinus elevation with autologous concentrated growth factors alone. Implant Dent 2014;23:168–174.
64. Gülşen U, Şentürk MF, Mehdiyev İ. Flap-free treatment of an oroantral communication with platelet-rich fibrin. Br J Oral Maxillofac Surg 2016;54:702–703.
65. Gargallo-Albiol J, Tattan M, Sinjab KH, Chan HL, Wang HL. Schneiderian membrane perforation via transcrestal sinus floor elevation: A randomized ex vivo study with endoscopic validation. Clin Oral Implants Res 2019;30:11–19.
66. Öncü E, Bayram B, Kantarci A, Gülsever S, Alaaddinoğlu EE. Positive effect of platelet rich fibrin on osseointegration. Med Oral Patol Oral Cir Bucal 2016;21:e601–e607.
67. Anitua E, Orive G, Pla R, Roman P, Serrano V, Andía I. The effects of PRGF on bone regeneration and on titanium implant osseointegration in goats: A histologic and histomorphometric study. J Biomed Mater Res A 2009;91:158–165.
68. Del Fabbro M, Bortolin M, Taschieri S, Ceci C, Weinstein RL. Antimicrobial properties of platelet-rich preparations. A systematic review of the current pre-clinical evidence. Platelets 2016;27:276–285.
69. Del Fabbro M, Corbella S, Ceresoli V, Ceci C, Taschieri S. Plasma rich in growth factors improves patients' postoperative quality of life in maxillary sinus floor augmentation: Preliminary results of a randomized clinical study. Clin Implant Dent Relat Res 2015;17:708–716.
70. Sohn DS, Lee JS, An KM, Choi BJ. Piezoelectric internal sinus elevation (PISE) technique: A new method for internal sinus elevation. Implant Dent 2009;18:458–463.
71. Sohn DS, Huang B, Kim J, Park I, Park CC. Utilization of autologous concentrated growth factors (CGF) enriched bone graft matrix (sticky bone) and CGF-enriched fibrin membrane in implant dentistry. J Implant Adv Clin Dent 2015;7(10):11–29.
72. Vandeweghe S, De Ferrerre R, Tschakaloff A, De Bruyn H. A wide-body implant as an alternative for sinus lift or bone grafting. J Oral Maxillofac Surg 2011;69:e67–e74.
73. Jung JH, Choi BH, Zhu SJ, et al. The effects of exposing dental implants to the maxillary sinus cavity on sinus complications. Oral Surg Oral Med Oral Pathol Oral Radiol Endod 2006;102: 602–605.
74. Jung JH, Choi BH, Jeong SM, Li J, Lee SH, Lee HJ. A retrospective study of the effects on sinus complications of exposing dental implants to the maxillary sinus cavity. Oral Surg Oral Med Oral Pathol Oral Radiol Endod 2007;103:623–625.
75. Ragucci GM, Elnayef B, Suárez-López Del Amo F, Wang HL, Hernández-Alfaro F, Gargallo-Albiol J. Influence of exposing dental implants into the sinus cavity on survival and complications rate: A systematic review. Int J Implant Dent 2019;5:6.
76. Hämmerle CH, Araújo MG, Simion M; Osteology Consensus Group 2011. Evidence-based knowledge on the biology and treatment of extraction sockets [published correction appears in Clin Oral Implants Res 2012;23:641]. Clin Oral Implants Res 2012;23(suppl 5):80–82.
77. Chen Z, Li J, Wang HL, Yu H. Initial bone volume changes after immediate implant placement associated with filling the gap using bovine bone in molar sites. Int J Oral Maxillofac Implants 2019;34:521–528.
78. Smith RB, Tarnow DP, Sarnachiaro G. Immediate placement of dental implants in molar extraction sockets: An 11-year retrospective analysis. Compend Contin Educ Dent 2019;40:166–170.
79. Akin R. A new concept in maintaining the emergence profile in immediate posterior implant placement: The anatomic harmony abutment. J Oral Maxillofac Surg 2016;74:2385–2392.
80. Liu L,Yu WH, Li XT, Zhao H, Yang JJ. Clinical application study of immediate implantation without bone grafting in maxillary molars: A clinical study with one-year follow up. Br J Oral Maxillofac Surg 2022;60:332–336.

5

IMMEDIATE IMPLANT PLACEMENT IN INFECTED MOLAR SITES

Massimo Del Fabbro
Sourav Panda
Silvio Taschieri

Immediate implants, ie, those placed into fresh extraction sockets, are becoming more and more common in clinical dentistry today as their usage helps to moderate the extensive bone resorption and shrinkage in alveolar ridge dimensions (both vertically and horizontally) known to take place after routine tooth extraction.[1] The approach can allow for optimal implant positioning as well as reduced total treatment time.

The concept is not new, having been first introduced using ceramic implants by Schulte and Heimke in 1976.[2] Following the epic publication by Adell et al[3] in 1981 in which human clinical results using the Brånemark-type titanium threaded implant were published, Anneroth and colleagues[4] reported that immediate placement of similar implants into mandibular incisor sockets of monkeys could be successful, at least if submerged healing was allowed. Then in 1989, Lazzara published a descriptive report of two clinical cases of immediate implant placement in fresh extraction sockets.[5] He stressed the importance of good primary stability and suggested that ideally the implant should be seated 2 mm subcrestally to minimize the impact of early crestal bone loss and allow the surrounding gingival tissues to grow over the site, producing a soft tissue seal during site healing. Somehow, that critical factor of implant placement depth was not always recognized in a lot of later work. The most coronal aspects of the buccal and linguopalatal socket walls are generally thin (< 2 mm), but they thicken more apically so that if subcrestal placement is employed, significant crestal resorption around the implant often can be avoided.

Interestingly, and once more ahead of his time, Lazzara did not promote hard tissue grafting of peri-implant gaps, but instead to minimize the perceived risk of soft connective tissue and/or epithelial downgrowth into these gaps, he suggested placing an ePTFE (expanded polytetrafluoroethylene) barrier (GORE-TEX, W. L. Gore) over the osteotomy, leaving it exposed and secured with sutures, but removed after 1 month. This choice of barrier material was an odd one because using it would have run the risk of wound infection through the expanded (ie, porous) PTFE, but this apparently wasn't an issue in these first patients as the barriers were not in place for that long. He listed the main advantages of immediate implantation from the surgical and prosthetic standpoints, foreseeing the subsequent evolution and more widespread application of the approach. Immediate implant placement offers both economic and social benefits. Treatment time is decreased and can be shortened further if nonsubmerged initial healing is employed, which later publications confirmed to be possible. Less evident (but no less important) advantages also demonstrated by later investigations included implant survival/success rates comparable with (and in some cases better than) earlier protocols placing implants only at healed extraction sites, enhanced hard and soft tissue volume maintenance, and prosthetically driven 3D implant positioning even if socket walls are compromised and in need of augmentation grafting.[6]

An important consideration with immediate implant placement, however, is the fact that many teeth slated for extraction can be enveloped with chronic infection arising from endodontic and/or periodontal pathology because the causative pathogenic microorganisms have the potential to hamper or delay normal bone healing and osseointegration if not effectively managed.[7–9] Teeth with an endodontic periradicular infection rarely may present with apical actinomycosis, most commonly caused by *Actinomyces* species. This is a chronic granulomatous infectious lesion, difficult to eradicate and characterized by suppuration, abscess formation, and draining sinus tracts. The clinical and radiographic presentation may be indistinguishable from common apical periodontitis, but the lesion is far more difficult to eradicate, sometimes requiring extended antibiotic treatment before an implant can be successfully placed.[10] Notwithstanding the presence of this rare type of infection, some reports have indicated that, in general, chronically infected tooth sites may not represent a contraindication for immediate implantation provided that complete eradication of granulation tissue and affected bone can be achieved.[9] A histomorphometric study in dogs showed that immediate implant placement at infected sites was feasible. The investigators induced infection experimentally at mandibular third and fourth premolars by exposing and infecting their pulpal tissue with autogenous dental plaque. After a 3-month interval, radiographs confirmed periapical infection of the test teeth, and thereafter, following tooth extraction and site debridement, implants were placed immediately. Controls included implants placed immediately following extraction of healthy premolars in the same animals. Both previously infected and control implants integrated satisfactorily. However, the control site implants did show significantly greater bone-to-implant contact histologically at the times examined ($P < .05$).[11]

Immediate placement of dental implants into debrided, previously infected root sockets can be challenging. Primary implant stability is as always crucial for successful osseointegration, and loss of supporting bone with compromise of one or more socket walls will increase the risk of failure, as can the need for and added risk of regenerative bone grafting procedures. Even delayed implant placement at sites where periodontal infection was the reason for extraction has been shown to result in significantly slower bone healing than where delayed implants were placed at healed sockets of previously periodontally disease-free teeth.[12] Other possible implications for the placement of immediate implants at infected extraction sites include whether the infection is acute or chronic in nature, whether debridement of infected tissue has been thorough enough, whether immediate or delayed implant loading will be undertaken, and whether appropriate antibiotic coverage has been used.[13,14] Some authors have even suggested that latent microbial deposits may remain in bone at apparently well-healed extraction sites, stressing once more how thorough debridement must be.[15,16] Consequently, the situation becomes more challenging in cases where immediate replacement of infected multirooted teeth is being considered because of the greater anatomical difficulty in accessing contaminated bone. Other considerations when contemplating immediate implant placement at molar sites include whether the infection is in close proximity to or has already reached the maxillary sinus floor, or whether debridement will endanger the integrity of mandibular nerve canal. This chapter describes some current clinical protocols for successfully placing immediate molar implants (IMIs) into chronically infected sockets.

Relevant Literature Review

Published systematic literature reviews with meta-analyses have indicated that placement of dental implants into infected extraction sockets may carry a small increased risk of failure compared with immediate implant insertion into noninfected fresh extraction sockets, with survival rates for the former being in the range of 95%.[13,14,17–19] In what seems to have been the most recent literature review on this topic,[19] the authors identified nine studies in which a pool of 2,281 sites were analyzed. Compared with noninfected sites that received immediate implants, infected sites showed no significant differences in implant survival rates (risk ratio [RR] = 0.99; 95% confidence interval [CI] = 0.98 to 1; *P* = .08). As well, no significant statistical differences were found in marginal bone level (mean difference = –0.03; 95% CI = –0.1 to 0.04; *P* = .41), marginal gingival level (mean difference = –0.07; 95% CI = –0.17 to 0.04; *P* = .23), probing depth (mean difference = 0.06; 95% CI = –0.24 to 0.36; *P* = .7), or modified bleeding index (mean difference = –0.00162196; 95% CI = –0.09 to 0.09; *P* = .97) at the latest follow-up. Interestingly, however, others have challenged these findings. For example, in their systematic review and meta-analysis, de Oliveira-Neto et al concluded that implants placed in infected sites had three times the risk of failing.[20] Clearly then, patient selection, presurgical protocols, and site debridement must be technique sensitive.

In preparation for writing this chapter, a further literature search was undertaken. A systematic search was conducted using electronic databases including MEDLINE, SCOPUS, CENTRAL, and EMBASE with the following keywords: immediate implants, infected sites, infected sockets, periodontal infection, endodontic failure, periapical lesion/pathology. Furthermore, key peer-reviewed dental journals were hand-searched to identify evidence regarding placement of immediate implants at infected sites. A total of 1,349 abstracts were screened to identify 27 articles reporting the outcomes of immediate implants placed into infected tooth sockets, with data including those from randomized controlled trials, prospective and retrospective cohort studies, and some case series reports. A brief summary of the most relevant findings follows, but as will be seen, not a lot of data exist for IMIs placed in infected molar sockets.

Casap et al[9] described a protocol for a case series of 30 immediate implants (mostly maxillary anterior sites with implant dimensions 10–16 mm long and 3.7–4.7 mm in diameter) placed into infected/debrided sockets of 20 patients. The pathologies encountered included subacute periodontal infections, endo-perio infections, chronic periodontitis, chronic periapical lesions, and one periodontal cyst. Patients were initiated on a daily dose of 1.5 g amoxicillin (or 0.9 g clindamycin in penicillin-sensitive patients) 4 days prior to surgery and continued for 10 days postoperatively. The protocol emphasized meticulous debridement of the infected tissues using curettes in combination with peripheral and periapical ostectomy of the alveoli using a combination of oval and round burs. Osteotomy drilling was extended into native bone 3 to 4 mm apically to ensure good primary implant stability. Guided bone regenerative grafting was done to fill any peri-implant gaps using xenograft particles (Bio-Oss, Geistlich) covered with screw-stabilized, titanium-reinforced ePTFE followed by soft tissue primary closure. Complications included early exposure of the ePTFE barriers in two patients (managed using frequent rinsing with 0.12% chlorhexidine) and one case of antibiotic-induced pseudomembranous colitis. One implant failed shortly after restoration, having developed inadequate integration.

Lindeboom et al[8] had the previous year (2006) published results from a prospective randomized study with 50 nonsmoking patients each with a single chronically infected tooth. Treatment involved either immediate implant placement or delayed implant placement after socket grafting and site healing. Thirty-two implants were placed in the anterior maxilla and another 18 at premolar sites, all being randomly assigned for either immediate or delayed implant placement. One hour before surgery, patients were given 600 mg clindamycin. Following tooth extraction, thorough degranulation of all sockets was performed, and samples were taken for microbiologic analysis. Implants were seated 2 mm below the cementoenamel junctions of adjacent teeth. Apical infection had resulted in loss of the buccal plate at all 50 sites, and this was managed with augmentation using autogenous corticocancellous bone (taken from either retromolar or chin donor sites) covered by a collagen membrane (Bio-Gide, Geistlich) and primary soft tissue closure. Larger-diameter implants

(5.5 or 6.5 mm) were placed at the immediate sites, and the minimally acceptable torque during placement of all implants had to be 25 Ncm. Cumulative implant survival rates at 6 months were 92% at the immediate implant placement sites compared with 100% at the grafted and delayed implant placement sites. Two implants in the immediate placement group had shown mobility at second-stage surgery and were removed. The remaining 48 implants all had survived at the 1-year follow-up. When the bacterial specimens collected at the time of extraction were cultured, no growth was seen in 9 of the 50 extracted teeth. In 21 immediate implant sites and 20 delayed implant sites, microorganisms could be cultured, the most prevalent bacteria being *Fusobacterium nucleatum* (70%) and *Peptostreptococcus micros* (42%). Bacteria were found in the sample from one failed immediate implant but not the other, suggesting that the failures could easily have been due to surgical technique rather than the presence of these bacteria.

A later (2011) prospective controlled clinical trial reported by Truninger et al[21] gave favorable results for immediate implants placed into sockets of teeth with established periapical pathology. In each of 13 patients requiring extraction of a tooth with apical pathology, immediate implants were placed, while in another group of 16 patients, implants were placed immediately into noninfected tooth sockets. The infected sites had presented with pain, periapical radiolucencies greater than 1 mm, suppuration, or a combination of these findings. The distribution of implants placed was restricted to incisors, canines, and premolars. Employing full mucoperiosteal flap elevation, teeth were extracted atraumatically and sockets debrided. Implants with dimensions best suited for each socket were chosen to obtain adequate stability while still achieving optimal prosthetic positioning. Guided bone regeneration (GBR) was performed using xenograft particles (Bio-Oss spongiosa particles) and resorbable collagen membranes (Bio-Gide). All patients received penicillin-type antibiotics for 5 days and rinsed with a 0.2% chlorhexidine digluconate solution. After transmucosal or semisubmerged healing, implants were loaded at 3 months and followed for 3 years, at which time all implants were still in place. Data from what appear to be the same patient cohort were later presented by Jung et al[22] after 5 years in function, and again all implants had survived.

Montoya-Salazar et al[23] analyzed results from a split-mouth study with 18 patients; in each, one implant had been immediately placed into an infected tooth socket and another into a control noninfected site. The infected sites presented with chronic endodontic and/or periodontal lesions. After tooth extraction, the infected sockets were debrided using curettes, cleaned with 90% hydrogen peroxide, irradiated with Er,Cr:YSGG laser, and irrigated with sterile saline. Implant osteotomies were extended 3 to 4 mm beyond the socket apices to ensure adequate stability. GBR to encourage fill of peri-implant bone gaps was performed using xenograft particles covered with titanium-reinforced ePTFE membranes, the latter being protected by primary soft tissue closure. Implants were uncovered and crowns placed at 4.5 months, and the 3-year survival rates were reported as 94.4% for the test implants (one implant failed between 2 and 3 years) and 100% for the controls, the differences not being statistically different. The authors concluded that immediate implant placement at infected tooth sites, at least at nonmolar sites, can be considered a safe, effective, and predictable treatment option when appropriate steps are taken to clean and decontaminate the sockets.

Blus et al[24] compared the impact of acute versus chronic infection versus no infection on immediate implant placement. In their prospective cohort study with 2-year follow-up, 86 patients received 168 immediate implants distributed into three groups: 85 noninfected, 36 acutely infected, and 47 chronically infected sites. Infection was considered chronic when the presentation was a periapical cyst or granuloma with absence of pain, fistula, pus, and/or active periodontitis. Infection was considered acute when periapical pathology also was associated with pain, presence of pus or a fistula for periodontally involved sites, or presence of pus at the apex of endodontically involved sites. All patients were prescribed amoxicillin with clavulanic acid (Augmentin, GlaxoSmithKline) to be taken as 1 g twice per day for 5 days starting 6 to 12 hours before surgery. Flapless, atraumatic extractions were performed with the aid of an ultrasonic surgical device, which was also used to debride infected sites. At the 1-year follow-up, it was reported that a total of three implants had failed, including one of the 85 belonging to the noninfected group (lost 3 weeks after placement) and two from the acute infection group (one failed after 2 months of healing and the other had been immediately loaded and failed after 1 month of function). Thus, the 1-year survival rates were 98.8%, 94.4%, and 100% respectively for the originally noninfected, acutely infected, and chronically infected sockets. These outcomes were reported as statistically nonsignificant, but considering the small sample size might be interpreted to mean that acute infection posed an elevated risk for immediate implantation. Others have suggested a less risky protocol for acutely infected teeth can be to extract, debride, and perform early implant placement (ie, after 4 to 6 weeks' healing).[25]

Hita-Iglesias et al[26] reported data from another prospective, split-mouth trial in which 168 immediate implants were placed in 60 patients at maxillary incisor, canine, and premolar sites. Each patient received a minimum of two implants, one in a fresh socket associated with chronic periapical disease (average lesion size between 4 and 8 mm) but without pain, fistula formation or suppuration, and the other(s) in a healthy fresh socket. All the test teeth had previously been unsuccessfully treated endodontically. To be included, all implant sites required the presence of adjacent teeth, uneventful extractions, and radiographic evidence of the presence of all walls as well as 3 to 4 mm of bone being available beyond the root apex to ensure adequate implant primary stability. Smokers were excluded, as were patients with a history of bruxism. Flapless surgery was employed, and since peri-implant gaps never exceeded 3 mm in a horizontal or vertical direction, gap grafting was not performed. Crowns were delivered after 4 months of nonsubmerged healing. In addition to implant losses, failure was also recorded if there was a recurrence of periapical disease, if vertical crestal bone loss in radiographs became greater than half the implant length, or if the implant had mobility. The implant survival rate was 98.2% for the total sample (n = 168). Of the three implants lost, two were from the test group, and one was from the control group (in the same patient as one of the former). Among the surviving test implants, 5 were also considered failures due to excessive bone loss (n = 3) or because of the recurrence of the periapical lesions (n = 2). Survival rates then were significantly lower in the test than control sites at 12 months postloading (90.8% vs 98.1%). It was notable that all test site infections (although chronic) were endodontic in origin, but no investigations were done to see if actinomycosis could have been the reason for any of the failures.

Zuffetti et al[27] reported on 193 implants (115 in the maxilla and 78 in the mandible) placed in sockets of infected teeth of various types, including 18 (9.3%) at maxillary and 47 (24.3%) at mandibular molar sites. Outcomes were compared with those of 334 implants placed immediately into noninfected sites (including those of 55 [16.4%] maxillary and 53 [15.9%] mandibular molar teeth). Clinic protocol included antibiotic prophylaxis using Augmentin 2 g 1 hour before surgery and then 1 g three times daily for 6 days (alternatively, 500 mg clarithromycin 1 hour before surgery and then 300 mg twice daily for 6 days with patients allergic to amoxicillin). Of the infected sockets, in 134 cases, the tooth extracted was suffering from periodontitis, while in the remaining 59, the infection was of endodontic origin. Flapless surgery was performed unless some bone regeneration was required, and the teeth were removed atraumatically using periotomes and forceps after separating roots of molars using rotary instrumentation. Thorough curettage was performed in all sockets first using manual curettes, but followed using Piezosurgery inserts (PS2, Mectron) and generous sterile saline irrigation. When possible, implants were placed 1 mm deeper than the level of the buccal alveolar crest, and xenograft particles (Bio-Oss) covered by collagen membranes (Bio-Gide) used to encourage fill of any peri-implant gaps. By the mean follow-up time of approximately 50 months, 10 implants had failed: 7 implants placed into noninfected sockets and 3 placed into originally infected sockets. In the noninfected group, five implant failures happened within 6 months of placement, one failed after 8 months, and one after 11 months. Two of the five failures were at molar sites in patients who smoked more than 10 cigarettes per day. This would represent a molar site failure rate of 1.8%. In the infected socket group, two implants failed within 6 months of placement, and one failed after 9 months; all three were at molar sites in nonsmokers (molar site failure rate of 4.6%). None of the failed implants showed any signs of concurrent infection. Overall, survival of immediate implants placed into infected sockets (98.4%) was reported as being not significantly different from those placed in noninfected sockets (97.9%). The authors concluded that immediate placement of implants into periodontally or endodontically infected tooth sockets appears to be a safe option.

Most recently, Narad et al[28] reported a case series of 15 nonsmoking patients in whom 24 implants were placed immediately into extraction sockets of nonmolar teeth affected by infections related to subacute periodontal infection, combined endo-perio lesions, or failed endodontic treatments of previously traumatically devitalized teeth. Antibiotic prophylaxis with a daily dose of 1.5 g amoxicillin (or 0.9 g clindamycin in penicillin-sensitive patients) was started 4 days preoperatively and continued for 7 days postoperatively. Following reflection of full-thickness mucoperiosteal flaps, the involved teeth were atraumatically extracted with minimal damage to the socket cortical walls. All sockets were meticulously debrided with curettes followed by intrasocket ostectomies using a rotary oval bur and vigorous sterile saline irrigation to remove contaminated bone. The debrided sockets were then prepared to receive implants of sufficient length (9 to 13 mm) to ensure that the osteotomies extended 2 to 4 mm apically into native bone. Any residual peri-implant gaps of greater than 2-mm width were filled with particulate allograft material, and releasing incisions added if need be to achieve primary soft tissue closure. It was reported that all implants appeared healthy at the 2-year follow-up exam.

One modification of the methods so far described for placing implants immediately into infected sockets is the addition of autologous blood-derived growth factors in the form of platelet-rich plasma (PRP) or platelet-rich fibrin (PRF)[29–32] (Fig 5-1). These preparations made chairside from the patient's venous blood can offer antimicrobial, anti-inflammatory, and concentrated growth factors (CGFs) known to accelerate vascularization and bone healing. A prospective cohort study by Del Fabbro et al[33] published in 2009 reported 1-year outcomes from 30 patients following placement of 61 immediate implants at various sites, including molars, all with chronic periapical lesions of endodontic or endo-perio origin. Twenty-six of the sites had endodontic while 35 had endo-perio lesions. Antibiotic usage was limited to a 2-g loading dose of amoxicillin and clavulanic acid (Augmentin) 1 hour before surgery. After tooth extraction, biopsies of the infected tissue were examined histologically and demonstrated characteristics typical of periapical granuloma in all cases. After careful socket debridement and osteotomy preparation, autologous platelet-derived growth factors in clot form (prepared chairside using the PRGF System [BTI Biotechnology Institute]) were inserted into the osteotomies immediately prior to implant insertion as was done in the case depicted in Fig 5-1 using CGF (autologous PRF clot prepared chairside using a Silfradent medifuge). For clarification, PRGF (plasma rich in growth factors) and CGF fibrin clots are more or less the same, ie, autologous fibrin clots containing significant levels of platelet-derived growth factors.[30] Implants also were coated with PRGF in liquid form, and following their placement, all gaps wider than 1 mm and/or dehiscence defects were filled with PRGF mixed with autogenous bone chips. Part of a PRGF clot also was sometimes used as a covering membrane before soft tissue suturing, again as was done in Fig 5-1f with CGF.[32] As an aside, PRGF or CGF fibrin clots also have been used as graft material when combining immediate maxillary molar implant placement with indirect sinus elevation.[34] Prosthetic loading of the implants (14 partial prostheses/26 single crowns) in Del Fabbro's study[33] was done after 3 to 4 months of site healing. Overall, the implant survival rate was 98.4% after 1 year of function (100% in the maxilla/96.8% in the mandible). However, survival was dependent on the original lesion type, with 100% survival at endo-perio sites but only 96.2% at purely endodontic infection sites. A subsequent follow-up of this study[35] with an expanded sample size (126 implants in total) compared the 5-year follow-up outcomes of postextraction implants placed in infected sites with or without PRGF and submitted to either immediate or delayed loading. Molar sites represented 38% of the 61 implants in the PRGF group and 29% of the 65 implants in the control group. The implant survival rates at the 5-year follow-up remained high and similar between groups (97.4% for PRGF/97.8% for controls), although soft tissue healing had been significantly faster at 3 and 7 days postsurgery with the PRGF-treated sites. It is noteworthy that the investigators used only a single loading dose of antibiotic for management of both infected and noninfected sites, unlike in most other studies where more extended antimicrobial intervention was used. Whether antibiotic usage might be totally eliminated when PRGF or CGF are used as standard protocol remains to be seen, but it may be

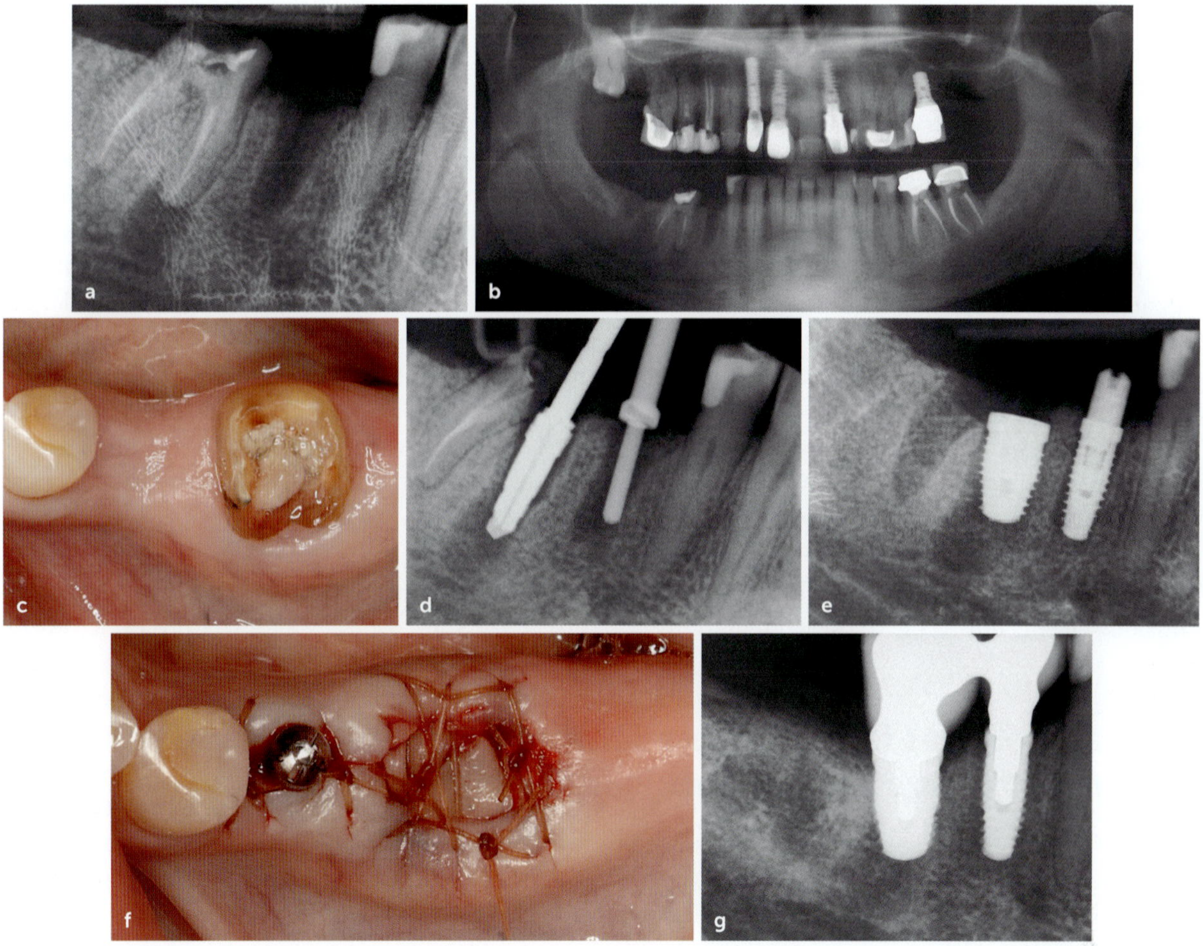

FIG 5-1 *(a)* This 66-year-old man presented for implant treatment to replace his recently extracted mandibular right second premolar and for an immediate molar implant at the first molar site. The molar had a failed endodontic treatment with a large chronic, asymptomatic periapical radiolucency and was deemed to be nonrestorable. *(b)* The patient's panoramic radiograph suggested that the lesion had not impacted the mandibular canal. *(c)* The preoperative clinical state of the mandibular right first molar. *(d)* After separating the molar roots, the mesial root was removed atraumatically without raising a mucoperiosteal flap, and the apical lesion was aggressively instrumented with curettes. The distal root was left in situ during osteotomy preparation to help to stabilize the bur. This intraoperative radiograph indicated the need to alter the implant orientations. *(e)* After completing the two osteotomies, the distal root was removed, and a large PRF clot with concentrated growth factors (CGF) prepared from the patient's own blood was packed into the molar osteotomy immediately before inserting the implant. A 10-mm-long × 6-mm-diameter T3 implant (Zimmer Biomet) was inserted into the mesial molar root socket, the larger diameter being needed to help in stabilizing the implant via contact with the osteotomy walls. The premolar site received a 11.5 × 4–mm T3 implant. *(f)* The insertion torque of the premolar implant allowed it to receive a healing abutment, but since the IMI had an insertion torque less than 25 Ncm, it received only a healing screw subsequently covered with another CGF clot. A third clot was placed in the distal root socket of the molar. *(g)* This periapical radiograph shows the restored implants 10 months after implant insertion. Bone remodeling has yet to be completed. (Surgery performed by Dr Quang Nguyen, University of Toronto.)

a useful question to investigate given the growing concern with microbial antibiotic resistance and emergence of "super-bugs." PRGF fibrin or CGF clots also can be used on their own to fill peri-implant gaps when all socket walls are intact or if need be (ie, when one or more socket walls are compromised) with added particulate graft material.[36]

In summary, while there are limited data for immediate implant placement at chronically infected molar sites, the treatment has shown favorable outcomes often not significantly different from those sites with implants placed immediately into noninfected molar sockets. Key factors for success include atraumatic tooth removal and deliberate aggressive debridement of infected soft and hard tissues. It may be necessary to have 3 to 4 mm of noninfected apical bone height to achieve adequate initial implant stability, and subcrestal implant placement will help to reduce the impact of expected postsurgical crestal bone loss. No standard antibiotic protocol exists for managing infected sites, and indeed whether antibiotic usage is needed provided that debridement is sufficient has not been investigated. Greenstein and Tarnow[37] have published a recent literature review on antibiotic regimens and suggested that a single loading dose is sufficient for implant placement in medically fit patients receiving implants in noninfected sites. Submerged site healing appears not to be needed. Nor is peri-implant gap grafting always needed, provided that adequate stability and good peri-implant flap adaptation is achievable around an appropriate healing abutment. The use of autologous PRF clots at the time of implant placement needs further investigation, as it may offer considerable advantage in combatting retained bacteria and accelerating vascularization and bone healing during initial osseointegration.[38]

Clinical Protocols for Immediate Implants in Infected Molar Sites

Careful planning in advance of placing IMIs is essential and should include 3D radiographic assessment using CBCT to reveal tooth and socket anatomies; the interseptal bone volume and its usefulness in stabilizing an IMI; the presence, thickness, and height of the buccal cortical plate; as well as the proximity of vital structures. Clinical assessment should include evaluation of the periodontal status of the condemned tooth and its neighbors as well as determination of whether the infection is quiescent. For mandibular molars, the distance between the root apices and the mandibular nerve canal should be no less than 4 mm. For maxillary molars, the presence of a substantial interradicular septum (IRS; type A) should be noted. The distance between the apical portion of the septum and the maxillary sinus should be sufficient to avoid invading the sinus domain by no more than 3 to 4 mm if indirect sinus floor elevation is planned, and the sinus should be healthy and functional.

While the absolute need for antibiotic usage has not been established, our protocol has been to administer 2 g of amoxicillin 1 hour before surgery.[37] Performing flapless surgery will help to minimize loss of alveolar bone during postoperative alveolar ridge remodeling. Decoronation of the molar and separation of all roots using rotary instruments and generous saline irrigation will facilitate their removal individually and atraumatically. Curettage of the alveolus after extraction, especially in the presence of apical lesions, must be carried out scrupulously and completely. Magnification devices and proper illumination will facilitate this crucial step, as will special drill kits such as the ultra-coarse diamond ones. These are specially engineered to quickly grab and remove granulation tissue and underlying affected bone as well as creating multiple bleeding points in the alveolus.

Some clinicians have included decontamination of infected sockets with Er,Cr:YSGG 2780-nm lasers,[39,40] or irrigation of the debrided sockets with peroxide or chlorhexidine,[41] but we have not included either of these extra steps, as there are no data confirming them to be beneficial compared to their nonuse. With maxillary molar sites, IMIs ideally will be positioned at the center of the IRS. A slight underpreparation (eg, 0.3 mm) of the osteotomy relative to the intended implant diameter will help to ensure adequate initial implant stability, achieving an initial torque of between 25 and 30 Ncm. Ideally, the implant platform should be positioned at least 1.5 mm subcrestally both buccally and palatally. Provided that there is sufficient IRS to stabilize the implant, localized indirect sinus floor elevation with osteotomes or specialized osseodensifying burs[42] can be used to allow implants of appropriate lengths to be used (see also chapters 7 and 11).

For mandibular molars, having a substantial IRS is much less likely, and therefore technique modifications such as drilling the osteotomy through the tooth before removing its roots and/or using a wider-diameter implant stabilized by the buccal and lingual bony buttresses (see also chapter 8) may be the preferred approach. With both maxillary and mandibular IMIs, it is important to have sufficient peri-implant keratinized soft tissue for long-term patient comfort and stable crestal bone. Generally, IMIs will be placed without raising a mucogingival flap, and if there is concern about the thickness and/or width of keratinized gingiva (both should be ≥ 2 mm), soft tissue grafting can be done at the time of implant placement using, for example, the so-called "socket seal" technique by covering the implant with a soft tissue graft from the patient's palate.[43] Alternatively, a membrane can be created by flattening autologous PRF clots (PRGF or CGF), placing them over the

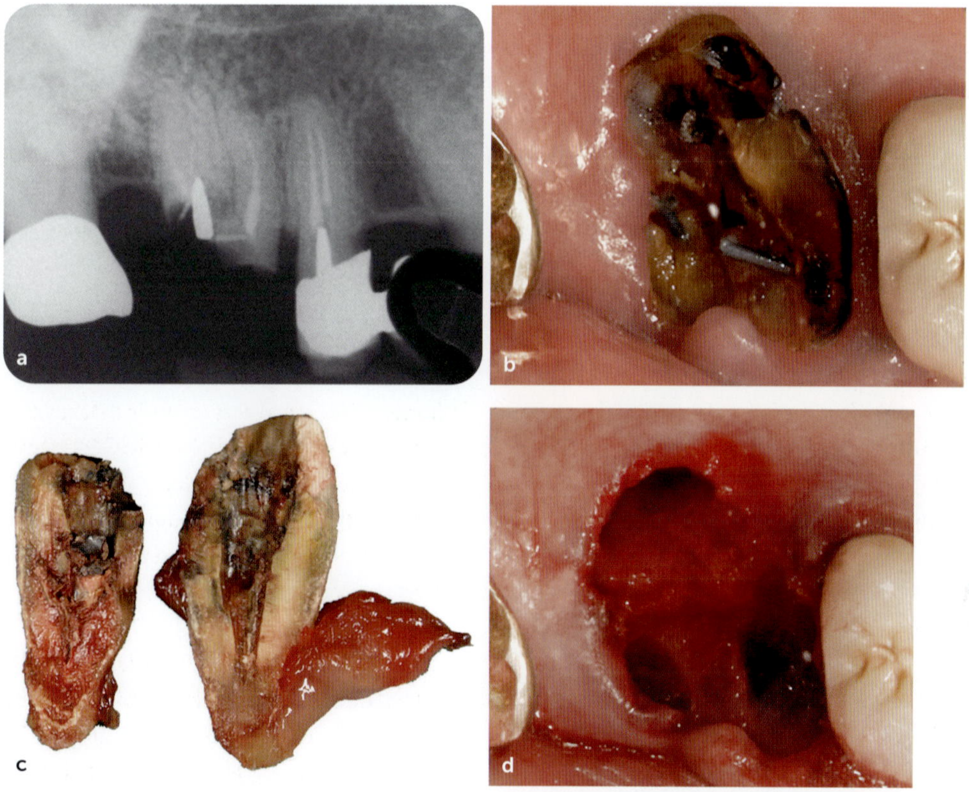

FIG 5-2 *(a)* A nonrestorable maxillary first molar required extraction. *(b)* This maxillary first molar showed failure of its endodontic treatment with a chronic rarefying osteitis, which in its chronicity had caused a periosteal reaction, lifting the sinus floor. *(c)* The tooth was sectioned and removed and clearly had been infected for some time. *(d)* Following extraction, the IRS bone that remained was considered type B.[46]

implant healing screw, and securing them with sutures.[35,36,44,45]

Sample Cases

Case 1: Chronically infected maxillary first molar

This patient presented with a failed endodontic treatment of a nonrestorable maxillary right first molar with a large apical radiolucency (Fig 5-2a). There were no signs of swelling or purulence. Using a flapless approach, the tooth was partially sectioned and removed atraumatically revealing type B interseptal/furcal bone[46] (Figs 5-2b to 5-2d). Following socket debridement, an implant was successfully placed into the IRS with dehiscences on the buccal and palatal aspects of the furcal bone. Despite the large gaps, no corrective grafting was done (Fig 5-2e). The site was covered with PRGF fibrin clots stabilized with sutures (Fig 5-2f). The 1- and 2-week postoperative clinical images are seen in Figs 5-2g and 5-2h, where soft tissue coverage is progressing well despite evidence that the patient had continued smoking cigarettes. A radiograph taken after 3 months of site healing (Fig 5-2i) showed the root sockets to be healing well. Figure 5-2j shows the clinical status of soft tissue healing at 5 months, at which time the reentry and restoration were performed. The definitive restoration is shown clinically and radiographically after 1 year in function in Figs 5-2k and 5-2l.

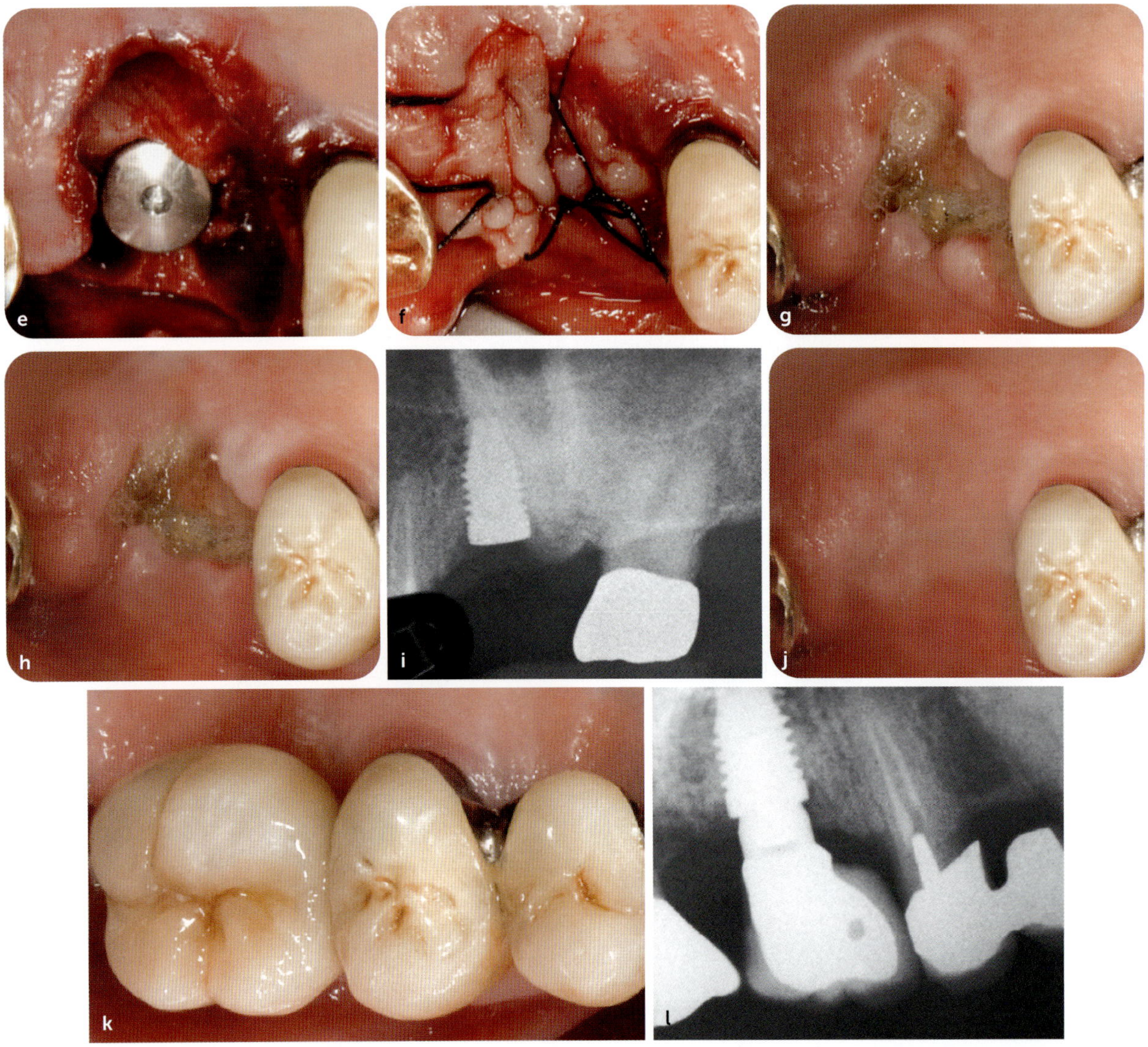

FIG 5-2 *(cont) (e)* An implant was successfully placed into the IRS bone with dehiscences mesially and distally. Despite the large gaps, no corrective grafting was done, and after placing a healing screw, the site was left to heal without sutures. *(f)* The remaining gaps were filled with several autologous PRF clots stabilized by sutures. *(g)* At the 1-week postoperative visit, the wound shows exuberant granulation tissue formation and coverage of the implant. Evidence of cigarette smoking can be seen, as soft tissue hyperkeratosis was the likely reason for superficial avascularity of the surface of the granulation tissue. *(h)* The continuing site healing at 2 weeks. *(i)* This radiograph taken 3 months postoperatively shows the root sockets to be healing well. The implant was placed without apical grafting, and in this film, you can see the layering effect of the new bone forming around the implant apex in the former area of periosteal reaction to the infection. *(j)* This clinical image shows the soft tissue healing at 5 months. Note that minimal change in buccopalatal dimension has occurred despite the fact that no gap grafting was done. *(k)* A clinical image of the implant restoration after 1 year in function. *(l)* The radiograph of the restored implant after 1 year in function shows stable crestal bone.

Case 2: Nonrestorable, nonvital mandibular first molar with periapical rarefactions

A 47-year-old woman presented with a necrotic mandibular left first molar exhibiting discomfort upon chewing. The preoperative radiograph showed some apical sclerosis, suggesting that the infection had been present for some time (Fig 5-3a). The crown was sectioned away to allow the two roots to be removed separately using a flapless technique. Despite the narrow IRS, drilling into it was possible (Fig 5-3b).

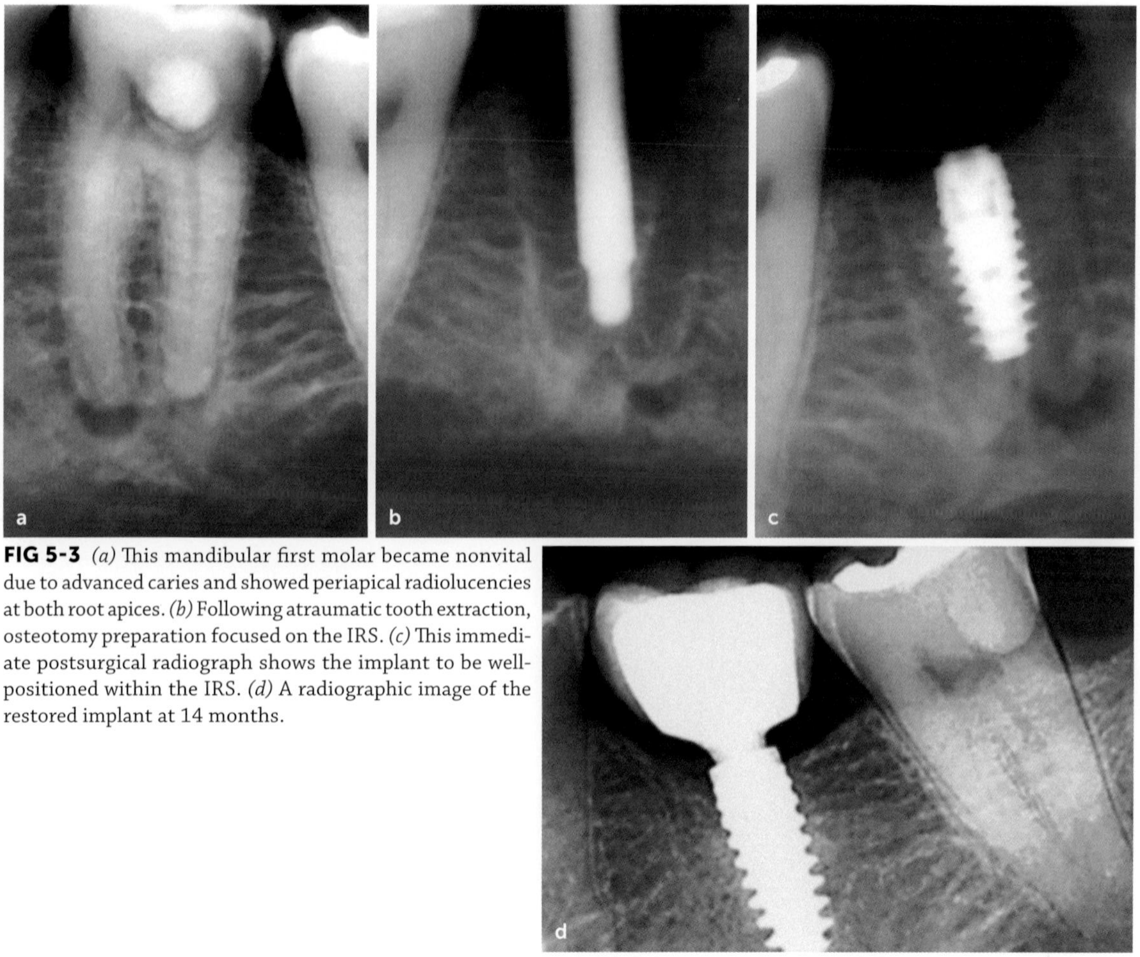

FIG 5-3 *(a)* This mandibular first molar became nonvital due to advanced caries and showed periapical radiolucencies at both root apices. *(b)* Following atraumatic tooth extraction, osteotomy preparation focused on the IRS. *(c)* This immediate postsurgical radiograph shows the implant to be well-positioned within the IRS. *(d)* A radiographic image of the restored implant at 14 months.

Once the osteotomy was completed, an implant with aggressive threads was inserted and largely contained by the IRS bone, thereby eliminating the need to involve bone apical to the former root apices for added stability (Fig 5-3c). The gaps and root sockets were filled with autologous PRF clots (PRGF)[47] prepared chairside from the patient's venous blood and covered with another PRGF clot flattened to form a membrane. After 4 months, the implant was restored, taking advantage of the platform-switch feature of the implant to minimize future bone loss. Figure 5-3d provides the radiographic status of the restored implant after 14 months in function.

Case 3: Mandibular molar with endodontic complications

This patient presented with a failed endodontic treatment on a mandibular second molar with radiographic evidence of a periapical lesion that had progressed quite close to the mandibular canal (Figs 5-4a and 5-4b). After atraumatic tooth removable and curettage, the operator elected to place the IMI into the distal root socket to maintain a healthy distance from the implant that had previously been placed at the first molar site. To avoid damaging the inferior alveolar nerve (IAN), the distal root apex was not instru-

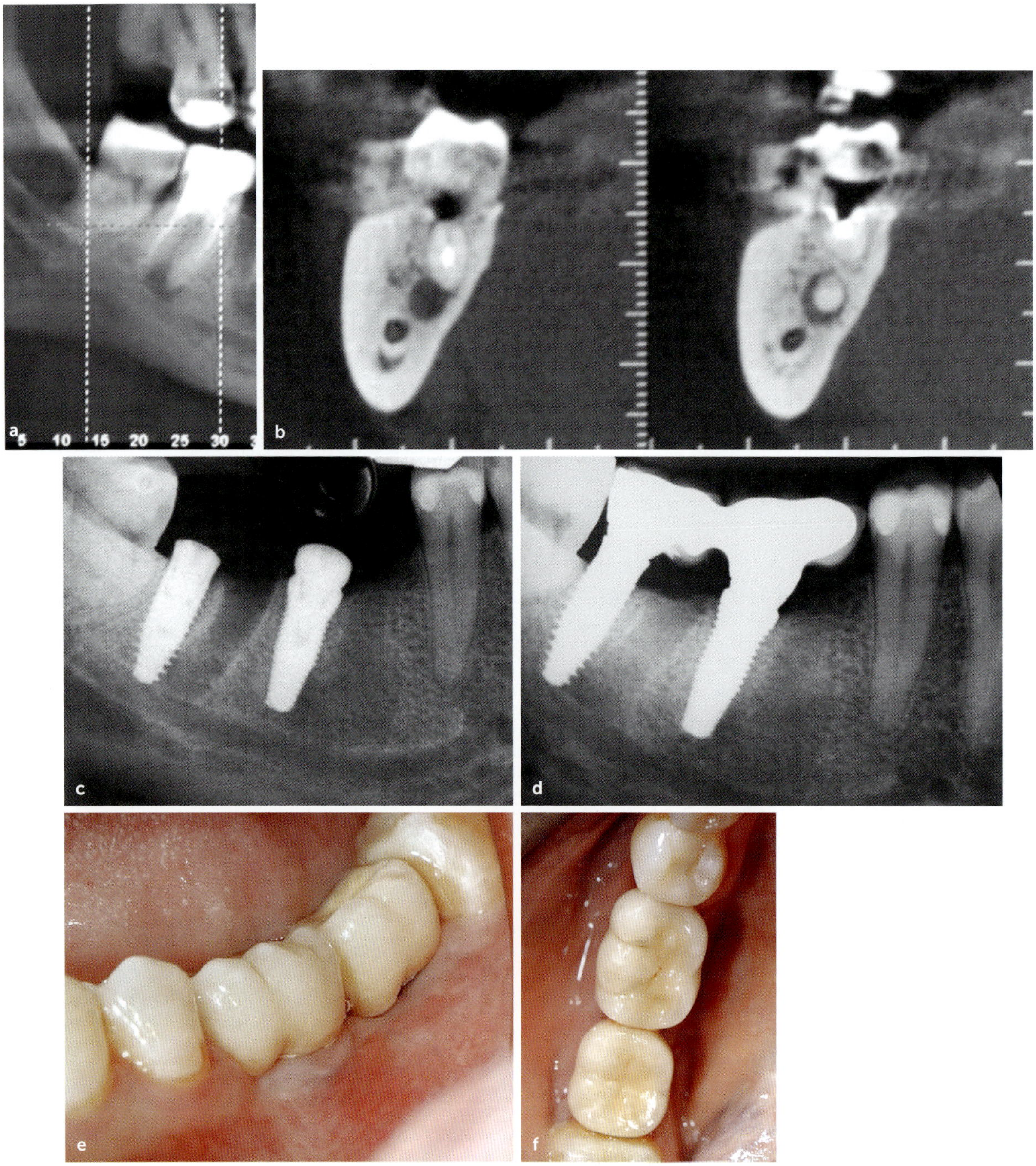

FIG 5-4 *(a)* The mandibular right second molar showed failure of its endodontic treatment with development of a periapical rarefaction in close proximity to the IAN. After failure of an attempt to perform a retreatment, the decision was made to extract and place an IMI. *(b)* These CBCT cuts confirm that the periapical lesion was quite close to the mandibular canal. *(c)* The operator opted to place the IMI in the distal root socket of the second molar, choosing a 12-mm-long implant with a 2-mm machined collar to leave it supracrestal and avoid damage to the mandibular nerve. *(d)* A posttreatment radiograph taken at 1 year in function. Note the stable crestal bone levels but slow healing of the mesial root socket of the second molar. The IMI used had a long machined collar to allow nonsubmerged healing. *(e and f)* The clinical situation after 1 year in function.

mented or drilled, leaving the implant to be secured laterally by the socket walls (Fig 5-4c). Platelet clots were used to fill the mesial root socket. The positioning of the IMI allowed a prosthesis design that could easily be cleaned by the patient (Figs 5-4d to 5-4f).

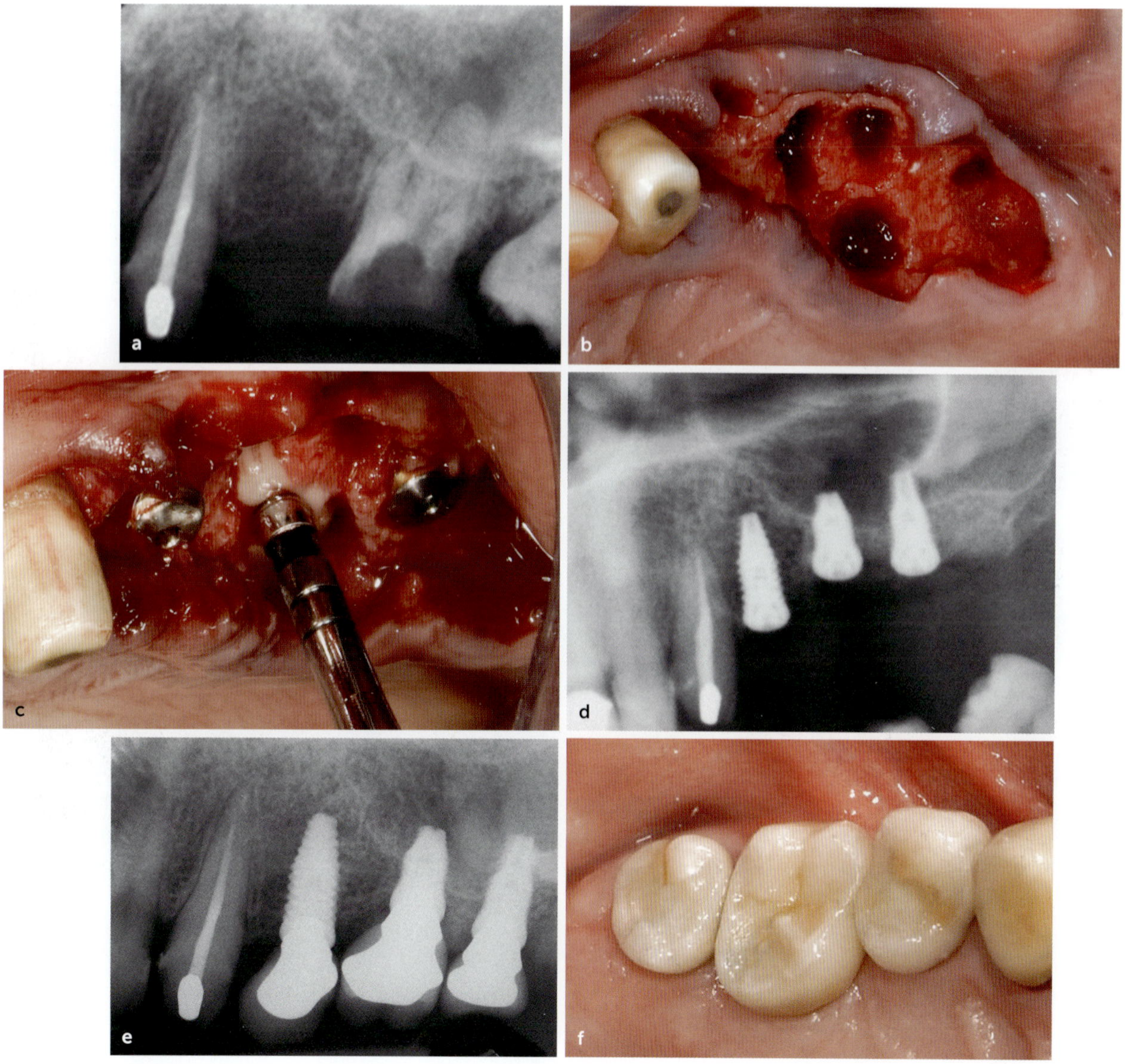

FIG 5-5 *(a)* This preoperative radiograph shows a maxillary second molar to be nonvital with an apical granuloma that has likely penetrated the sinus floor. *(b)* Following removal of the teeth, the IRS of the second molar appears adequate in volume to receive an IMI. *(c)* Immediate implants were placed using routine procedures at the premolar and third molar sites, following which an autologous PRF clot was inserted using osteotomes into the second molar site before doing an indirect sinus floor elevation. *(d)* The immediate postoperative radiograph image verifying that the second molar implant has penetrated the sinus floor. *(e)* A radiograph at 12 months in function showing the implants with separate, nonsplinted crowns and all with platform switching to help in stabilizing crestal bone levels. Bone has formed around the implant apex in response to the sinus membrane elevation and insertion of the autologous PRF clot. *(f)* An occlusal view of the definitive implant crowns.

Case 4: Nonvital maxillary first molar with chronic infection that appears to have penetrated the sinus floor

This patient presented with hopeless teeth in the maxillary left quadrant, including her second premolar and second and third molars. The second molar had a large periapical lesion affecting its palatal root that seemed to have penetrated into the maxillary sinus (Fig 5-5a). Once the teeth were removed, the second molar was seen to have an IRS suitable for an IMI (Fig 5-5b). After partially preparing an osteotomy in the IRS, a PRF clot was inserted to act as an interface as the sinus floor was upfractured by osteotomes (Fig 5-5c), following which the implant was inserted (Figs 5-5d to 5-5f). The purpose of using the clot was to provide antibacterial and bone-promoting benefits in healing the compromised sinus.

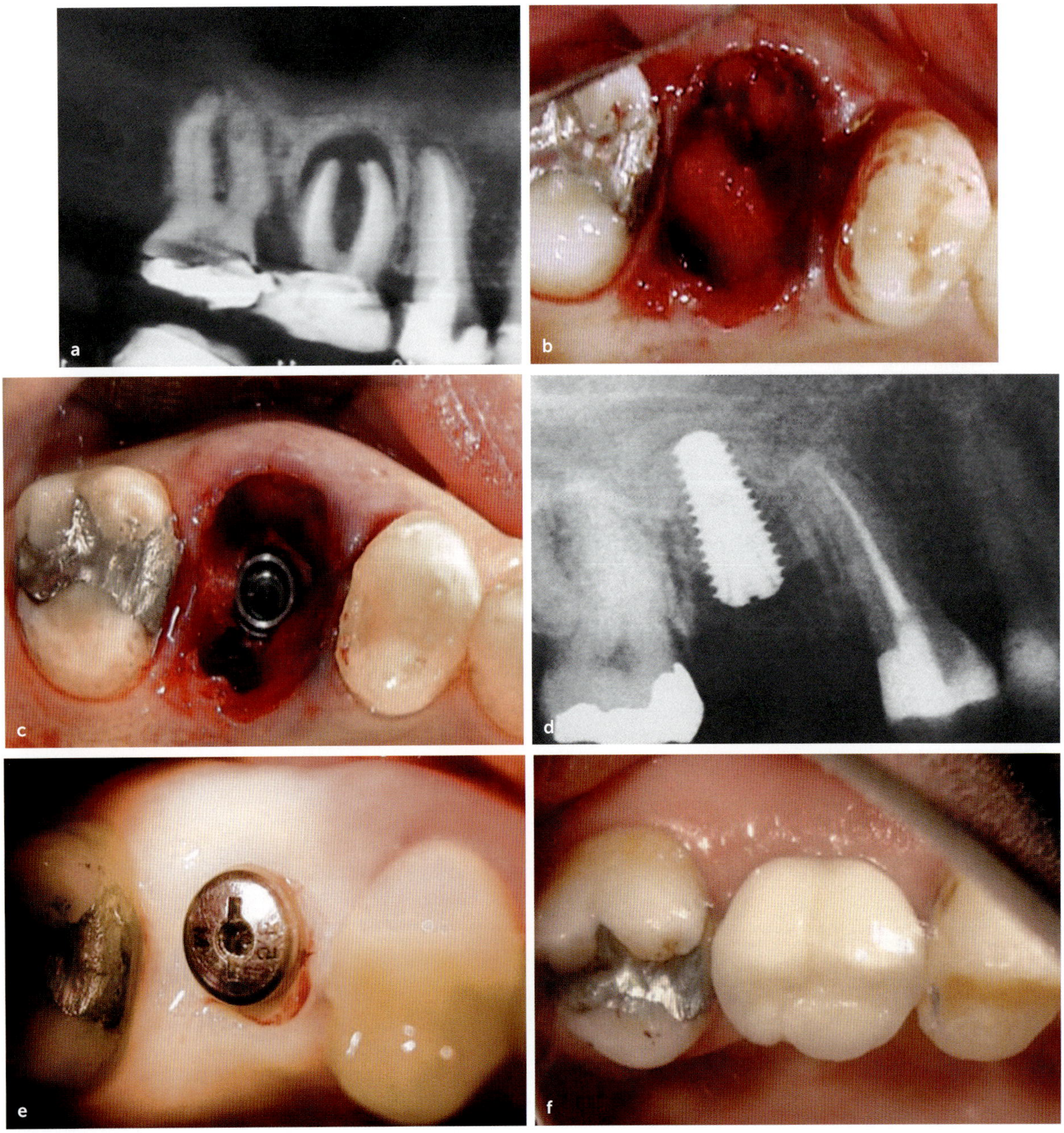

FIG 5-6 *(a)* This maxillary first molar showed failure of its endodontic treatment with a large chronic rarefying osteitis, which in its chronicity had caused a periosteal reaction, lifting the sinus floor. *(b)* Following extraction, the IRS that remained was considered type B.[46] *(c)* An implant was successfully placed into the IRS bone with dehiscences buccally and palatally. No corrective grafting was done, and after placing a healing screw, the site was left to heal without sutures. *(d)* This radiograph taken 32 months postoperatively shows the root sockets to be healing well. Although the implant was placed without apical grafting, one can see a layering effect of the new bone forming around the implant apex in the former area of periosteal reaction to the infection. *(e)* This clinical image shows the soft tissue healing at 3 months. Note that minimal change in buccopalatal dimension has occurred despite the fact that no gap grafting was done. *(f)* The clinical image 1 year after implant restoration showing excellent buccal tissue contour.

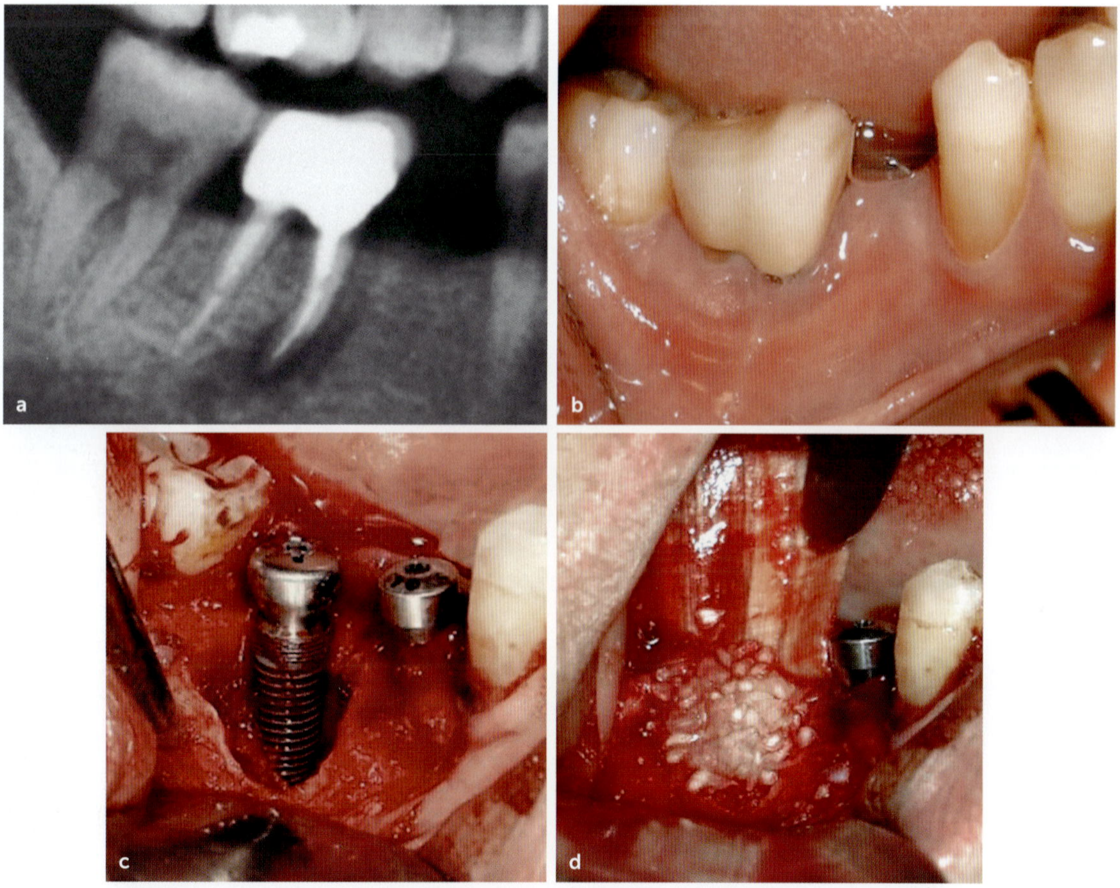

FIG 5-7 *(a)* This infected endodontically treated molar was condemned. *(b)* Clinically, there was evidence of a draining sinus buccally. *(c)* It was possible to stabilize the implant in the type B septum despite the total loss of buccal bone. *(d)* GBR using particulate allograft and a resorbable membrane was needed to reconstruct the damaged alveolar ridge buccal to the implant. →

Case 5: Maxillary first molar with chronic infection and sinus floor reaction

This patient presented with a failed endodontic treatment of the maxillary right first molar that had led to a large apical radiolucency (Fig 5-6a). There were no signs of swelling or purulence. The apical pathology had been present long enough to put pressure on the sinus floor and cause a periosteal bone reaction. Using a flapless approach, the tooth was removed without difficulty, revealing a type B IRS (Fig 5-6b).[46] Following socket debridement, an implant was successfully placed into the IRS with dehiscences on the buccal and palatal aspects of the furcal bone. No gap grafting was done, and after placing a healing screw, the site was left to heal without sutures (Fig 5-6c). A radiograph taken after 3 months' site healing (Fig 5-6d) showed the root sockets to be healing well. The implant had been placed without apical grafting, and in Fig 5-6d, one can see the layering effect of new bone forming around the implant apex in the former area of periosteal reaction to the infection. At this time (Fig 5-6e), the keratinized soft tissues can be seen to be abundant and healthy, and the clinical image of the restored implant is shown in Fig 5-6f.

Case 6: Infected molar managed with an IMI in combination with GBR

Figure 5-7 demonstrates a case using GBR to help stabilize an IMI placed in type B IRS.

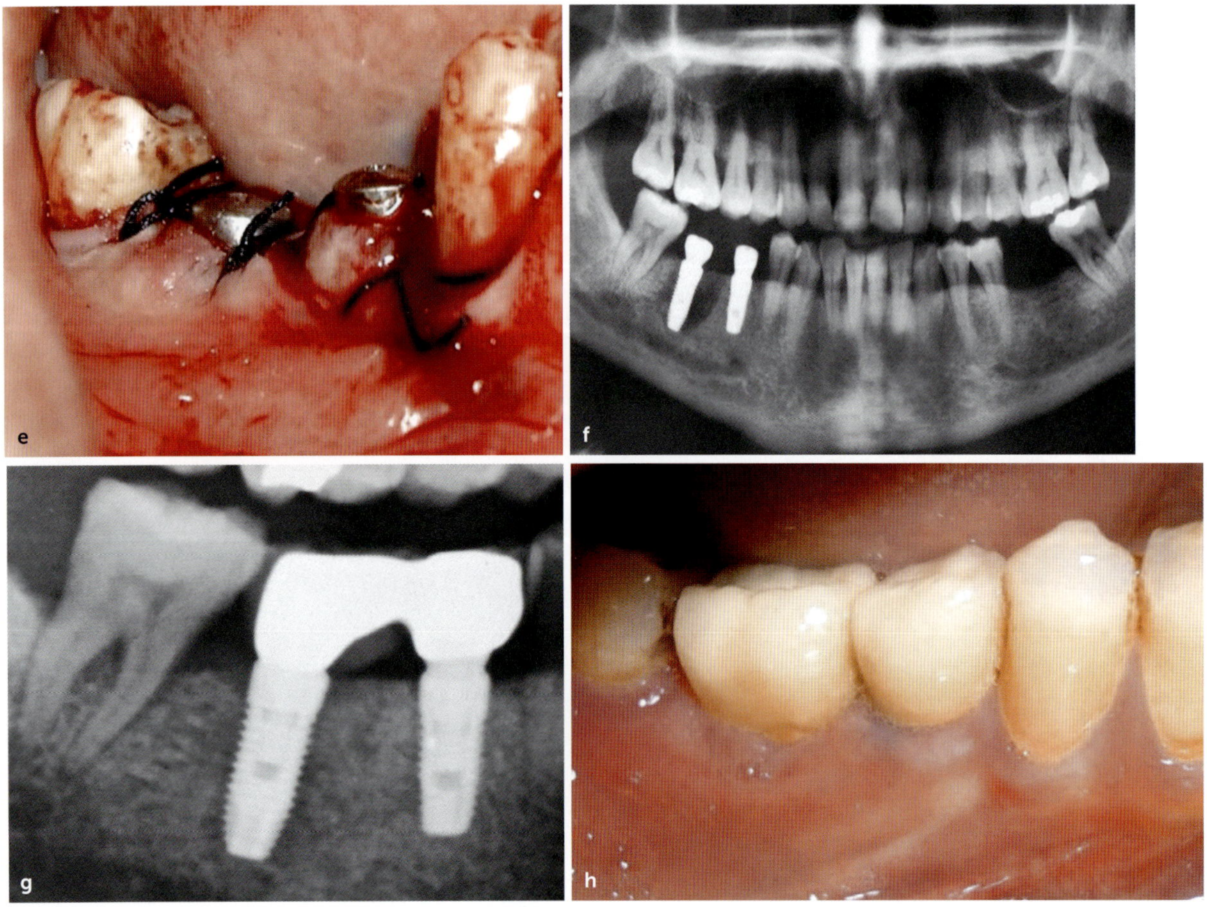

FIG 5-7 *(cont) (e)* A large-diameter healing abutment was used to help in securing the membrane and to allow nonsubmerged healing with nonocclusal loading. *(f)* A panoramic radiograph taken immediately following the surgery shows the extent of the defect managed with GBR. A second implant was used to replace the second premolar during the same procedure. *(g)* This radiograph at 1 year in function shows ongoing bone remodeling in the formerly infected socket. *(h)* A clinical photograph of the implant-supported two-unit prosthesis after 1 year in function. (Case provided by Dr Ali Akbar Khoshkhounejad, Tehran, Iran.)

Conclusion

Despite early concerns about placing immediate implants into chronically infected tooth sockets, multiple studies have shown this not to be a significant contributor to complications or implant failure. Chronic large endodontic infections may be the most likely to fail, probably due to their specific microbial populations. However, certain issues must still be addressed with controlled clinical investigations, such as when to use systemic antibiotics, whether laser socket decontamination is of significant value, if topical antimicrobial agents such as chlorhexidine should be used to irrigate the sites, and whether introduction of autologous PRF preparations should become routine procedure.

KEY POINTS

- Most published data relate to largely asymptomatic chronically infected sites.
- Investigation into the cause of the infection hopefully will help to determine it as primarily endodontic, root fracture, primarily periodontic, or combined endo-perio.
- For large, long-standing endodontic lesions, consideration should be given to the possibility of *Actinomyces* infections with microbiologic sampling of the lesions.
- Generally, although not confirmed to be necessary by published controlled study data, systemic antibiotic usage is undertaken preoperatively, oftentimes for several days before tooth extraction, especially with large periapical lesions.
- As with all IMIs, flapless surgery, separation of molar roots, and atraumatic extraction are recommended.
- After extraction, meticulous socket debridement is necessary using both curettes and large-diameter rotary burs.
- Decontamination with chlorhexidine solution or using lasers has been proposed but is not substantiated in random controlled clinical studies.
- Consideration should be given to slightly underpreparing osteotomies (eg, 0.3 mm) to ensure high initial stability.
- Inserting autologous PRF clots to the osteotomies immediately before implant placement will provide some further antibacterial impact and encourage faster bone healing.
- As always, high initial implant stability is crucial for success.

References

1. Schropp L, Wenzel A, Kostopoulos L, Karring T. Bone healing and soft tissue contour changes following single-tooth extraction: A clinical and radiographic 12-month prospective study. Int J Periodontics Restorative Dent 2003;23:313–323.
2. Schulte W, Heimke G. The Tübinger immediate implant [in German]. Quintessenz 1976;27(6):17–23.
3. Adell R, Lekholm U, Rockler B, Brånemark PI. A 15-year study of osseointegrated implants in the treatment of the edentulous jaw. Int J Oral Surg 1981;10:387–416.
4. Anneroth G, Hedström KG, Kjellman O, Köndell PA, Nordenram A. Endosseus titanium implants in extraction sockets. An experimental study in monkeys. Int J Oral Surg 1985;14:50–54.
5. Lazzara RJ. Immediate implant placement into extraction sites: Surgical and restorative advantages. Int J Periodontics Restorative Dent 1989;9:332–343.
6. Werbitt MJ, Goldberg PV. The immediate implant: Bone preservation and bone regeneration. Int J Periodontics Restorative Dent 1992;12:206–217.
7. Villa R, Rangert B. Early loading of interforaminal implants immediately installed after extraction of teeth presenting endodontic and periodontal lesions. Clin Implant Dent Relat Res 2005;7(suppl 1):S28–S35.
8. Lindeboom JA, Tjiook Y, Kroon FH. Immediate placement of implants in periapical infected sites: A prospective randomized study in 50 patients. Oral Surg Oral Med Oral Pathol Oral Radiol Endod 2006;101:705–710.
9. Casap N, Zeltser C, Wexler A, Tarazi E, Zeltser R. Immediate placement of dental implants into debrided infected dentoalveolar sockets. J Oral Maxillofac Surg 2007;65:384–392.
10. Angaji M, Brar J. Implant therapy and apical actinomycosis: Case report. J Can Dent Assoc 2011;77:b124.
11. Chang SW, Shin SY, Hong JR, et al. Immediate implant placement into infected and noninfected extraction sockets: A pilot study. Oral Surg Oral Med Oral Pathol Oral Radiol Endod 2009;107:197–203.
12. Ahn JJ, Shin HI. Bone tissue formation in extraction sockets from sites with advanced periodontal disease: A histomorphometric study in humans. Int J Oral Maxillofac Implants 2008; 23:1133–1138.
13. Waasdorp JA, Evian CI, Mandracchia M. Immediate placement of implants into infected sites: A systematic review of the literature. J Periodontol 2010;81:801–808.
14. Corbella S, Taschieri S, Tsesis I, Del Fabbro M. Postextraction implant in sites with endodontic infection as an alternative to endodontic retreatment: A review of literature. J Oral Implantol 2013;39:399–405.
15. Nelson S, Thomas G. Bacterial persistence in dentoalveolar bone following extraction: A microbiological study and implications for dental implant treatment. Clin Implant Dent Relat Res 2010; 12:306–314.
16. Deporter DA. Complications after implant site ridge preservation and delayed implant placement: A case report. Clin Adv Periodontics 2014;4:14–18.

17. Chrcanovic BR, Martins MD, Wennerberg A. Immediate placement of implants into infected sites: A systematic review. Clin Implant Dent Relat Res 2015;17(suppl 1):e1–e16.
18. Zhao D, Wu Y, Xu C, Zhang F. Immediate dental implant placement into infected vs. non-infected sockets: A meta-analysis. Clin Oral Implants Res 2016;27:1290–1296.
19. Saijeva A, Juodzbalys G. Immediate implant placement in non-infected sockets versus infected sockets: A systematic review and meta-analysis. J Oral Maxillofac Res 2020;11:e1.
20. de Oliveira-Neto OB, Lemos CA, Barbosa FT, de Sousa-Rodrigues CF, Camello de Lima FJ. Immediate dental implants placed into infected sites present a higher risk of failure than immediate dental implants placed into non-infected sites: Systematic review and meta-analysis. Med Oral Patol Oral Cir Bucal 2019;24: e518–e528.
21. Truninger TC, Philipp AO, Siegenthaler DW, Roos M, Hämmerle CH, Jung RE. A prospective, controlled clinical trial evaluating the clinical and radiological outcome after 3 years of immediately placed implants in sockets exhibiting periapical pathology [published correction appears in Clin Oral Implants Res 2011; 22:235]. Clin Oral Implants Res 2011;22:20–27.
22. Jung RE, Zaugg B, Philipp AO, Truninger TC, Siegenthaler DW, Hämmerle CH. A prospective, controlled clinical trial evaluating the clinical radiological and aesthetic outcome after 5 years of immediately placed implants in sockets exhibiting periapical pathology. Clin Oral Implants Res 2013;24:839–846.
23. Montoya-Salazar V, Castillo-Oyagüe R, Torres-Sánchez C, Lynch CD, Gutiérrez-Pérez JL, Torres-Lagares D. Outcome of single immediate implants placed in post-extraction infected and non-infected sites, restored with cemented crowns: A 3-year prospective study. J Dent 2014;42:645–652.
24. Blus C, Szmukler-Moncler S, Khoury P, Orrù G. Immediate implants placed in infected and noninfected sites after atraumatic tooth extraction and placement with ultrasonic bone surgery. Clin Implant Dent Relat Res 2015;17(suppl 1):e287–e297.
25. Prati C, Zamparini F, Pirani C, Gatto MR, Piattelli A, Gandolfi MG. Immediate early and delayed implants: A 2-year prospective cohort study of 131 transmucosal flapless implants placed in sites with different pre-extractive endodontic infections. Implant Dent 2017;26:654–663.
26. Hita-Iglesias C, Sánchez-Sánchez FJ, Montero J, et al. Immediate implants placed in fresh sockets associated with periapical pathology: A split-mouth design and survival evaluation after 1-year follow-up. Clin Implant Dent Relat Res 2016;18:1075–1083.
27. Zuffetti F, Capelli M, Galli F, Del Fabbro M, Testori T. Post-extraction implant placement into infected versus non-infected sites: A multicenter retrospective clinical study. Clin Implant Dent Relat Res 2017;19:833–840.
28. Narad C, Lingraj JB, Aulakh KK, Handa K, Kotrashetti SM, Pinto PX. Assessment of primary stability of the implant placed in prepared infected extraction sockets. J Oral Biol Craniofac Res 2018;8:154–157.
29. Dohan Ehrenfest DM, Andia I, Zumstein MA, Zhang CQ, Pinto NR, Bielecki T. Classification of platelet concentrates (platelet-rich plasma-PRP, platelet-rich fibrin-PRF) for topical and infiltrative use in orthopedic and sports medicine: Current consensus, clinical implications and perspectives. Muscles Ligaments Tendons J 2014;4:3–9.
30. Borsani E, Bonazza V, Buffoli B, et al. Biological characterization and in vitro effects of human concentrated growth factor preparation: An innovative approach to tissue regeneration. Biol Med (Aligarh) 2015;7:256.
31. Rodella LF, Favero G, Boninsegna R, et al. Growth factors, CD34 positive cells, and fibrin network analysis in concentrated growth factors fraction. Microsc Res Tech 2011;74:772–777.
32. Sohn DS, Huang B, Kim J, Park I, Park CC. Utilization of autologous concentrated growth factors (CGF) enriched bone graft matrix (sticky bone) and CGF-enriched fibrin membrane in implant dentistry. J Implant Adv Clin Dent 2015;7(10):11–29.
33. Del Fabbro M, Boggian C, Taschieri S. Immediate implant placement into fresh extraction sites with chronic periapical pathologic features combined with plasma rich in growth factors: Preliminary results of single-cohort study. J Oral Maxillofac Surg 2009;67:2476–2484.
34. Taschieri S, Del Fabbro M. Postextraction osteotome sinus floor elevation technique using plasma-rich growth factors. Implant Dent 2011;20:418–424.
35. Taschieri S, Lolato A, Ofer M, Testori T, Francetti L, Del Fabbro M. Immediate post-extraction implants with or without pure platelet-rich plasma: A 5-year follow-up study. Oral Maxillofac Surg 2017;21:147–157.
36. Zhou J, Li X, Sun X, et al. Bone regeneration around immediate placed implant of molar teeth with autologous platelet-rich fibrin: Two case reports. Medicine (Baltimore) 2018;97(44): e13058.
37. Greenstein G, Tarnow D. Effectiveness of antibiotics to reduce early implant loss in systemically healthy patients. Compend Contin Educ Dent 2020;41:102–110.
38. Brucoli M, Sonzini R, Bosetti M, Boffano P, Benech A. Plasma rich in growth factors (PRGF) for the promotion of bone cell proliferation and tissue regeneration. Oral Maxillofac Surg 2018; 22:309–313.
39. Crippa R, Aiuto R, Guardincerri M, Peñarrocha Diago M, Angiero F. Effect of laser radiation on infected sites for the immediate placement of dental implants. Photobiomodul Photomed Laser Surg 2020;38:186–192.
40. Kakar A, Kakar K, Leventis MD, Jain G. Immediate implant placement in infected sockets: A consecutive cohort study. J Lasers Med Sci 2020;11:167–173.
41. Jofre J, Valenzuela D, Quintana P, Asenjo-Lobos C. Protocol for immediate implant replacement of infected teeth. Implant Dent 2012;21:287–294.
42. Huwais S, Mazor Z, Ioannou AL, Gluckman H, Neiva R. A multicenter retrospective clinical study with up-to-5-year follow-up utilizing a method that enhances bone density and allows for transcrestal sinus augmentation through compaction grafting. Int J Oral Maxillofac Implants 2018;33:1305–1311.
43. Landsberg CJ. Implementing socket seal surgery as a socket preservation technique for pontic site development: Surgical steps revisited: A report of two cases. J Periodontol 2008;79: 945–954.
44. Al Nashar A, Yakoob H. Evaluation of the use of plasma rich in growth factors with immediate implant placement in periodontally compromised extraction sites: A controlled prospective study. Int J Oral Maxillofac Surg 2015;44:507–512.
45. S Medikeri R, Meharwade V, M Wate P, V Lele S. Effect of PRF and allograft use on immediate implants at extraction sockets with periapical infection: Clinical and cone beam CT findings. Bull Tokyo Dent Coll 2018;59:97–109.
46. Smith RB, Tarnow DP. Classification of molar extraction sites for immediate dental implant placement: Technical note. Int J Oral Maxillofac Implants 2013;28:911–916.
47. Anitua E, Piñas L, Alkhraisat MH. Long-term outcomes of immediate implant placement into infected sockets in association with immediate loading: A retrospective cohort study. J Periodontol 2016;87:1135–1140.

6

VERTICAL RIDGE AUGMENTATION IN CONJUNCTION WITH IMMEDIATE IMPLANT PLACEMENT

Dong-Seok Sohn

Conventional Ridge Augmentation Solutions

Severe vertical bone defects and resorptive loss of alveolar ridge anatomy commonly result following extraction of chronically infected and/or cracked molars. If this loss of bony support cannot be minimized using socket preservation grafting at the time of tooth removal, augmentation grafting procedures most likely will be needed should the patient wish to have their lost teeth replaced with dental implant restorations. Various grafting approaches have been developed to overcome these vertical bony deficiencies, including distraction osteogenesis (DO),[1,2] guided bone regeneration (GBR) using resorbable or nonresorbable barrier membranes,[3,4] sandwich augmentation (SA) with interpositional bone grafting,[5,6] allogeneic/autogenous onlay block bone grafts,[7,8] titanium mesh–assisted bone augmentation,[9] or in the case of simultaneous dental implant placement, the autogenous bone ring technique.[10,11] Each of these procedures has advantages, disadvantages, and potential complications, so the choice of technique used is often based primarily on the surgeon's previous experiences.

Distraction osteogenesis

DO was first described in 1905 by Codivilla, when he reported lengthening of a femur by axial distraction forces.[12] DO is the biologic process of new bone formation between bone segments gradually separated by incremental traction forces. It is a relatively simple and predictable operative technique, and it provides a method to regain both hard and soft tissues without the need for grafting[13] while maintaining vitality of the distracted segment.[14] However, it does require special training on the part of the surgeon and daily patient adjustments of the distraction device (highly dependent on compliance). DO can result in improper control of force vectors, malpositioning of the distracted segment, and pain associated with tensional force applications. As well, when applying DO for vertical augmentation, long edentulous periods and the number of surgical interventions required are considered disadvantages.

Sandwich augmentation

SA with interpositional bone grafting requires that a local pedicle bone segment be freed with osteotomy cuts and moved crestally,[2] and it can result in a vertical gain in bone height of 6 to 10 mm.[15] It requires the preservation of the lingual or palatal periosteum to maintain vascular supply to the segmented bone to maintain viability and minimize resorption of the transpositioned bone.[6,16] Compared with DO, SA requires less patient compliance and is less costly. However, neither DO nor SA allow simultaneous dental implant placement. Furthermore, neither technique can achieve simultaneous horizontal alveolar ridge augmentation. Some generally transient (~ 6 weeks' duration) nerve damage with paresthesia likely related to manipulation of the mental nerve during flap elevation is also common with SA.[17]

Autogenous block grafting

Onlay autogenous block bone grafting has been utilized and is considered a reliable surgical procedure for the reconstruction of vertical alveolar defects.[6,15,18,19] However, this approach is at high risk of graft exposure related to soft tissue flap dehiscence during healing, resulting in infection and graft failure. Successful grafts are also at high risk of late resorption, likely because of poor revascularization during their consolidation.[20,21] Other drawbacks include temporary mental paresthesia, technical limitations, morbidity at donor sites, and long edentulous healing intervals.[22-24] To overcome some of these issues, allogeneic or xenogeneic blocks have been utilized instead of autogenous ones, but these have unproven long-term outcomes once implants are subsequently added to the formula.[25]

Guided bone regeneration

Vertical GBR augmentations employing particulate bone allogeneic or xenogeneic graft materials and various barrier membranes or titanium mesh are considered predictable with some advantages compared to SA, DO, and block bone grafting. Considerable simultaneous gain in both horizontal and vertical dimensions can be achieved with minimal risk of complications and shorter edentulous periods compared with DO, SA, and block grafting.[26,27] Titanium mesh in particular to cover particulate grafts gives reliable vertical bone gain due to effective space maintenance. However, because the graft particles needed are only osteoconductive, bone regeneration is slow, and again long edentulous periods are needed before dental implant placement can be undertaken.

Ring Blocks with Bone and Dentin

The use of autogenous bone blocks shaped like rings is another way to gain simultaneous increases in alveolar bone height and width. These ring-shaped blocks can be prepared with central osteotomies meant to house an implant, allowing simultaneous implant placement in large extraction site defects.[10,11] The technique reduces treatment time but comes with the disadvantage of needing a donor site. Generally, the ring block is harvested from the chin using a trephine bur, making the procedure moderately invasive. Therefore, the use of allogeneic ring blocks has been suggested as an alternative.[28,29] However, allogeneic block bone grafts demonstrate faster resorption during healing, potential cracking due to masticatory forces, and poor integration compared with autogenous block bone grafts.[30]

Most recently, demineralized and microperforated autogenous tooth ring blocks prepared from the patient's own extracted tooth or teeth have been put forward as alternatives to autogenous bone rings (Fig 6-1). Once demineralized and microperforated, these ring grafts are especially valuable since, as well as providing a 3D scaffold for new bone formation, they are genetically compatible with the host, will release helpful growth factors such as BMPs (bone morphogenetic proteins) during site healing, will become ingrown and well-integrated with host bone, and will ultimately be replaced with continued bone remodeling during functional loading[31-34] (Fig 6-2).

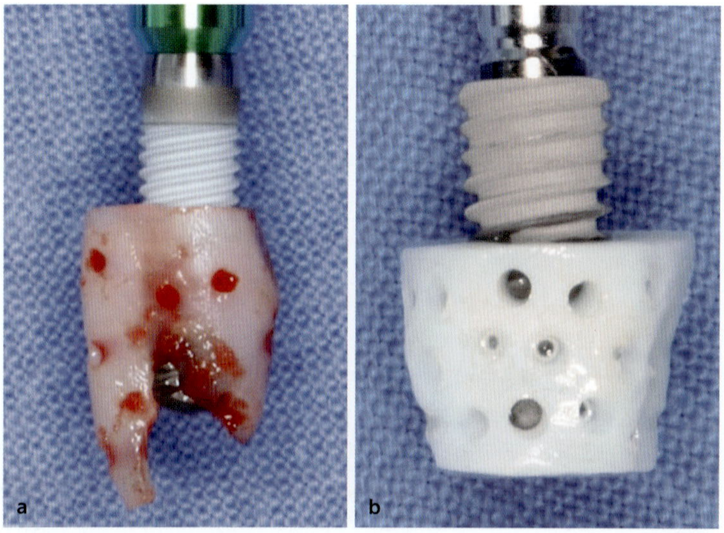

FIG 6-1 *(a)* A tooth ring prepared from an extracted premolar. *(b)* A ring graft prepared from an extracted molar.

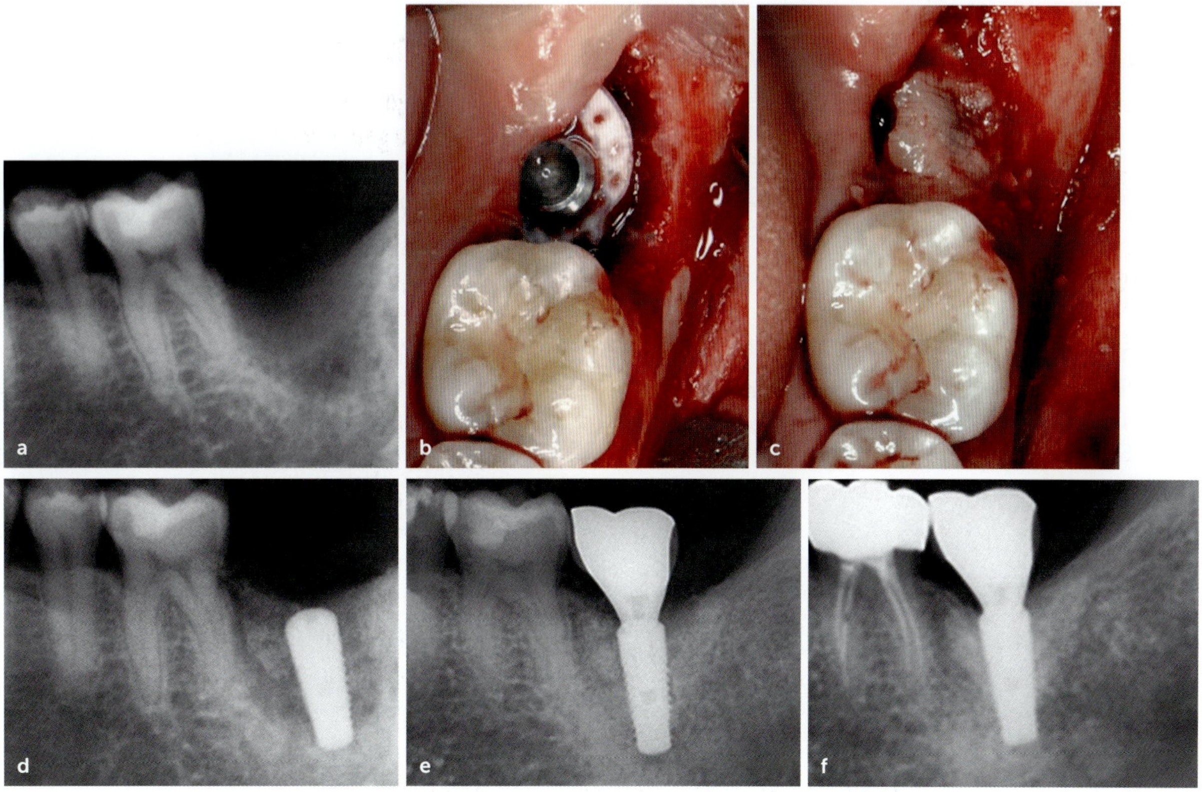

FIG 6-2 *(a)* The immediate postextraction periapical radiograph at a mandibular second molar site. *(b)* Following 6 weeks of initial site healing to allow for soft tissue closure over the extraction site, a tooth ring block prepared from the extracted tooth was engaged with a dental implant and installed in the defect. *(c)* Decalcified particulate tooth graft material also prepared from the extracted tooth was used to fill the peri-implant/ring graft residual defects and covered with platelet-rich fibrin clots prepared from the patient's own blood[34] prior to repositioning and suturing the soft tissue flaps. *(d)* A periapical radiograph taken immediately after placement of the implant/tooth ring combination. *(e)* The baseline radiograph taken at the time of delivery of the implant crown. *(f)* A periapical radiograph taken at the recall visit after 6 years in function. (Surgery performed by Dr Insook Park, Daegu, South Korea.)

Demineralized tooth dentin was introduced as an alternative to autogenous bone grafts when it was recognized that it has both osteoinductive and osteoconductive properties,[35–37] as well as a similar chemical composition to human bone.[38] Like bone, dentin has a high content of type I collagen that becomes exposed after appropriate demineralization, acting as a scaffold for new bone formation.[39–42] As well, unlike nondemineralized dentin, demineralized dentin releases valuable osteogenic growth factors when used as a graft material.[43,44] Appropriate demineralization of dentin lowers its high hydroxyapatite crystallinity, which enhances osteoblast adhesion and increases the resorption rate of the dentin biomaterial.[45–48] Demineralization of dentin at room temperature takes time, but it can be accelerated under vacuum pressure and ultrasonic vibrations in specialized machines while still maintaining its collagen architecture and original protein content.[43] Demineralization time in these machines must be carefully controlled and should not exceed 30 minutes, as this will lead to collapse of the collagen scaffold and loss of dentinal tubular structures.[43] As a result, the resorption rate of the graft will be too fast due to its low content of hydroxyapatite, and poor bone regeneration will be the result due to poor space maintenance at the grafted site. A study has determined that 15 minutes of demineralization under vacuum and ultrasonic vibration is appropriate for preparing particulate dentin particles as an osteoinductive graft material. In contrast, for the preparation of dentinal tooth-bone block grafts, 60 minutes of demineralization is required.[48]

Preparation of demineralized particulate tooth graft biomaterial

After extraction of hopeless or impacted teeth, all soft tissues, calculus, caries, pulp tissue, and restorations must be eliminated using high-speed burs under coolant. The remaining tooth structure is then crushed with a sterile mallet until it has been reduced to a powder of 0.8- to 1-mm particle size. Further processing, including demineralization, washing, and sterilization, then takes place in a vacuum-ultrasonic device (eg, VacuaSonic CosmoBioMedicare). As stated, the optimal demineralization time for preparing particulate graft biomaterial in the machine using 0.6N HCl is 15 minutes. Sterilization of the graft in the machine is achieved using a peracetic acid–ethanol solution and followed by washing with phosphate-buffered saline all in the vacuum-ultrasonic device. Once prepared, the demineralized dentin particulate graft intended for use on the same day is stored at 4°C until needed. If the material is not intended for use on the same day as the tooth extraction, it should be stored at −20°C in a freezer until needed.

Preparation of tooth block grafts

As with the preparation of particulate graft, all soft tissue and foreign materials attached to the extracted tooth or teeth must be removed completely using rotary burs with coolant to prevent heat denaturalization of dentin proteins. The tooth can then be dissected into two pieces with a rotary disk, again under coolant. Several micro-holes (~ 0.5 mm wide) are then drilled into each tooth block using a small round bur to allow vascular invasion of the graft following its insertion into the bone defect. These perforated tooth blocks then are demineralized for 60 minutes using 0.6N HCl and sterilized in the vacuum-ultrasonic device, turning them into malleable blocks. Thinner (ie, ~ 2-mm thickness) laminate sheets of demineralized dentin can also be prepared (see Case 3 on page 108). Storage conditions are the same as with the particulate preparations.

Preparation of tooth rings

After thorough cleaning of the extracted tooth or teeth as described previously, a mid-root horizontal section of tooth structure can be prepared as a 4- to 6-mm-thick tooth ring. The remaining portions of the extracted tooth then can be turned into particulate graft material. Meanwhile, the tooth ring is microperforated with a fissure or round bur under coolant again to allow blood vessel invasion. A central opening into the tooth ring to receive a dental implant is created with appropriate implant drills. Underpreparation is recommended to ensure that the implant will fit snugly into the ring. Thereafter, the rings are processed in the machine following the same protocol as that used for block tooth-bone biomaterials.

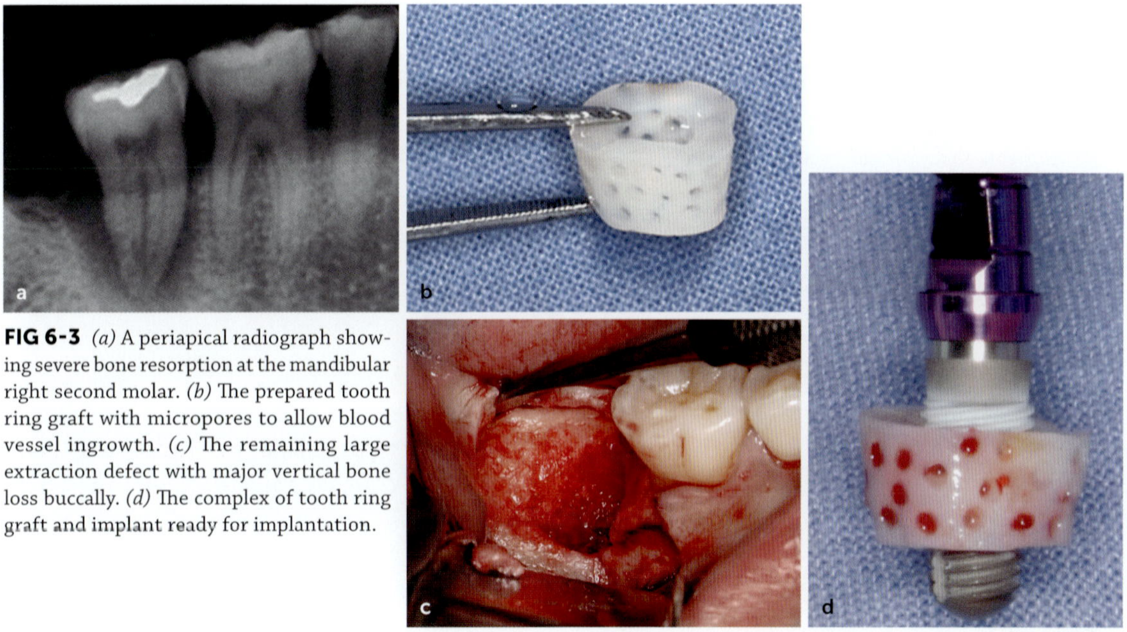

FIG 6-3 *(a)* A periapical radiograph showing severe bone resorption at the mandibular right second molar. *(b)* The prepared tooth ring graft with micropores to allow blood vessel ingrowth. *(c)* The remaining large extraction defect with major vertical bone loss buccally. *(d)* The complex of tooth ring graft and implant ready for implantation.

Sample Cases

Case 1

A healthy 50-year-old man complained of severe mobility and pain associated with his mandibular right second molar. The tooth was condemned due to advanced periodontal attachment loss and Class III mobility (Fig 6-3a). Extraction and early implant placement with a demineralized tooth ring graft was planned, as significant vertical socket augmentation was needed. After cleaning the tooth with a high-speed bur and copious coolant, it was sectioned into three pieces (the crown, midsection of the root, and apical root portion) using a disk. The crown and apical root portions were crushed with a sterile mallet and processed as particulate graft as already described. The midsection of the root was hollowed through the center with an implant drill to allow engagement of a dental implant. Microperforations were also drilled into the ring block (to allow blood vessel invasion), followed by demineralization and sterilization as described previously (Fig 6-3b). The prepared biomaterials were then stored at –20°C until needed.

Six weeks after extraction, healthy soft tissue closure was achieved, allowing implant surgery to be performed using sticky tooth particulate grafting. For preparation of this graft biomaterial, a sample of the patient's venous blood was drawn from the forearm into blood collection tubes (Vacutainer, Becton Dickinson). One sample drawn into a citrate-coated (anticoagulant; white-capped) tube was used to prepare autologous fibrin glue (AFG), while samples in four silica/glass-coated (red-capped; no anticoagulant) tubes were used to obtain fibrin clots containing concentrated growth factor (CGF).[34] The tubes were immediately centrifuged in a specifically programmed centrifuge (Medifuge, Silfradent). The AFG sample was centrifuged for 2 minutes, and after removing this one tube, the remaining four red-capped tubes were centrifuged for a further 14 minutes to allow clotting. The straw-colored fluid in the white-capped tube was withdrawn into a syringe and mixed with the previously prepared particulate tooth graft to form "sticky tooth particulate" biomaterial.

Full-thickness flaps were raised at the former extraction site, and all granulation tissue was removed with a piezoelectric scraper cooled with physiologic saline. The large defect showed major bone loss buccally (Fig 6-3c). A slightly underprepared osteotomy then was prepared for an 11.5×4.7–mm implant (Tapered Screw-Vent, Zimmer Biomet). Before implant placement, the prepared tooth ring was engaged with the implant fixture (Fig 6-3d). This complex of implant

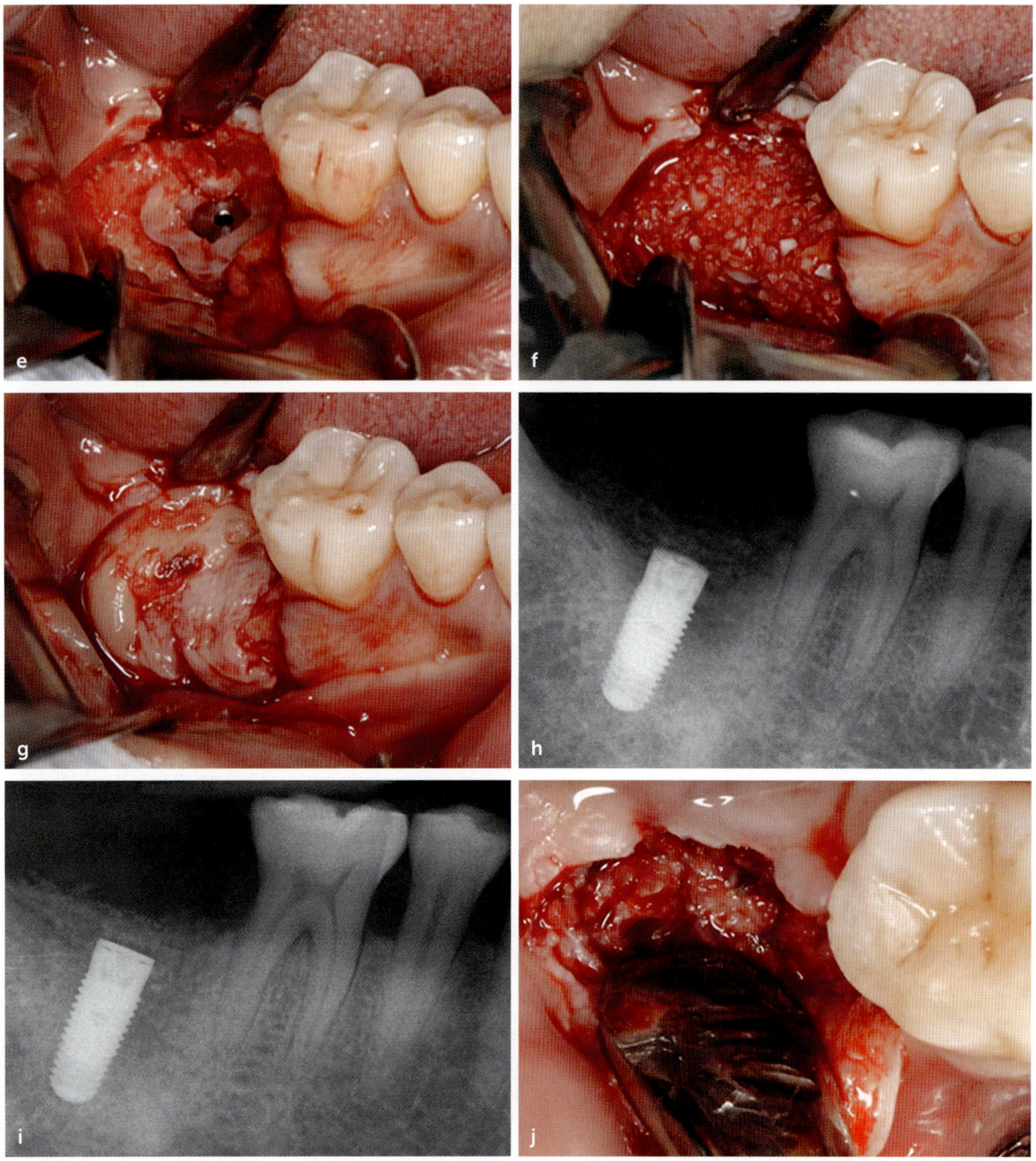

FIG 6-3 *(cont) (e)* The complex of ring graft and implant was placed and secured apically into the defect. Note that the implant platform was positioned ~ 1 mm deeper than the top of the ring graft. Note also the vertical augmentation of the buccal wall. *(f)* All gaps between the socket defect and ring graft were filled with sticky particulate tooth biomaterial. *(g)* The site was covered with CGF membranes followed by tension-free flap closure. *(h)* The immediate postoperative radiograph. *(i)* A radiograph taken after 5 months of healing. *(j)* Uncovering after 5 months of healing revealed growth of new bone over the cover screw, at which time a provisional crown was connected to the implant.

and ring then was positioned into the osteotomy with apical engagement of the implant, making sure that its platform was seated 1 to 2 mm below the ring's upper limit (Fig 6-3e). All remaining gaps between the socket and the ring graft were filled with the prepared sticky tooth biomaterial (Fig 6-3f). Thereafter, the CGF clots, which had been compressed in a sterile metal box to form membranes, were placed over the grafted site to accelerate wound healing (Fig 6-3g). Finally, primary closure with tension-free suturing was achieved to allow good healing and complication-free regeneration. A postoperative radiograph can be seen in Fig 6-3h. After 5 months of site healing (Fig 6-3i), reentry surgery was performed, revealing that new bone had covered the top of the implant (Fig 6-3j). A zirconia restoration was subsequently delivered (Figs 6-3k and 6-3l). The radiograph in Fig 6-3m shows the situation after 1 year in function.

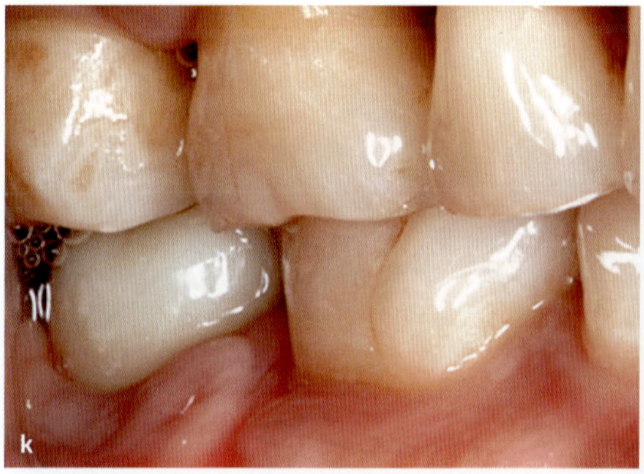

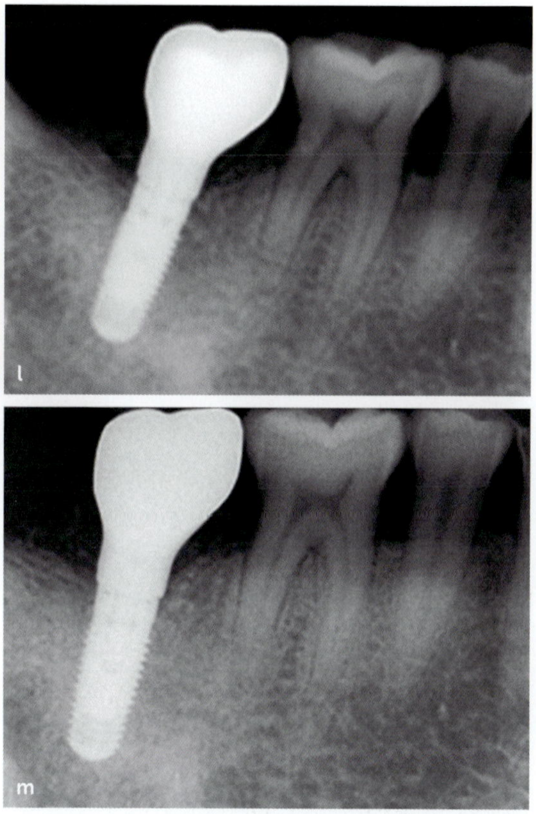

FIG 6-3 *(cont) (k)* A definitive restoration was delivered after 2 months with the provisional crown. *(l)* A periapical radiograph taken at delivery of the definitive restoration. *(m)* Note the bone remodeling after 1 year of clinical function with the definitive restoration.

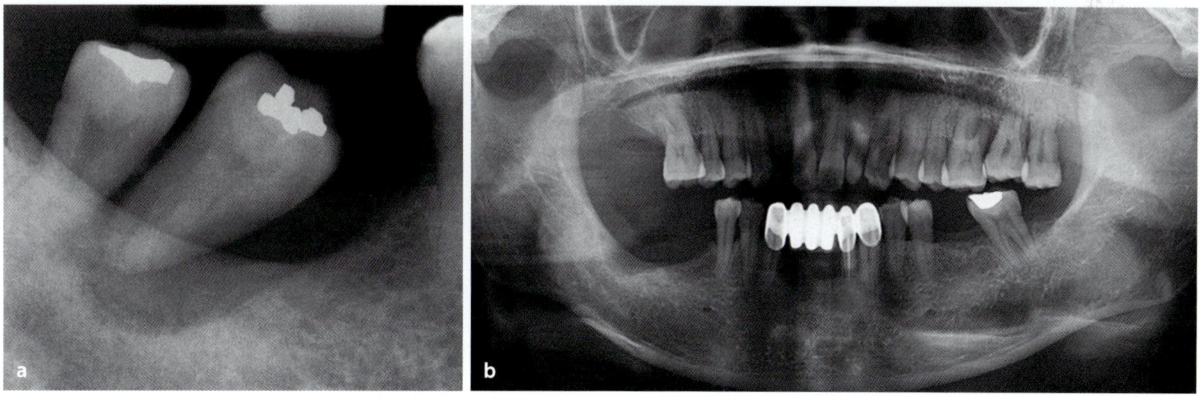

FIG 6-4 *(a)* The mandibular right first and second molars presented with severe bone loss. *(b)* A panoramic radiograph shows the severe bone loss that was left after extraction of the molars in the right mandible.

Case 2

In a second case, a 57-year-old woman presented with a chief complaint of difficulty in chewing at the right posterior mandible. Her right first and second molars revealed severe mobility and alveolar bone loss due to periodontal disease (Figs 6-4a and 6-4b). The plan was to place two immediate molar implants. Particulate tooth graft biomaterial was prepared as already described for immediate use. After graft preparation was complete, samples of the patient's venous blood were collected in vacutainers to allow preparation of both sticky tooth graft and CGF membranes. All granulation tissues were removed from the sockets

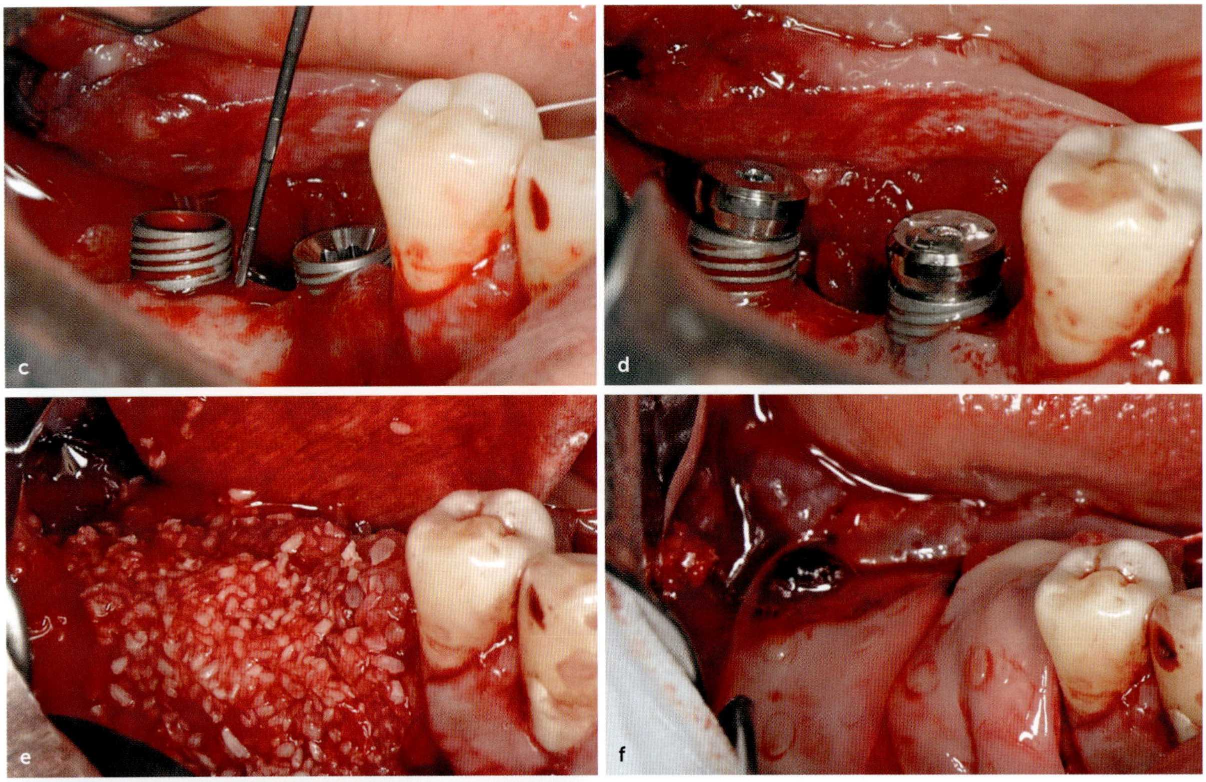

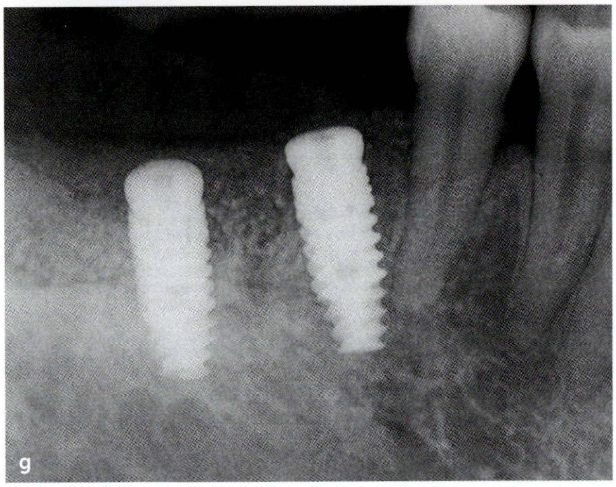

FIG 6-4 *(cont) (c)* Two immediate molar implants were placed. Final positioning of first molar implant platform was 1 mm subcrestal to the distal proximal bone height of the second premolar. The implant stability was good because underpreparation was performed. *(d)* Healing abutments (2-mm height) were added and torqued at 10 Ncm. These low-profile abutments were meant to act as tenting screws to prevent vertical collapse of the particulate bone graft. *(e)* Sticky particulate tooth was grafted over the implants. Unlike standard particulate graft materials, sticky tooth particles will not migrate, as they are firmly bound together with autologous fibrin glue. *(f)* The particulate graft was first covered with a commercially available collagen barrier material and subsequently covered again using two CGF fibrin membranes. *(g)* The immediate postoperative radiograph. →

using a piezoelectric-driven bone scraper (Surgybone, Silfradent). Slightly undersized osteotomies then were prepared for two 10 × 4.65–mm threaded implants (I.C.E. Implant, AlphaBio Simplantology) such that the implant platforms would be positioned 1 mm subcrestally in relation to the distal bone height at the second premolar (Fig 6-4c). This left a 3-mm vertical bone defect interproximally between the two implants and approximately a 6-mm vertical defect distal to the second molar implant. Short healing abutments (2 mm long) were placed to act as tenting support (Fig 6-4d) followed by grafting with the prepared sticky tooth biomaterial (Fig 6-4e). A 30 × 40–mm collagen membrane (LysoGide, Oscotec) was placed over the graft followed by two CGF membranes (Figs 6-4f and 6-4g). Following tension-free wound closure, healing was uneventful, allowing uncovering using an apically repositioned flap after 4 months (Figs 6-4h to 6-4j). The definitive zirconia two-unit fixed restoration was delivered after 6 weeks of progressive loading with a provisional restoration (Figs 6-4k and 6-4l). Marginal bone was stable after 3 years in function (Fig 6-4m).

FIG 6-4 *(cont) (h)* A CBCT scan taken after 4 months of site healing suggested substantial new bone height. *(i)* A periapical radiograph obtained after 4 months of healing also showed favorable ridge augmentation. *(j)* At the 4-month reentry surgery, favorable ridge augmentation was observed. *(k)* Restoration was with a two-unit fixed prosthesis. *(l)* A radiograph taken at delivery of the definitive restoration. *(m)* A radiograph of the two immediate molar implants after 3 years of clinical function.

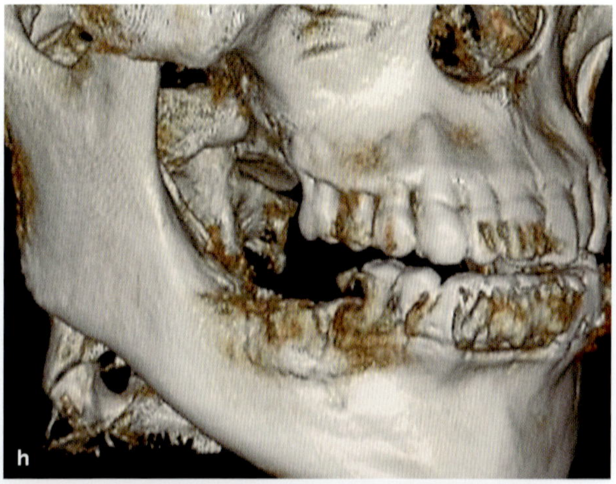

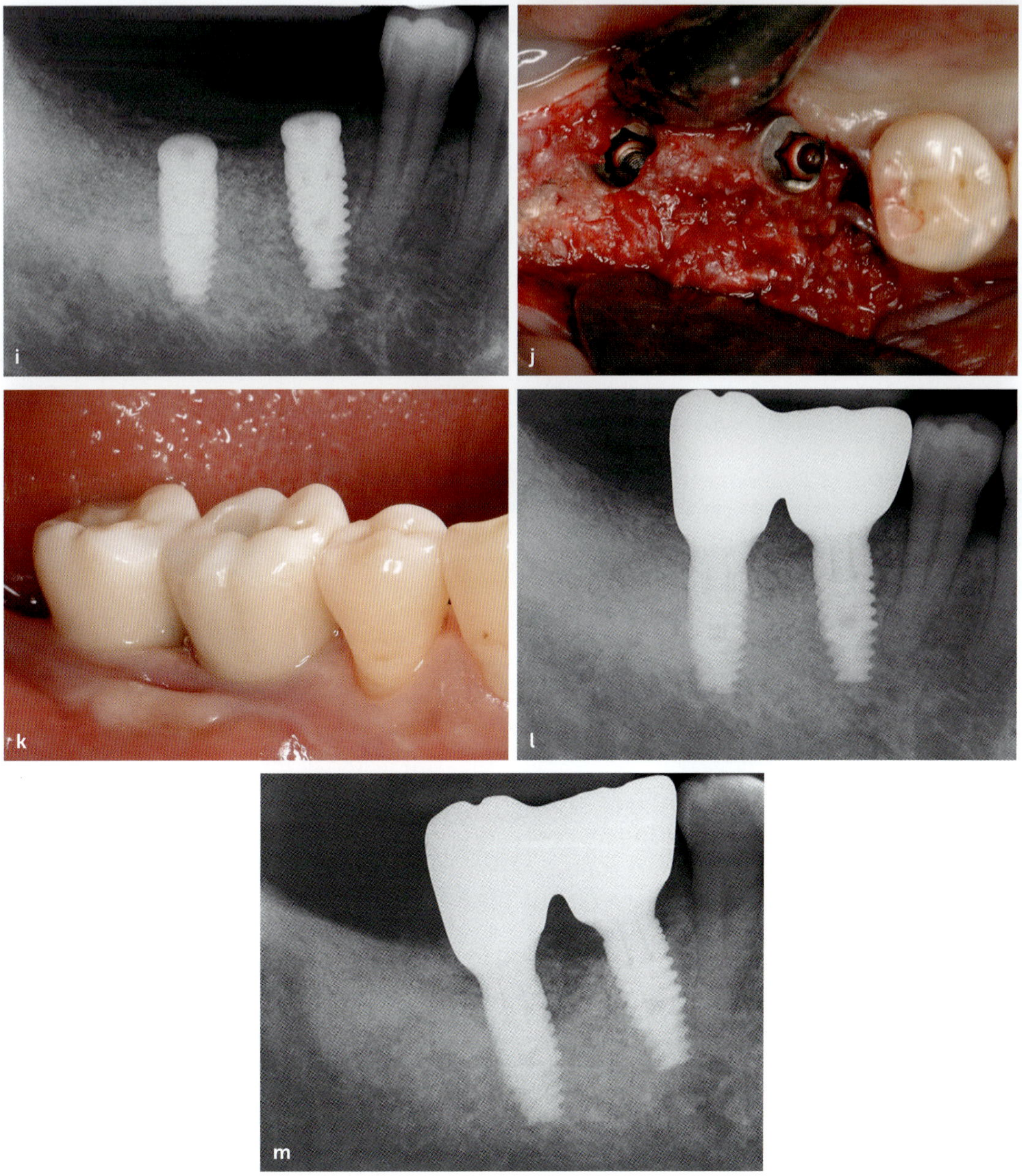

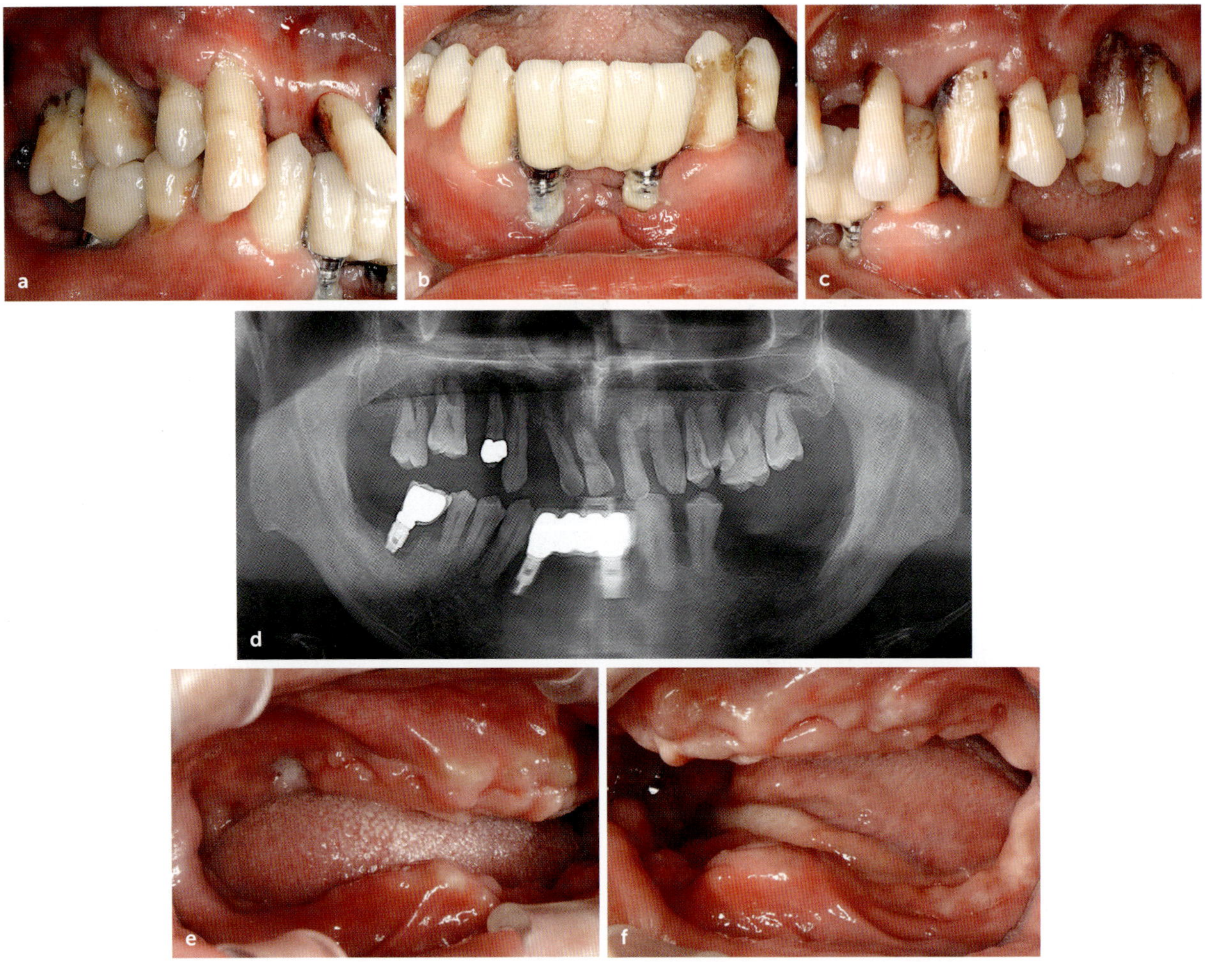

FIG 6-5 *(a to c)* Intraoral photographs taken at the first visit. Note the poor oral hygiene. The patient requested immediate function after extraction of the hopeless teeth. *(d)* The pretreatment panoramic radiograph showed generalized severe bone loss and three previously installed failing dental implants. *(e and f)* Soft tissue healing was allowed for 8 weeks. →

Case 3

A final case documents immediate molar implant placement and simultaneous vertical ridge augmentation using a laminate plate of demineralized autologous tooth biomaterial and sticky tooth graft biomaterial. A 44-year-old man presented with the complaint of generalized tooth mobility and difficulty chewing. He had suffered from severe chronic periodontitis for many years. Gross calculus deposits were seen throughout the dentition, which also showed severe generalized bone loss, pathologic tooth migration, and three failing dental implants (Figs 6-5a to 6-5d). Impressions were taken beforehand in order to prepare transitional immediate full dentures, and when the dentures were ready, the extractions were done, and the dentures with soft liners were inserted. All extracted teeth were used to prepare particulate tooth graft biomaterial as well as laminate plates of the same material. The laminate plates were prepared similarly to the block grafts but with a thickness of only ~ 2 mm.

After 8 weeks of soft tissue healing (Figs 6-5e and 6-5f), radiographs were obtained once more (Figs 6-5g to 6-5j). These images documented the severe postextraction anatomical defects. Following full-thickness flap elevations in the left mandible, severe vertical and horizontal bone deficiencies were observed (Fig 6-5k). After removal of all granulation tissues, a Bone-Pen Kit (Acrodent) was utilized to assist in initial preparation of the osteotomies (Figs 6-5l and 6-5m). An autogenous bone collector (ACM, NeoBiotech)

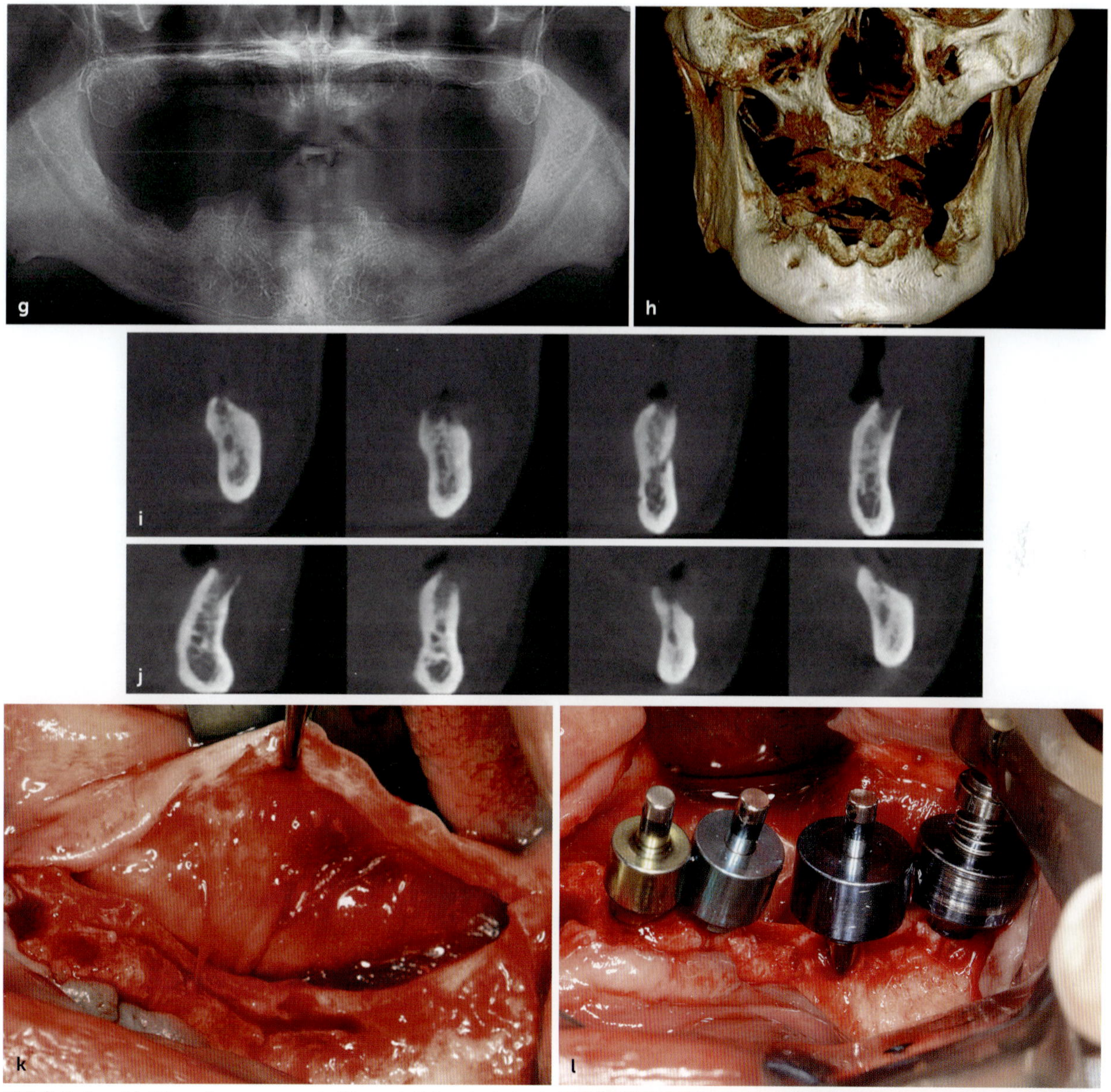

FIG 6-5 *(cont) (g)* Note the severe vertical bony deficiencies in both arches at 8 weeks of soft tissue healing. *(h)* The 3D radiographic image again confirmed the severe vertical bone defects in the posterior mandible. *(i)* The cross-sectional CBCT images at the right posterior mandible. *(j)* The cross-sectional CBCT images at the left posterior mandible. *(k)* Note the severe 3D bony defects in the left posterior mandible after full-thickness flap elevations. *(l and m)* A BonePen Kit was used for the initial osteotomy site preparations to attempt parallelism of the implants.

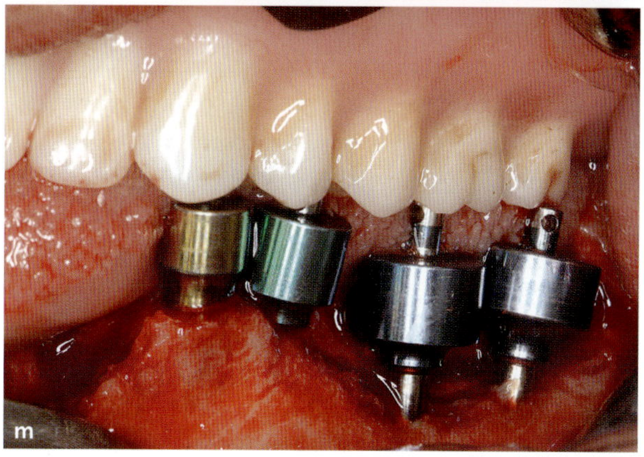

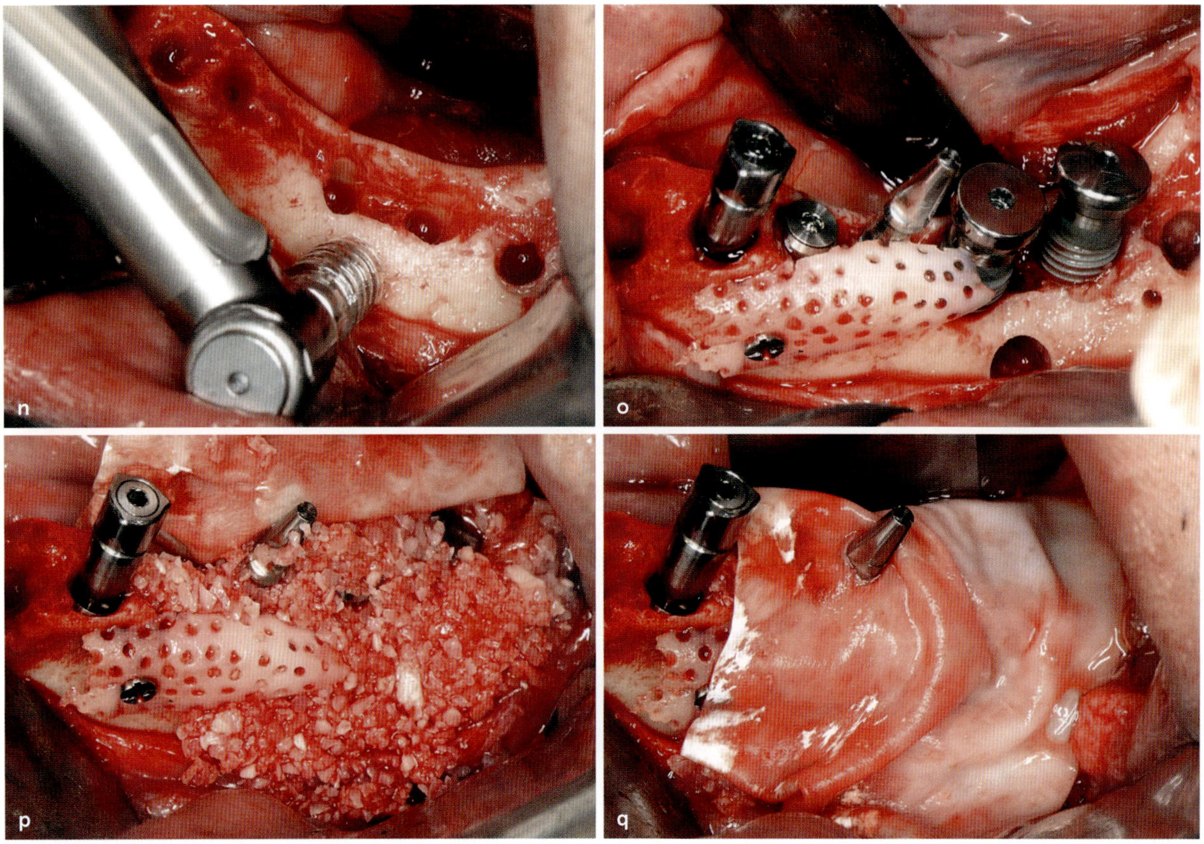

FIG 6-5 *(cont) (n)* An ACM device was utilized to perform large decortications on the buccal cortex at the molar implant sites. The harvested autogenous bone was used to supplement the tooth-derived biomaterials. *(o)* While the premolar implants were submerged ~ 1 mm subcrestally, approximately 6 mm of vertical exposure was left at the molar sites. A laminate (plate-form) tooth block was stabilized with one microscrew. This created a box-like effect to assist with containment of the particulate tooth biomaterial/autogenous bone composite graft. Note that 3-mm-long healing abutments were placed on the molar implants to act as vertical tenting devices. A mini implant was placed between two of the implants to support an immediate transitional fixed restoration. *(p)* A composite of sticky particulate tooth biomaterial and collected autogenous bone was grafted over the vertical defects. *(q)* A collagen barrier was used to cover the grafted site. Bone tacks were not used to stabilize the membrane.

was used to decorticate the buccal cortical bone and collect autogenous bone chips (Fig 6-5n). Osteotomy preparation was such that the final sites were slightly underprepared to assist with implant stabilization. Two implants were placed at the former premolar sites with seating ~ 1 mm subcrestally, while the two implants placed at the former molar sites were placed 2 mm subcrestal to their proximal bone heights but with approximately 6 mm of each of the two molar implants left exposed elsewhere (Fig 6-5o). Healing abutments 3 mm in height were added to the molar implants to act as tenting devices. Meanwhile, one mini implant was placed between the two premolar implants. A tooth block graft that had been prepared as a laminate (bone plate) in the VacuaSonic machine was fixed with one microscrew on the buccal surface of the premolar area. This allowed for a boxing effect to maintain the collected autogenous bone particles and sticky particulate tooth biomaterial (Fig 6-5p). Thereafter, the site was covered with a collagen membrane (Fig 6-5q; LysoGide) followed by tension-free primary soft tissue closure.

Surgery was then continued in the right posterior mandible. Implants were placed with good stability at the two premolar and two molar sites, while two mini implants were placed—one between the two premolars and one between the second premolar and first molar implants (Fig 6-5r). These two mini implants and the one in the left mandible were meant to provide support for an immediate transitional fixed restoration needed during the healing period. Sticky particulate tooth biomaterial was used to cover all of the peri-implant defects (Fig 6-5s) and was subsequently covered using a collagen barrier at the molar

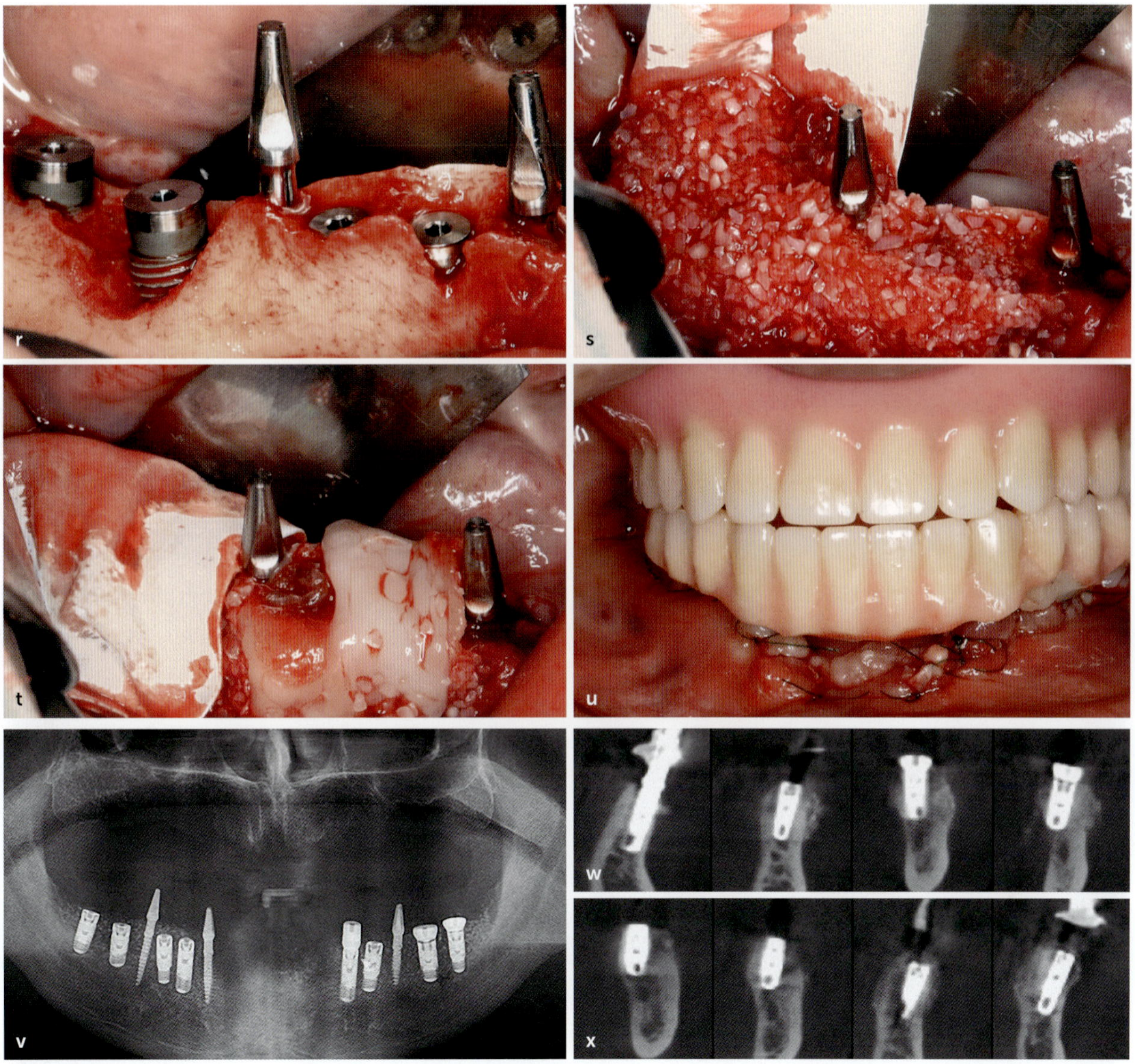

FIG 6-5 *(cont) (r)* Note the vertical bony defect at the molar implants and the horizontal defect at the premolar implants. Two mini implants were placed at the same time to help in the support of an immediate transitional fixed restoration. *(s)* Sticky particulate tooth biomaterial was added. *(t)* A collagen barrier was used to cover the molar implant sites, while CGF membranes covered the premolar implant sites. *(u)* An immediate fixed restoration was fabricated by modifying the patient's full denture. *(v)* An immediate postoperative panoramic radiograph confirms the implant positions and extensive augmentation. *(w)* The cross-sectional CBCT images of the left posterior mandible after 13 weeks of healing. *(x)* The cross-sectional CBCT images at the right posterior mandible after 13 weeks of healing.

sites and CGF membranes at the premolar sites (Fig 6-5t). Primary closure was achieved without tension, and the patient's denture was modified and cemented onto the three mini implants (Fig 6-5u). Healing was uneventful. The immediate postoperative panoramic radiograph shows the implant positioning and extensive grafting (Fig 6-5v). After 13 weeks of healing (Figs 6-5w and 6-5x), reentry surgery was undertaken, revealing favorable vertical and horizontal augmentation outcomes (Figs 6-5y and 6-5z). Excess bone over the cover screw at the right premolar implant was removed with a bone chisel and sent for histologic evaluation (Fig 6-5aa). The definitive implant-supported restorations are shown in Figs 6-5bb and 6-5cc, and the radiographs in Figs 6-5dd and Fig 6-5ee were taken at the recall visit at 1 year in function.

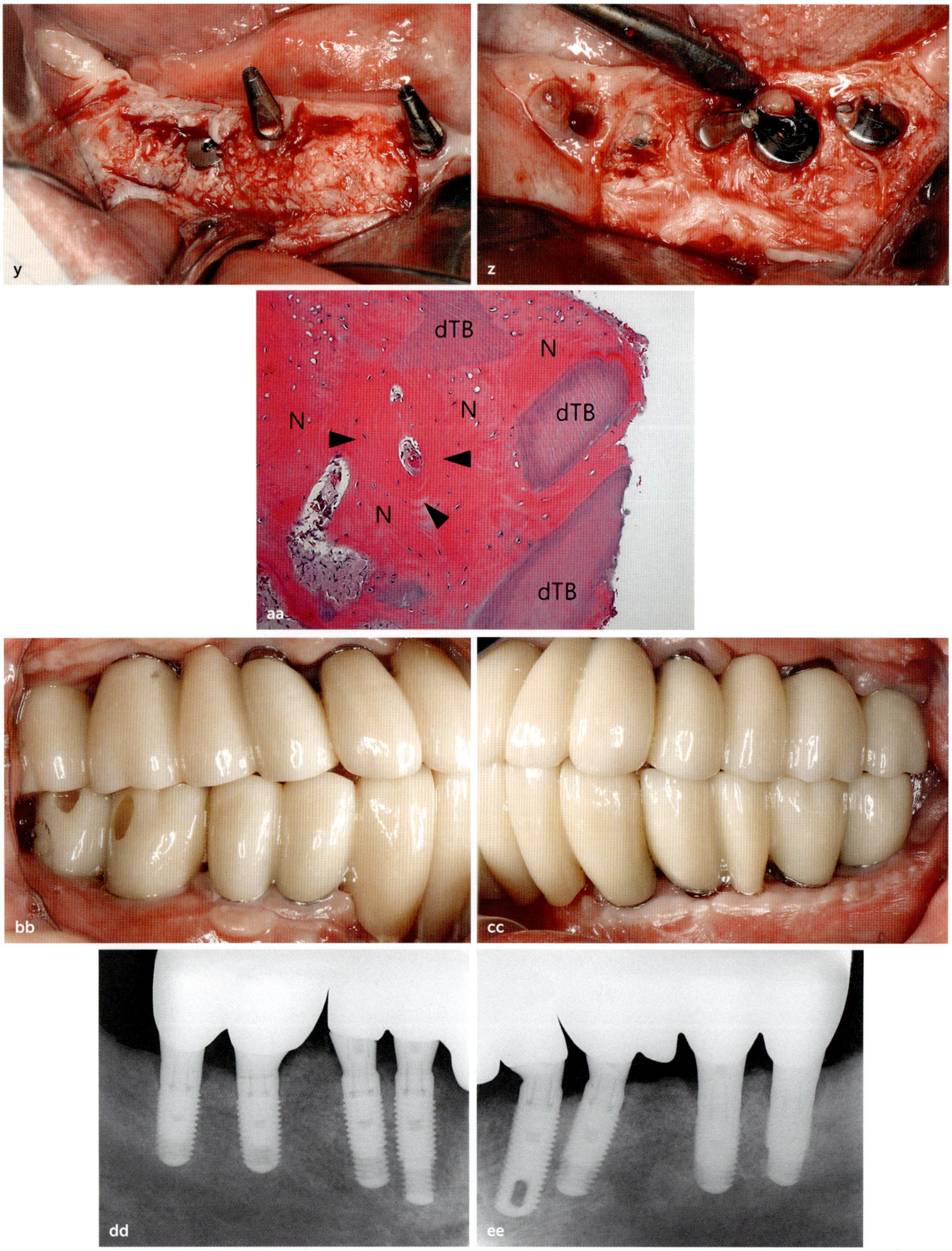

FIG 6-5 *(cont) (y and z)* The uncovering was done after 13 weeks of healing, showing very good bone regeneration. *(aa)* Histologic evaluation of the biopsy revealed highly active new bone formation in response to the grafted tooth biomaterial. Note the haversian canal in the newly formed lamellar bone *(arrowheads)*. dTB = demineralized particulate human tooth bone; N = newly formed bone. (Hematoxylin and eosin stain; magnification ×100). *(bb and cc)* The definitive fixed restorations were provided by Dr Kyu-Bok Lee (Daegu, South Korea). *(dd and ee)* Periapical radiographs obtained at the recall visit at 1 year in function.

Conclusion

3D ridge augmentation at the time of dental implant placement can be predictably achieved using demineralized particulate and block tooth-ring graft biomaterials. These biomaterials are genetically compatible with the donor/recipient and have been documented to have osteoinductive properties. Combining the particulate graft with autologous fibrin glue and covering the sites with autologous CGF fibrin clots prepared from the patient's own venous blood further enhances the regenerative potential. This grafting procedure combined with simultaneous dental implant placement and tension-free soft tissue flap closure markedly reduces treatment time and the number of surgical interventions needed to place implants in patients with severe alveolar bone defects.

KEY POINTS

- Hopeless or impacted teeth can be used to prepare tooth dentin biomaterials in particulate, ring-shaped blocks or laminate sheets.
- Following partial demineralization, these genetically compatible biomaterials have both osteoconductive and osteoinductive properties.
- Combining particulate dentin autograft with autologous fibrin glue prepared from the patient's own blood can create a "sticky graft" that is easy to use.
- Covering the "sticky graft" of dentin with autologous fibrin clots (CGF/PRF) as barrier materials further enhances hard and soft tissue regeneration when used in conjunction with immediate implants.
- Regeneration of deficient vertical bone height at immediate molar extraction sites can be predictably achieved at the time of immediate implant placement.

References

1. Block MS, Chang A, Crawford C. Mandibular alveolar ridge augmentation in the dog using distraction osteogenesis. J Oral Maxillofac Surg 1996;54:309–314.
2. Lee HJ, Ahn MR, Sohn DS. Piezoelectric distraction osteogenesis in the atrophic maxillary anterior area: A case report. Implant Dent 2007;16:227–234.
3. Tinti C, Parma-Benfenati S. Vertical ridge augmentation: Surgical protocol and retrospective evaluation of 48 consecutively inserted implants. Int J Periodontics Restorative Dent 1998;18:434–443.
4. Simion M, Jovanovic SA, Tinti C, Benfenati SP. Long-term evaluation of osseointegrated implants inserted at the time or after vertical ridge augmentation. A retrospective study on 123 implants with 1-5 year follow-up. Clin Oral Implants Res 2001;12:35–45.
5. Jensen OT, Kuhlke L, Bedard JF, White D. Alveolar segmental sandwich osteotomy for anterior maxillary vertical augmentation prior to implant placement [published correction appears in J Oral Maxillofac Surg 2006;64:997]. J Oral Maxillofac Surg 2006;64:290–296.
6. Sohn DS, Shin HI, Ahn MR, Lee JS. Piezoelectric vertical bone augmentation using the sandwich technique in an atrophic mandible and histomorphometric analysis of mineral allografts: A case report series. Int J Periodontics Restorative Dent 2010;30:383–391.
7. Vermeeren JI, Wismeijer D, van Waas MA. One-step reconstruction of the severely resorbed mandible with onlay bone grafts and endosteal implants. A 5-year follow-up. Int J Oral Maxillofac Surg 1996;25:112–115.
8. Novell J, Novell-Costa F, Ivorra C, Fariñas O, Munilla A, Martinez C. Five-year results of implants inserted into freeze-dried block allografts. Implant Dent 2012;21:129–135.

9. Poli PP, Beretta M, Cicciù M, Maiorana C. Alveolar ridge augmentation with titanium mesh. A retrospective clinical study. Open Dent J 2014;8:148–158.
10. Stevens MR, Emam HA, Alaily ME, Sharawy M. Implant bone rings. One-stage three-dimensional bone transplant technique: A case report. J Oral Implantol 2010;36:69–74.
11. Omara M, Abdelwahed N, Ahmed M, Hindy M. Simultaneous implant placement with ridge augmentation using an autogenous bone ring transplant. Int J Oral Maxillofac Surg 2016;45: 535–544.
12. Codivilla A. The classic: On the means of lengthening, in the lower limbs, the muscles and tissues which are shortened through deformity 1905. Clin Orthop Relat Res 2008;466:2903–2909.
13. Chiapasco M, Romeo E, Casentini P, Rimondini L. Alveolar distraction osteogenesis vs. vertical guided bone regeneration for the correction of vertically deficient edentulous ridges: A 1-3-year prospective study on humans. Clin Oral Implants Res 2004;15:82–95.
14. Rachmiel A, Srouji S, Peled M. Alveolar ridge augmentation by distraction osteogenesis. Int J Oral Maxillofac Surg 2001;30: 510–517.
15. Jensen OT. Alveolar segmental "sandwich" osteotomies for posterior edentulous mandibular sites for dental implants. J Oral Maxillofac Surg 2006;64:471–475.
16. Moon JW, Choi BJ, Lee WH, An KM, Sohn DS. Reconstruction of atrophic anterior mandible using piezoelectric sandwich osteotomy: A case report. Implant Dent 2009;18:195–202.
17. Sohn DS. Piezoelectric surgery for atrophic mandible: Vertical ridge augmentation with sandwich osteotomy technique and interpositional allograft. In: Tolstunov L (ed). Vertical Alveolar Ridge Augmentation in Implant Dentistry: A Surgical Manual. Hoboken: John Wiley & Sons, 2016:121–131.
18. Misch CM. The harvest of ramus bone in conjunction with third molar removal for onlay grafting before placement of dental implants. J Oral Maxillofac Surg 1999;57:1376–1379.
19. Clementini M, Morlupi A, Canullo L, Agrestini C, Barlattani A. Success rate of dental implants inserted in horizontal and vertical guided bone regenerated areas: A systematic review. Int J Oral Maxillofac Surg 2012;41:847–852.
20. Maiorana C, Beretta M, Salina S, Santoro F. Reduction of autogenous bone graft resorption by means of Bio-Oss coverage: A prospective study. Int J Periodontics Restorative Dent 2005;25: 19–25.
21. Nguyen TTH, Eo MY, Kuk TS, Myoung H, Kim SM. Rehabilitation of atrophic jaw using iliac onlay bone graft combined with dental implants. Int J Implant Dent 2019;5:11.
22. Sbordone L, Toti P, Menchini-Fabris GB, Sbordone C, Piombino P, Guidetti F. Volume changes of autogenous bone grafts after alveolar ridge augmentation of atrophic maxillae and mandibles. Int J Oral Maxillofac Surg 2009;38:1059–1065.
23. Scheerlinck LM, Muradin MS, van der Bilt A, Meijer GJ, Koole R, Van Cann EM. Donor site complications in bone grafting: Comparison of iliac crest, calvarial, and mandibular ramus bone. Int J Oral Maxillofac Implants 2013;28:222–227.
24. Aloy-Prósper A, Peñarrocha-Oltra D, Peñarrocha-Diago M, Peñarrocha-Diago M. The outcome of intraoral onlay block bone grafts on alveolar ridge augmentations: A systematic review. Med Oral Patol Oral Cir Bucal 2015;20:e251–e258.
25. Motamedian SR, Khojaste M, Khojasteh A. Success rate of implants placed in autogenous bone blocks versus allogenic bone blocks: A systematic literature review. Ann Maxillofac Surg 2016;6:78–90.
26. Cucchi A, Vignudelli E, Napolitano A, Marchetti C, Corinaldesi G. Evaluation of complication rates and vertical bone gain after guided bone regeneration with non-resorbable membranes versus titanium meshes and resorbable membranes. A randomized clinical trial. Clin Implant Dent Relat Res 2017;19:821–832.
27. Elnayef B, Monje A, Gargallo-Albiol J, Galindo-Moreno P, Wang HL, Hernández-Alfaro F. Vertical ridge augmentation in the atrophic mandible: A systematic review and meta-analysis. Int J Oral Maxillofac Implants 2017;32:291–312.
28. Giesenhagen B, Martin N, Donkiewicz P, et al. Vertical bone augmentation in a single-tooth gap with an allogenic bone ring: Clinical considerations. J Esthet Restor Dent 2018;30:480–483.
29. Giesenhagen B, Martin N, Jung O, Barbeck M. Bone augmentation and simultaneous implant placement with allogenic bone rings and analysis of its purification success. Materials (Basel) 2019;12:1291.
30. Deluiz D, Oliveira LS, Pires FR, Tinoco EM. Time-dependent changes in fresh-frozen bone block grafts: Tomographic, histologic, and histomorphometric findings. Clin Implant Dent Relat Res 2015;17:296–306.
31. Park IS. Ridge augmentation using block type of autogenous tooth bone graft material in severe alveolar bone resorption of single tooth: A case report. J Korean Assoc Oral Maxillofac Plast Reconstr Surg 2012;34:462–465.
32. Kim YK, Pang KM, Yun PY, Leem DH, Um IW. Long-term follow-up of autogenous tooth bone graft blocks with dental implants. Clin Case Rep 2017;5:108–118.
33. Kabir MA, Murata M, Akazawa T, Kusano K, Yamada K, Ito M. Evaluation of perforated demineralized dentin scaffold on bone regeneration in critical-size sheep iliac defects. Clin Oral Implants Res 2017;28:e227–e235.
34. Sohn DS, Huang B, Kim J, Park I, Park CC. Utilization of autologous concentrated growth factors (CGF) enriched bone graft matrix (sticky bone) and CGF-enriched fibrin membrane in implant dentistry. J Implant Adv Clin Dent 2015;7(10):11–29.
35. Yeomans JD, Urist MR. Bone induction by decalcified dentine implanted into oral, osseous and muscle tissues. Arch Oral Biol 1967;12:999–1008.
36. Bessho K, Tagawa T, Murata M. Purification of rabbit bone morphogenetic protein derived from bone, dentin, and wound tissue after tooth extraction. J Oral Maxillofac Surg 1990;48: 162–169.
37. Inoue T, Deporter DA, Melcher AH. Induction of cartilage and bone by dentin demineralized in citric acid. J Periodontal Res 1986;21:243–255.
38. Pashley DH. Dentin: A dynamic substrate—A review. Scanning Microsc 1989;3:161–176.
39. Huggins CB, Urist MR. Dentin matrix transformation: Rapid induction of alkaline phosphatase and cartilage. Science 1970; 167(3919):896–898.
40. Murata M, Kawai T, Kawakami T, et al. Human acid-soluble dentin with BMP-2 accelerates bone induction in subcutaneous and intramuscular tissues. J Ceram Soc Jap 2010;118:438–441.
41. Park M, Mah YJ, Kim DH, Kim ES, Park EJ. Demineralized deciduous tooth as a source of bone graft material: Its biological and physicochemical characteristics. Oral Surg Oral Med Oral Pathol Oral Radiol 2015;120:307–314.
42. Deporter DA, Komori N, Howley TP, et al. Reconstituted bovine skin collagen enhances healing of bone wounds in the rat calvaria. Calcif Tissue Int 1988;42:321–325.
43. Kim ES. Autogenous fresh demineralized tooth graft prepared at chairside for dental implant. Maxillofac Plast Reconstr Surg 2015;37:8.

44. Xu X, Sohn DS, Kim HG, Lee SJ, Moon YS. Comparative histomorphometric analysis of maxillary sinus augmentation with deproteinized bovine bone and demineralized particulate human tooth graft: An experimental study in rabbits. Implant Dent 2018;27:324–331.
45. Gomes MF, Abreu PP, Morosolli AR, Araújo MM, Goulart Md. Densitometric analysis of the autogenous demineralized dentin matrix on the dental socket wound healing process in humans. Braz Oral Res 2006;20:324–330.
46. Lee KH, Kim YK, Cho WJ, Um IW, Murata M, Mitsugi M. Autogenous tooth bone graft block for sinus augmentation with simultaneous implant installation: A technical note. J Korean Assoc Oral Maxillofac Surg 2015;41:284–289.
47. Kim YK, Lee JH, Um IW, Cho WJ. Guided bone regeneration using demineralized dentin matrix: Long-term follow-up. J Oral Maxillofac Surg 2016;74:515.e1–515.e5159.
48. Park SM, Kim DH, Pang EK. Bone formation of demineralized human dentin block graft with different demineralization time: In vitro and in vivo study. J Craniomaxillofac Surg 2017;45:903–912.

7

OSSEODENSIFICATION FOR IMMEDIATE MOLAR IMPLANT PLACEMENT

Salah Huwais
Samvel Bleyan
Rodrigo Neiva

As stressed in earlier chapters in this book, placement of immediate dental implants into molar fresh extraction sites is doable, but it should be considered a challenging procedure even for experienced clinicians.[1,2] While excellent survival outcomes have been reported in systematic literature reviews,[3,4] the main hurdles have been shown to be the difficulty in achieving adequate implant primary stability in the optimal implant position, increased risk of infection, minimizing alveolar ridge shrinkage, and maintaining adequate keratinized soft tissue to ensure long-term implant health and patient comfort.[5,6]

In their systematic review of immediate molar implant (IMI) performance, Ketabi et al[4] identified 15 papers published between November 2008 and May 2015 that included a total of 768 IMIs inserted in 757 patients. However, they reported that the majority of these studies were considered to be either prospective case series or retrospective case reports. They stressed that at the time there were no published reports of IMI performance from double-blind randomized controlled clinical trials comparing IMIs with implants placed at previously healed molar sites. The same authors later summarized what they found regarding indications and contraindications for IMIs, including proper case selection. Factors to be considered included the reason for tooth extraction; the remaining socket anatomy in terms of the condition of its walls; the dimensions of the interradicular septum (IRS) bone; the choice of an implant of appropriate geometry, length, and diameter; the depth and 3D positioning of implant placement; the size and location of remaining peri-implant gaps; and the amount and quality (ie, thickness and width) of remaining keratinized soft tissues. As well, sufficient remaining native bone apically to stabilize the implant may be crucial, particularly in mandible.

High primary stability is a prerequisite to reduce implant micromotion during the early healing phase.[7,8] However, initial stability with IMIs can be unpredictable and is often lower than with delayed molar implant placement.[9]

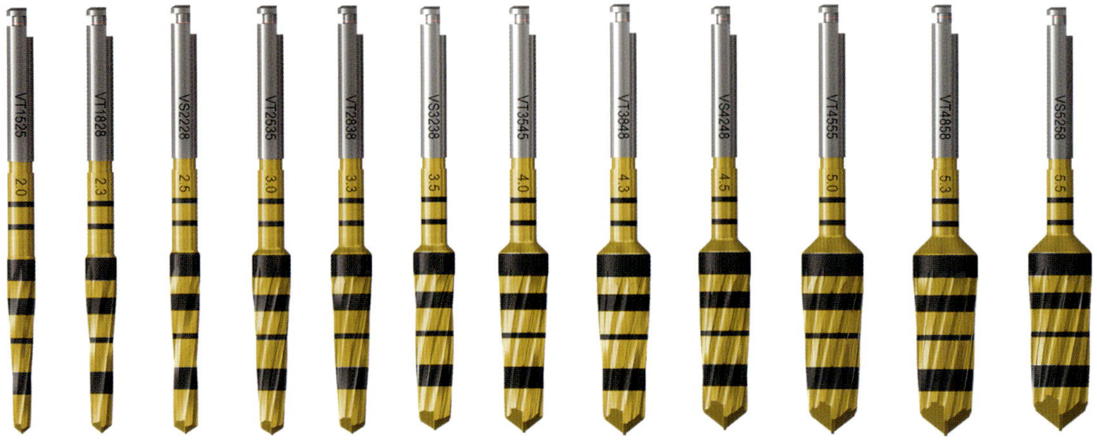

FIG 7-1 Densah burs (Versah) range in maximum diameter from 2.5 to 5.8 mm and are used in reverse mode to create osteotomies by osseodensification.

As well, maxillary molar implants generally achieve lower insertion torque values (ITVs) than mandibular sites due to lower bone density. Walker et al[10] reported the implant survival rate in immediate mandibular molar sites to be 86% when initial ITV was low (≤ 15 Ncm), but 90% to 96% when initial ITV was medium to high (30 to 50 Ncm). Often, low initial stability in molar extraction sockets dictates the need for wider-body implants and/or for primary full soft tissue closure to promote predictable healing.[11]

Molar septum preservation during extraction is a key element needed to achieve implant stability, and this preservation is achieved with unpredictable results utilizing standard drills.[12–14] Adequate septum width is essential for achieving implant stability. A minimum septum mesiodistal width of 3 mm or more is reported as an essential required element for successful expansion and adequate implant placement.[13–15] Therefore, the preservation and the expansion of the septal bone is an important factor for this treatment modality. Historically, rotary expanders, osteotomes, and specialized piezoelectric tips have been utilized to expand the septum in mandibular and maxillary molar extraction sites as well as to elevate the sinus floor and sinus membrane prior to immediate implant placement.[3,14–22]

How Osseodensification Works

One recent instrumentation method was introduced by Huwais and Meyer[23] for the achievement of adequate stability, both primary and secondary, using osteotomy site preparation via "osseodensification." Rather than removing or excavating bone as is the case with standard implant drilling, osseodensification preserves bone by compacting it along the surface of the developing osteotomy, tripling the bone-to-implant contact.[23,24] Large animal histologic studies have demonstrated that the high stability on the day of implant placement using osseodensification is maintained throughout the osseointegration process, and that the retained compacted bone can act as nucleating surfaces for osteoblastic bone deposition, facilitating the bridging of bone and implant surface regardless of the implant macro or micro geometry.[25]

Osseodensification is facilitated using specially designed burs (Versah) that are run in reverse (counterclockwise or CCW) mode generally at 800 to 1,200 rpm (Figs 7-1 and 7-2). They increase peri-implant bone density and bone-to-implant contact with associated substantial increases in primary stability of the implant.[23] This increase in primary stability is facilitated by the compaction/autografting of bone particles into the trabecular space, creating an elastic strain. This in turn results in a spring-back effect of bone toward the implant body, enhancing its primary stability without the traditional need to undersize the osteotomy diameter.[23,26,27] Osseodensification burs are used under copious saline irrigation and are thought to deform bone via viscoelastic and plastic mechanisms. The recommended technique is for the surgeon to utilize a constant, well-controlled "modu-

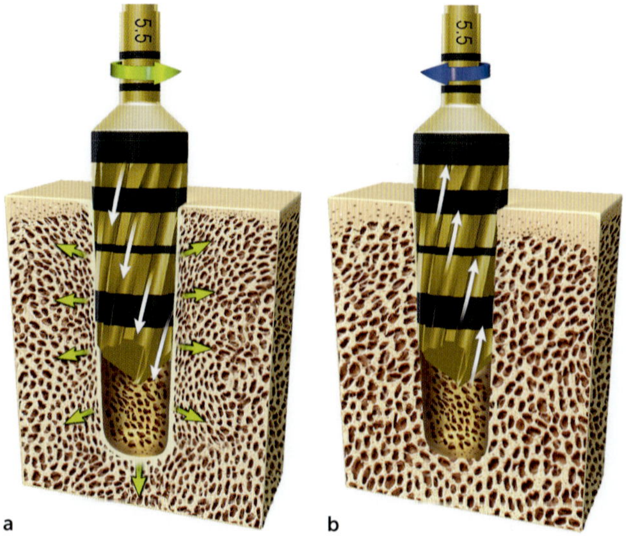

FIG 7-2 Densah burs are dual-action tools. They can be used with standard surgical implant engines with adequate irrigation to produce osseodensification when rotating in the noncutting direction (CCW), ie, densifying mode *(a)*, or to excavate bone when rotating in the cutting direction (CW), ie, cutting mode *(b)*. In either mode, the burs are run at 800 to 1,200 rpm.

lating" motion of the bur within the osteotomy, creating a hydraulic pressure wave ahead of the point of contact while avoiding untoward overheating of bone. The irrigation fluid being forced into the osteotomy will also result in autografting of bone particles into the trabecular space along the inner surface of the osteotomy, further densifying its walls.[23,27] This is in contrast to the situation with standard drilling (ie, clockwise or CW) protocols where bone particles are either extracted out of the osteotomies by the irrigation fluid or remain in the drill flutes.

Literature on Osseodensification

Osseodensification facilitates a controlled plastic deformation of trabecular bone.[23] This allows for trabecular bone expansion outwardly to produce the osteotomy. This combination of plastic deformation and the compaction/autografting facilitates implant placement with sufficient stability in sites with less-than-optimum bone quantity and quality (eg, IMI sites). Trisi et al[28] studied densification histologically, reporting that they were able to place and successfully integrate 5-mm-diameter implants into bone ridges in sheep iliac crest that were originally only 5 mm in width. More recently, Koutouzis et al[29] studied human clinical outcomes using osseodensification to facilitate plastic ridge expansion at healed edentulous sites with different alveolar ridge widths. In their retrospective case series, implant sites were divided into four groups according to their initial buccolingual/palatal ridge widths, as follows:

- G1: 3–4 mm
- G2: 5–6 mm
- G3: 7–8 mm
- G4: 10–11 mm

G1 ridges demonstrated the largest amount of ridge expansion (75%), followed by G2 (28%), G3 (17%), and G4 (0%). The authors concluded that G4 ridges had enough trabecular bone content to absorb the hydraulic wave generated by the densifying burs without showing any physical plastic expansion. In contrast, G1 (3–4 mm) ridges had insufficient trabecular bone in their cores to fully absorb the hydraulic wave generated, needing maximum plastic physical expansion. At each site, an implant equal in diameter or slightly wider (up to 0.7 mm wider) than the final bur was inserted, and any hard and/or soft tissue grafting deemed necessary was done with primary flap closure where needed. In total, 28 implants were placed in 21 patients (12 women and 9 men). Two implants failed to integrate, likely due to a low trabecular-to-cortical bone ratio, while the remainder became integrated and were restored, making the success rate 92.8%. It was concluded that the minimum ridge width required for predictable plastic expansion through osseodensification is 4 mm, of which at least 2 mm should be trabecular bone.

In addition to plastic expansion of ridges, clinical short- and long-term studies have demonstrated that osseodensification achieves enhanced implant stability and high implant success rates regardless of implant micro and macro geometry in several clinical scenarios, including immediate and early loading.[30–34] Tanello et al[31] reported results of a multicenter retrospective 5-year follow-up clinical study in which osseodensification protocols were used in both the maxilla and the mandible to place 254 implants with six different geometries in 184 patients. High implant primary and secondary stabilities were reported regardless of implant design, with an overall success rate of 97.7%. Additional clinical studies have reported on implant placement in conjunction with crestal sinus elevation and grafting, again with high success rates utilizing osseodensification.[33,35,36]

Preoperative CBCT scans are essential in determining whether or not osseodensification can assist in placing mandibular IMIs while also reducing the risk of surgical damage to the mandibular canal and/or lingual plate of bone. It has been suggested that at least 4 mm of bone apical to mandibular molar root apices will be required to achieve adequate primary stability of an IMI,[37] but this requirement is less of an issue if osseodensification is being planned. Mandibular first molars most commonly have type B sockets,[38] and IMIs placed here will most likely achieve the required stability within the confines of an expanded IRS and not necessarily require the usual 4 mm of native apical bone. In the posterior maxilla, the principle of osseodensification offers even greater advantage. Bone density generally is low here and can benefit from compaction. Further, maxillary first molars commonly have type A sockets,[38] making them ideal for densification—often without need to elevate the associated sinus floor. However, if sinus floor elevation is needed, it can easily and atraumatically be dealt with using specific osseodensification protocols. Support for this application and its clinical protocols comes from a recent multicenter retrospective clinical study.[35]

Surgical Considerations

As discussed elsewhere in this book, IMI placement is best done using flapless surgery, coronectomy, and then gentle removal of each molar root separately.[39,40] Avoiding elevation of a flap, particularly on the buccal aspect, will minimize disruption of its periosteal blood supply, which in turn will reduce the risk of crestal bone loss as well as preserve keratinized soft tissues. Following their systematic review and meta-analysis of 1,106 IMIs, Ragucci et al[41] concluded that more marginal bone loss occurred with flap reflection, especially in conjunction with thin gingival biotype cases. Depth of implant placement also has an impact on crestal bone loss, with the preferred approach being to place the implant prosthetic table 1 to 2 mm subcrestally on the buccal aspect.[42] The usual protocol for placing a mandibular molar IMI using osseodensification is illustrated in Fig 7-3.[44]

Anatomical Considerations

Generally, socket anatomy permitting, in order to achieve optimal placement, IMIs are best placed into the IRS bone. Smith and Tarnow[38] presented a classification of molar socket anatomy based on the dimensions of the remaining IRS bone after the tooth has been atraumatically extracted. In this classification, type A sockets were defined as those with sufficient bulk and width of IRS to stabilize and totally house the coronal aspect of the chosen implant. Type B sockets were those with sufficient bulk and width of IRS to stabilize but not fully house the implant, while type C were denoted as those with insufficient IRS to stabilize an IMI. Osseodensification is of value with both types A and B. With type A sockets, it can increase the density of the IRS osteotomy walls to enhance implant stability, while type B sockets can be expanded to house more of the implant periphery within the septal bone. As discussed elsewhere in this book, type C sockets, most commonly seen at mandibular second molar sites, are best treated with wider-diameter implants or with socket preservation and delayed implant placement (see chapters 1 and 3). The authors of this chapter also recently conducted a multicenter clinical study utilizing osseodensification to place implants into 145 molar septal sites (87 mandible, 58 maxilla) in 131 patients (90 female, 41 male). Initial septum width ranged from 2.5 to 4.1 mm with an average width of 3.3 mm (ie, generally type B sockets).[44] Maxillary septa were wider than mandibular ones. Osteotomy widths generated using osseodensification became 3.8 to 5.5 mm, with an average of

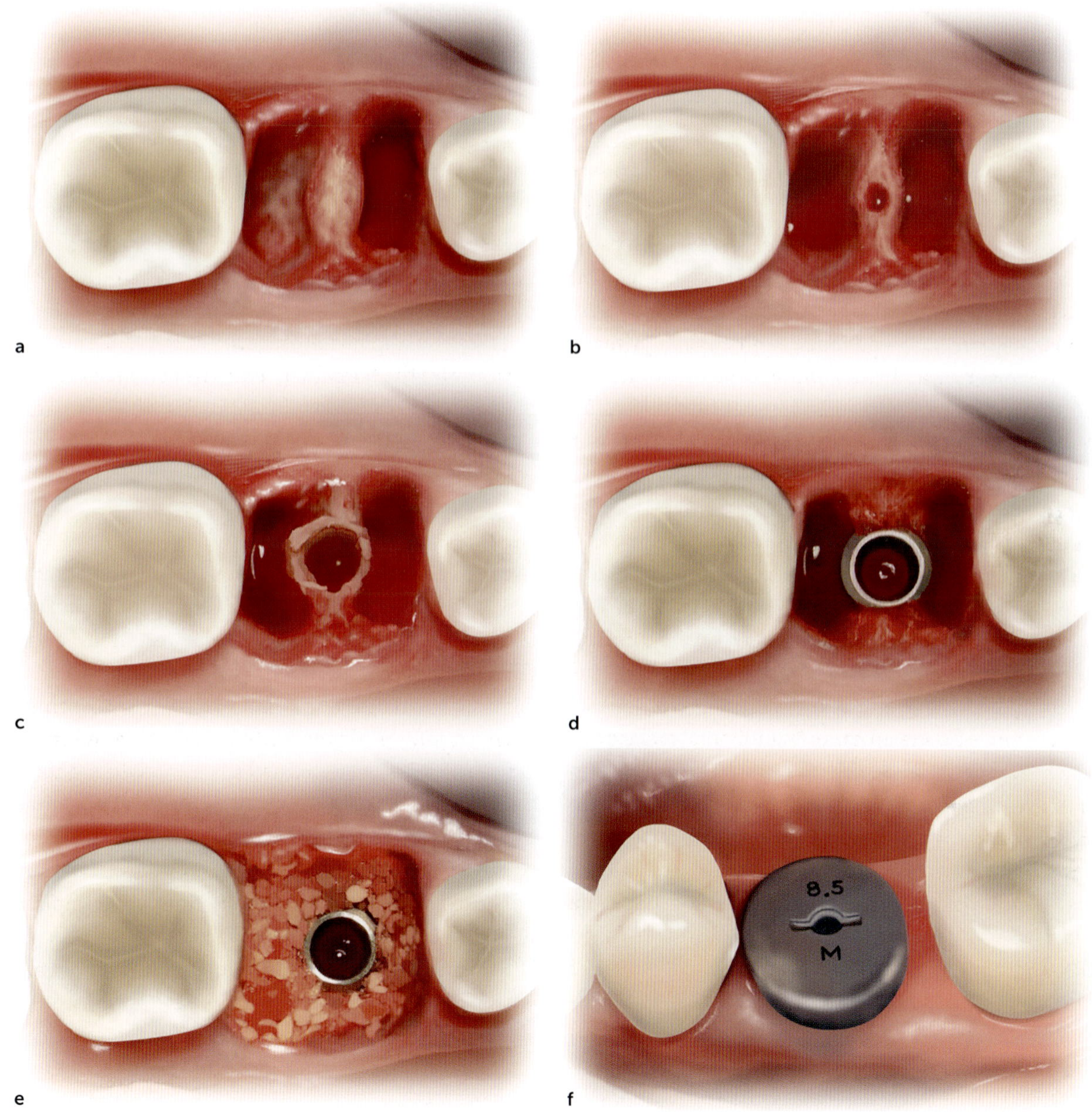

FIG 7-3 *(a)* Step 1: Separate the molar roots at the furcation without compromising the integrity of the IRS to permit their separate and atraumatic removal. *(b)* Step 2: After degranulating the socket as needed, use a pilot drill of 1.3 to 1.6 mm in diameter in CW mode (or a piezoelectric surgery tip) to begin preparation of the osteotomy into the IRS, continuing to a depth 1 mm beyond that of the planned implant length. This extra 1-mm depth will be needed to accommodate the bone shavings forced apically by subsequent burs, which will be run in reverse (CCW) mode. *(c)* Step 3: Depending on the implant type and diameter, follow the corresponding Densifying Reference Guide (https://versah.com/implant-system-drilling-protocols/), starting with the smallest diameter (2.0-mm) Densah bur, again to a depth 1 mm beyond the intended implant length. For site expansion, Densah burs must be operated in reverse mode (CCW) with drill speed 800–1,200 rpm and copious irrigation. Subsequent Densah burs should increase the osteotomy diameter in the smallest possible increments to avoid overstressing the bone during its expansion (ie, from 2.0 mm to 2.3 mm to 2.5 mm to 3.0 mm). The final bur can be chosen to be equal to or slightly larger in diameter relative to the major diameter of the selected implant, remembering that the expanded osteotomy walls will spring back once the final bur is removed. *(d)* Step 4: Implant placement can then be at an equicrestal or subcrestal position, depending on the implant design. *(e)* Step 5: Graft any remaining peri-implant gaps with a bone graft material if needed, preferably using an allograft with a high cancellous-to-cortical bone ratio. Consider sealing the site with biologics like an autologous platelet-rich fibrin (PRF) clot[43] or a collagen plug, and place a large-diameter healing abutment to help in protecting the grafted gaps. *(f)* Step 6: A large stock or wide custom healing abutment must be placed to seal the grafted extraction socket.

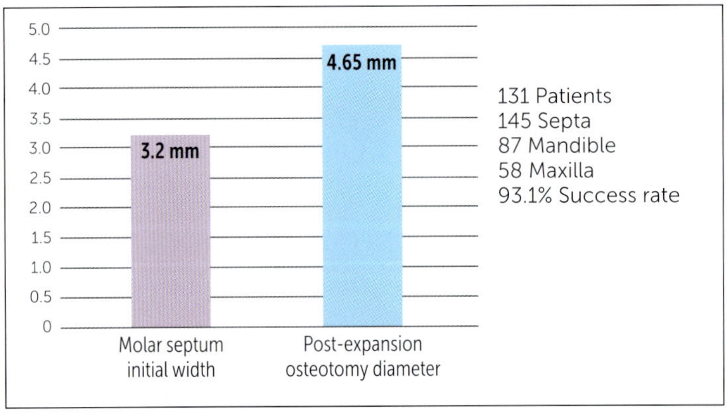

FIG 7-4 Molar septum expansion via osseodensification at 145 sites in 131 patients with follow-up of 12 to 60 months. The mean preoperative septal width was 3.2 mm, and this was increased with densification to a mean of 4.65 mm.[44]

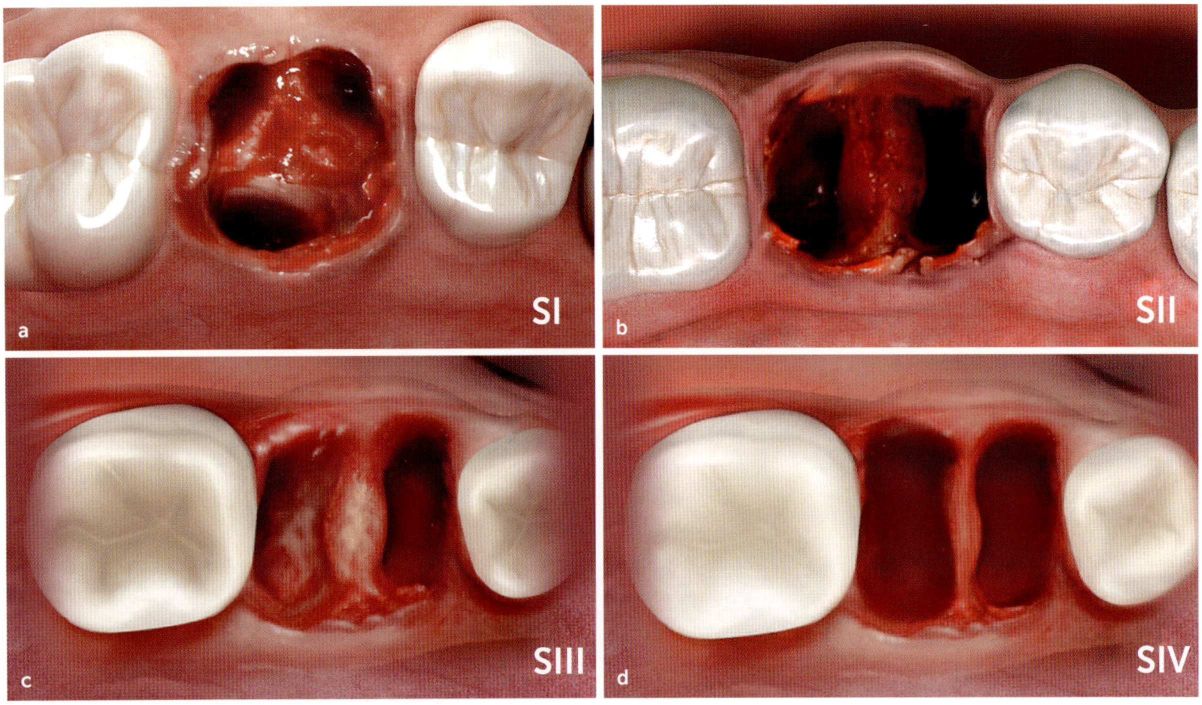

FIG 7-5 *(a)* SI IRS width > 4 mm. *(b)* SII IRS width 3 to 4 mm. *(c)* SIII IRS width 2 to 3 mm. *(d)* SIV IRS width < 2 mm or none. Based on the new classification, type SIII can be converted to type SII and type SII to type SI using osseodensification.

4.65 mm (Fig 7-4). Implant stability was measured by both ITVs and implant stability quotient (ISQ) values. ITV was higher in the mandible (35 to 60 Ncm) than the maxilla (20 to 60 Ncm) with a mean of 41.1 Ncm. ISQ values were taken at surgery (range of 60 to 82) and at the time of the restorative impression (range of 70 to 88). Implants were fully loaded between 3 and 9 months (average of 4.7 months) postimplantation. Ten implants failed at the restorative phase, resulting in a 93.1% implant survival rate.

Implant failures appeared to be associated with the use of nonsealing narrow-diameter immediate healing abutments. Osseodensification instrumentation facilitated bone preservation and expansion in septa with widths as small as 2.5 mm and adequate implant stability. Osseodensification also may facilitate septum bone preservation and conversion of type C molar sockets to type B and type B sockets to type A. The authors suggested a further classification of molar IRS into four types based on their widths. SI IRS was defined as having widths > 4 mm while SII widths were 3 to 4 mm. SIII IRS widths were proposed to be 2 to 3 mm and SIV < 2 mm or missing (Fig 7-5). Based on the new classification, type SIII can be converted to type SII and type SII to type SI using osseodensification.

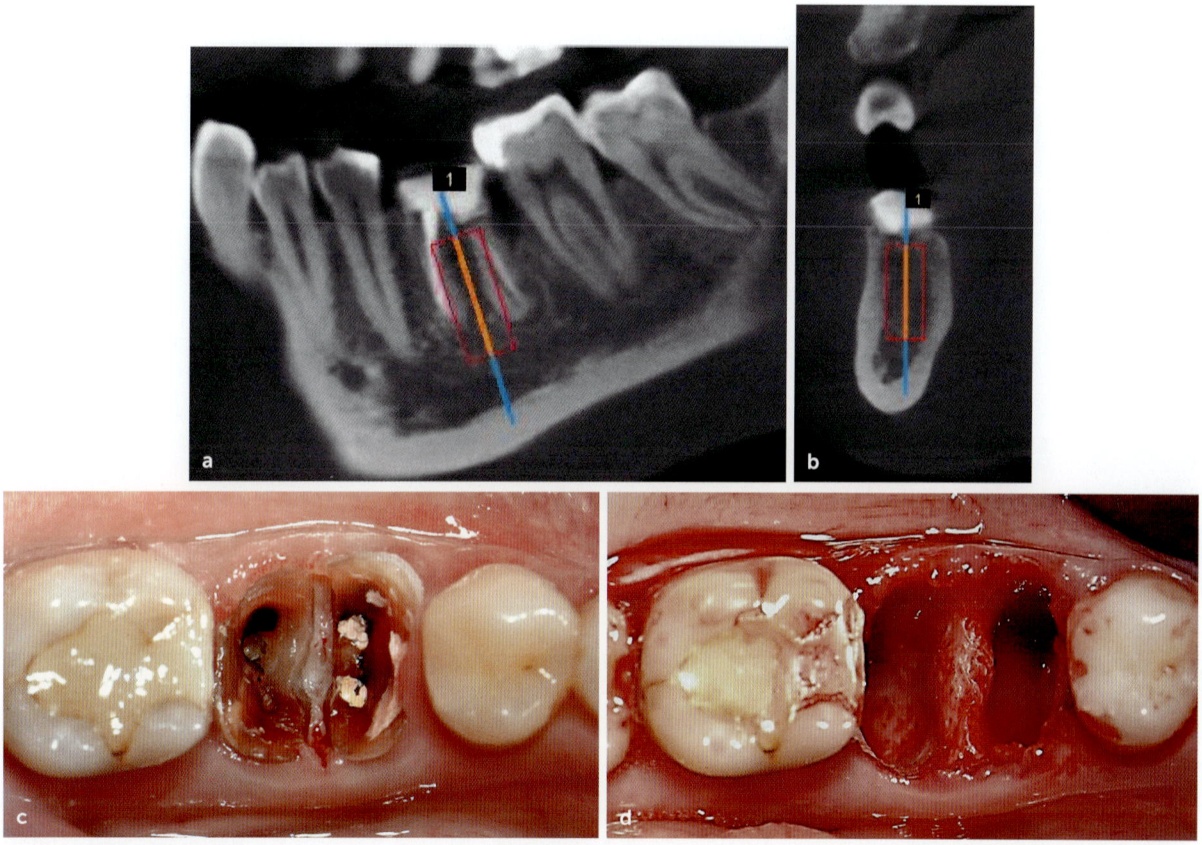

FIG 7-6 *(a)* A mandibular left first molar was deemed hopeless and a candidate for an IMI. This sagittal radiographic view and its coronal counterpart suggested a type B IRS and adequate bone to receive a 12 × 4.5–mm IMI utilizing septal expansion with osseodensification burs. *(b)* A coronal CBCT image of the furcal bone of the tooth in question. *(c)* The clinical presentation of the tooth after removal of the restoration and separation of the two roots through the furcation. *(d)* The two roots were removed atraumatically without a need to raise a mucoperiosteal flap, with preservation of the type B IRS.

Sample Cases

Case 1: Mandibular molar with type B socket

Case 1 displays the procedure performed at a mandibular type B socket according to the Smith and Tarnow classification.[38] The patient was a 47-year-old nonsmoker with controlled hypertension presenting with a loose restoration in an endodontically treated mandibular left first molar. After removal of the restoration, the tooth was deemed hopeless due to a root fracture. CBCT scanning suggested suitability for placement of an IMI (Figs 7-6a and 7-6b). The two roots were separated and removed individually without raising a soft tissue flap (Figs 7-6c and 7-6d). The implant chosen was a 12 × 4.5–mm Dentium Superline, and using the Densah bur reference guide for this implant type and its dimensions (Fig 7-6e), the osteotomy was begun in the IRS. Accordingly, after the pilot bur had been used in cutting mode to a depth of 13 mm (Figs 7-6f and 7-6g), a sequence of five burs with progressive, small increases in bur diameter (Densah burs VT1525, VT1828, VT2535, VT2838, and finally VT3545) was used, all in CCW mode, to create an osteotomy within the IRS (Figs 7-6h to 7-6l). Implant insertion followed (Fig 7-6m) with an initial torque of 30 Ncm and an ISQ value of 74.

To complete the procedure, all remaining peri-implant gaps were filled with an allograft of 70% cancellous and 30% cortical bone particles (Fig 7-6n; Osteogenics). Immediately prior to surgery, a sample

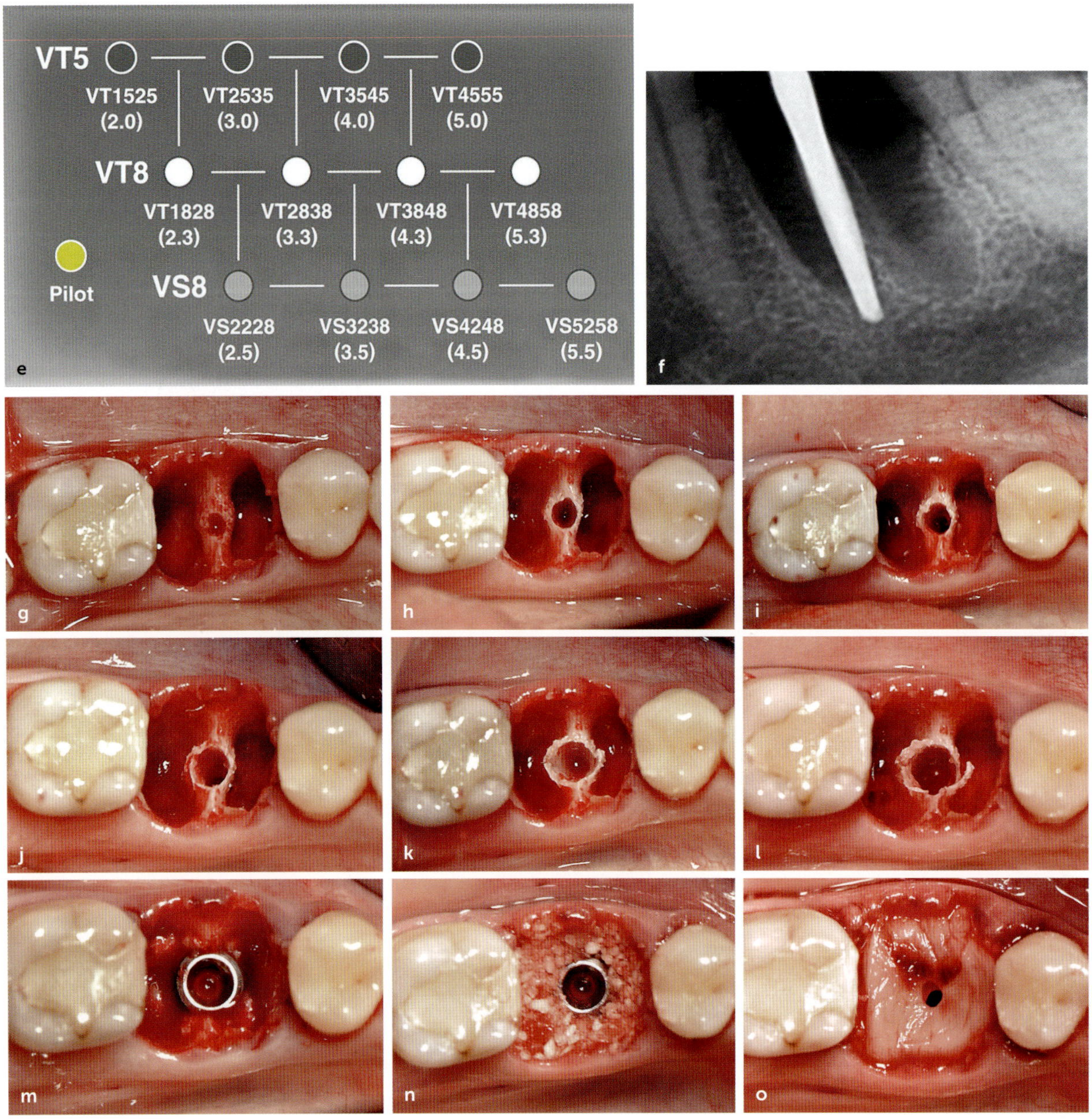

FIG 7-6 *(cont) (e)* Reference guide for inserting a 12 × 4.5–mm Dentium Superline implant using Densah burs with small-increment increase. *(f)* An intraoperative periapical radiograph shows Densah Bur VT1525 expanding the initial osteotomy depth of 13 mm. An osteotomy was created for a 12 × 4.5–mm Dentium Superline implant in a type B socket IRS using the following osseodensification bur sequence. *(g)* Pilot bur in CW mode to a depth of 13 mm. *(h)* Densah bur VT1525 (2.0) in CCW mode to 13 mm. *(i)* Densah bur VT1828 (2.3) in CCW mode to 13 mm. *(j)* Densah bur VT2535 (3.0) in CCW mode to 13 mm. *(k)* Densah bur VT2838 (3.3) in CCW mode to 13 mm. *(l)* Densah bur VT3545 (4.0) in CCW mode to 13 mm. Because of the small increases in Densah bur and osteotomy diameter, the expanding IRS remained intact throughout. *(m)* At the time of implant placement, the initial torque was recorded at 30 Ncm, while resonance frequency testing showed an ISQ value of 74. *(n)* The peri-implant gaps were filled with allograft to help in minimizing socket shrinkage during site healing. *(o)* An autogenous leukocyte- and PRF clot[43] was flattened and used as a barrier membrane to seal the site prior to placing a large-diameter healing abutment.

of venous blood had been taken from the patient and centrifuged to create leukocyte- and platelet-rich fibrin (L-PRF) clots.[43,45] This biologic membrane was then used to cover the implant and graft particles before a wide-diameter healing abutment was connected to the implant (Fig 7-6o). The healing abutment was 8.5 mm in diameter and helped to protect the grafted gaps (Figs 7-6p and 7-6q). A postoperative CBCT scan

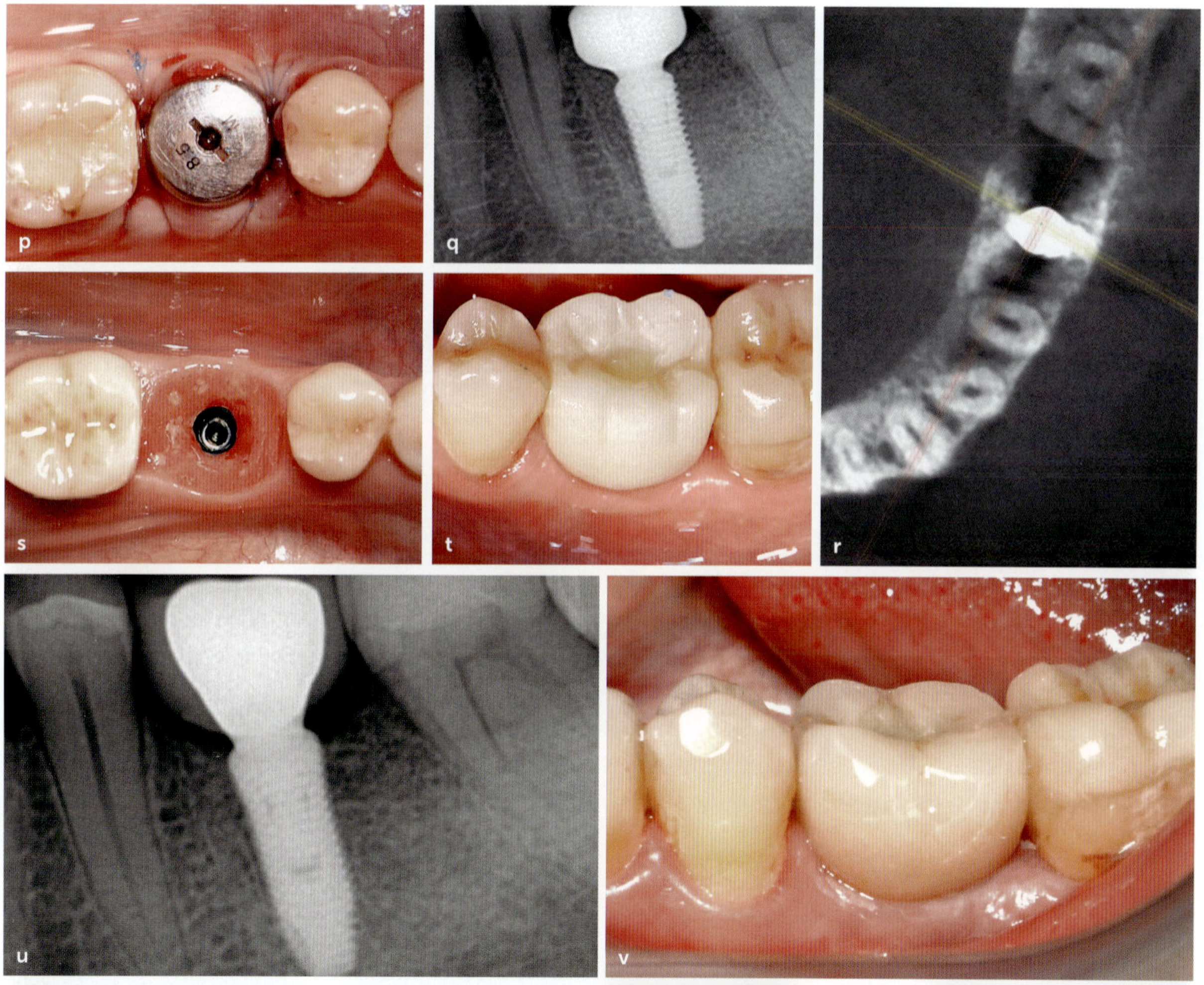

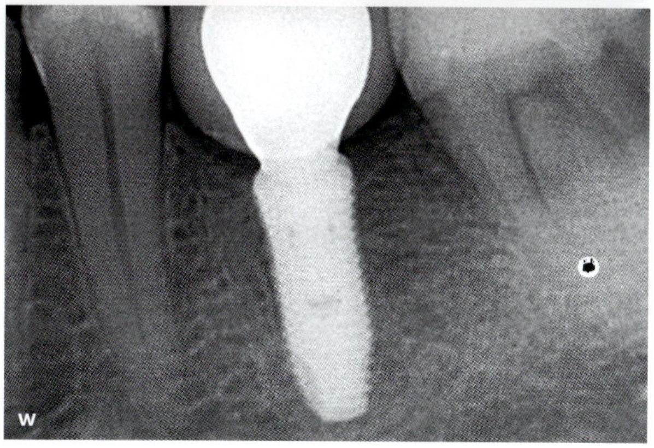

FIG 7-6 *(cont) (p)* An 8.5-mm-diameter healing abutment was connected to the implant and interrupted sutures placed interproximally to stabilize the papillae. Note that the large healing abutment provides a protective seal for the underlying grafted peri-implant gaps. *(q)* The immediate postoperative radiograph of the implant with the healing abutment. *(r)* A postoperative CBCT scan shows the implant to be in the optimal prosthetic position for a molar crown. *(s)* After 4 months' healing, the implant was ready for restoration. The ISQ value 1 month earlier had been 79. *(t)* The definitive restoration 4 months following insertion. *(u)* The radiographic appearance at 4 months postrestoration. *(v)* The clinical appearance after 4 years in function. *(w)* The radiographic appearance after 4 years in function. Note that platform switching has helped to minimize crestal resorption.

showed the implant to be in the optimal prosthetic position for a molar crown (Fig 7-6r).

After 3 months of healing, the implant had an ISQ value of 79 and was considered ready for restoration (Fig 7-6s). A porcelain-fused-to-metal crown was delivered 1 month later and is shown after 4 months in function in Figs 7-6t and 7-6u, and again after 4 years in function in Figs 7-6v and 7-6w.

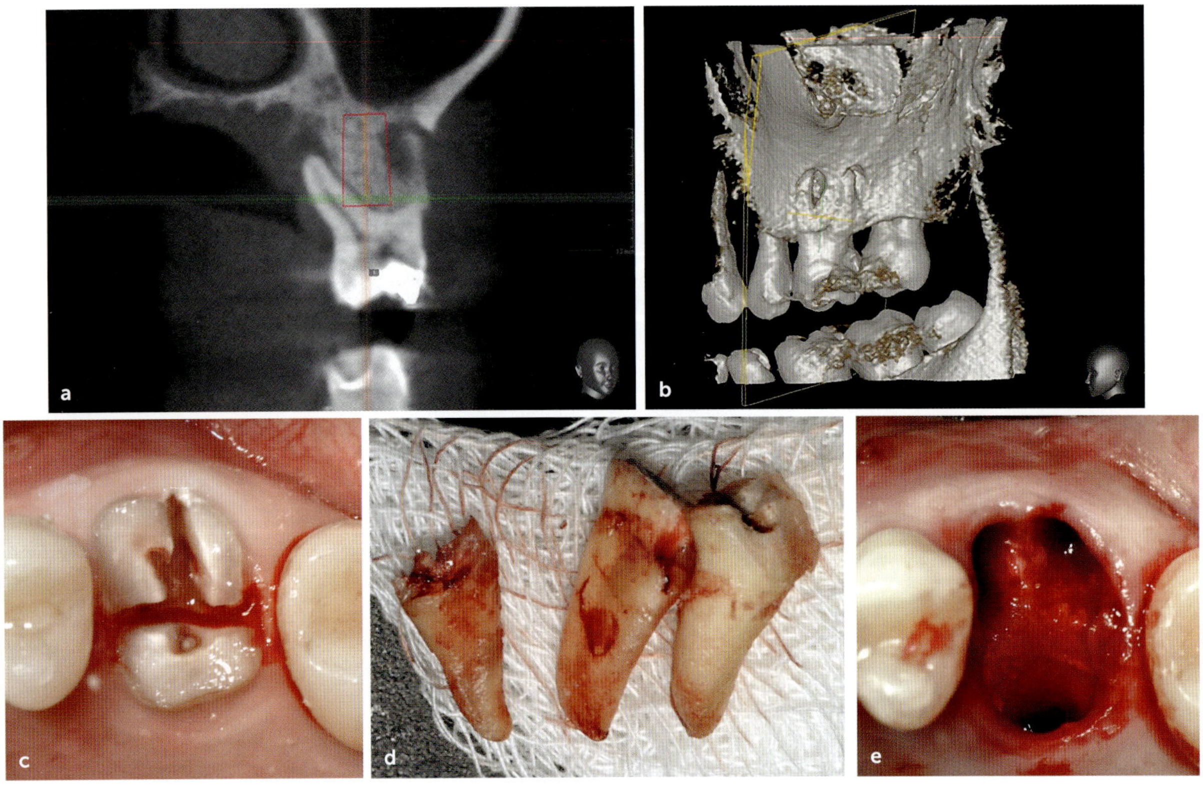

FIG 7-7 *(a)* The maxillary left first molar showed periapical infection with extensive bone loss buccally and palatally. *(b)* This 3D image confirms loss of buccal bone at the apices of the roots of the first molar. *(c)* The tooth was decoronated and sectioned to allow removal of each of the three roots separately. *(d)* The three roots were removed intact without raising a mucoperiosteal flap. *(e)* After removal of the roots, a type A IRS remained, with its narrowest diameter being 4 mm and with intact socket soft tissue walls. →

Case 2: Maxillary molar with type A socket

A second case shows the management of a type A maxillary IRS[38] at a left first molar site in a 53-year-old nonsmoker with no significant medical history. The tooth was nonvital with a large periapical abscess as well as buccal and palatal bone loss (Figs 7-7a and 7-7b). Possible treatment options (all with extraction of the tooth) were discussed, and the patient opted for an IMI. The implant chosen was a 10 × 4.5–mm Anyridge (MegaGen) implant. The tooth was decoronated using a high-speed bur and sectioned at the level of its furcation to allow separation of the three roots for individual removal atraumatically (Figs 7-7c and 7-7d). No soft tissue flap was elevated. Once the tooth roots had been removed, a large type A IRS remained, with its narrowest diameter being 4 mm (Fig 7-7e).

Osseodensification was planned to preserve and expand the septum, and the osteotomy was begun using a 1.6-mm-diameter pilot drill in cutting mode (Fig 7-7f). The drilling depth was 10 mm. Unlike the situation in the mandible, where the bone is generally denser, there is no need to drill to a deeper depth than the actual implant length being used in the posterior maxilla. Densification then was begun using the bur VT1525 (2.0) in reverse mode followed by a periapical radiograph that confirmed close proximity to the sinus floor (Fig 7-7g). Further development of the osteotomy was achieved using Densah burs VT2535 (3.0), VT2838 (3.3 mm), and VT3545 (4.0) all to the same depth of 10 mm (Fig 7-7h). A torqueing force of 40 Ncm was required to seat the implant (Fig 7-7i), and a subsequent radiograph confirmed that the sinus floor had not been breached (Fig 7-7j). While some clinicians[46] consider grafting of gaps around an IMI placed in a type A IRS to be unnecessary, the treating clinician elected to place an allograft mixture of 70% cancellous and 30% cortical bone particles (Fig 7-7k). Because the implant had an ITV of 40 Ncm and ISQ value of 77, it was decided to place an immediate custom chairside provisional composite crown to

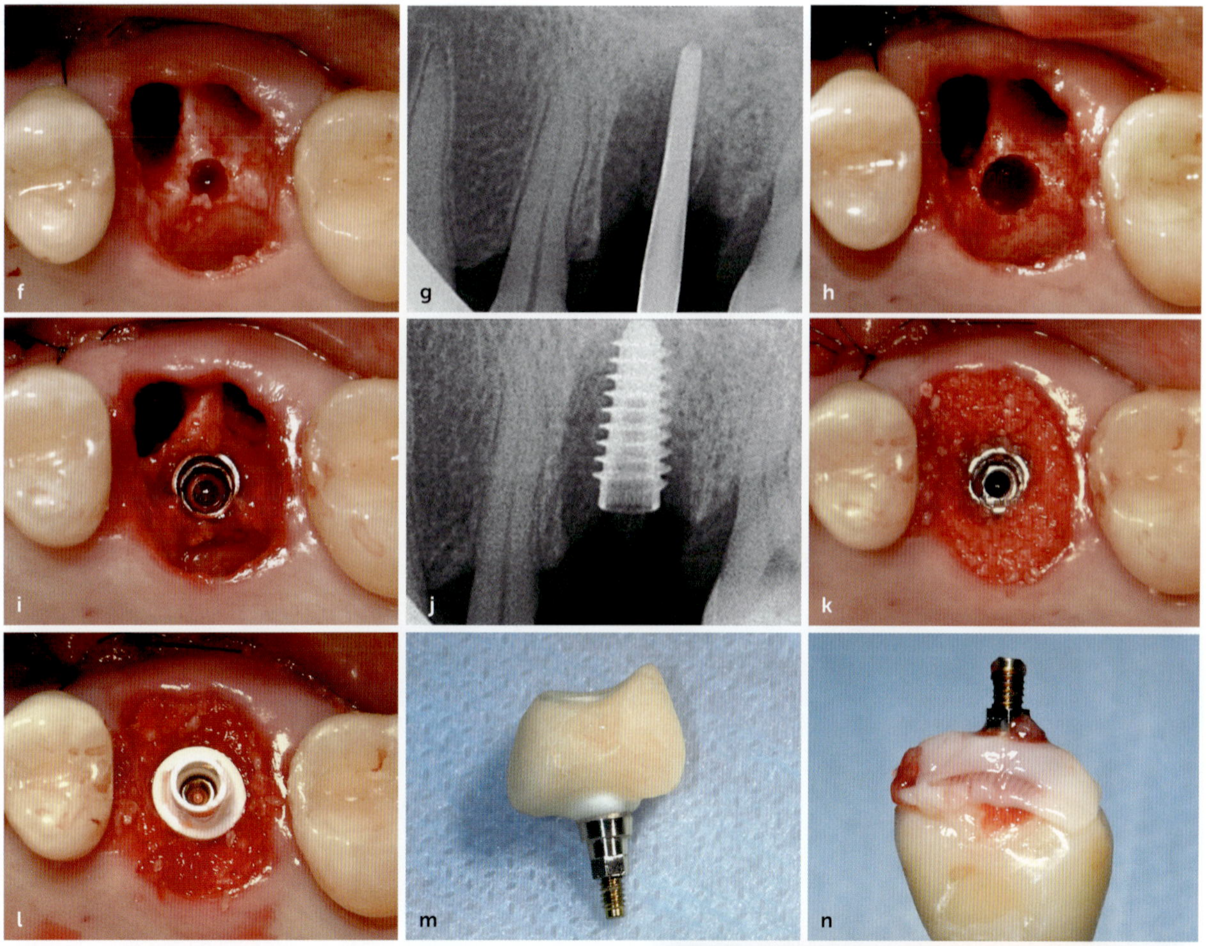

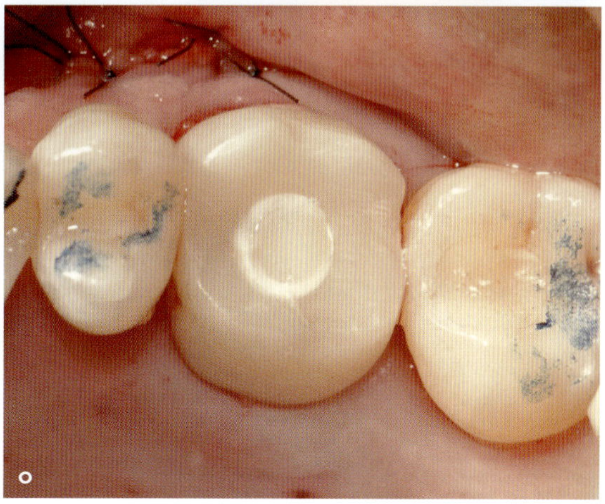

FIG 7-7 *(cont) (f)* A pilot drill was used to establish the initial osteotomy depth of 10 mm. *(g)* A radiograph taken after using the first densification bur confirmed that the sinus floor remained intact. *(h)* After using the required sequence of densifying burs, the osteotomy was seen to have been expanded and fully contained in the type A IRS. *(i)* The insertion torque required to seat the 10 × 5-mm implant was 40 Ncm. *(j)* A radiograph taken after implant insertion confirmed ideal positioning for a molar crown. *(k)* Allograft was placed in the peri-implant gaps with slight overfill to compensate for possible shrinkage during healing. *(l)* The implant had an insertion torque of 40 Ncm and ISQ value of 77, and with this degree of stability, it was decided to place an immediate custom chairside fully contoured composite healing abutment. *(m)* The healing abutment was fabricated and adjusted to allow for immediate, nonocclusal loading while protecting the graft material. *(n)* An autogenous PRF clot that had been prepared from the patient's venous blood was stretched over the retention screw and base of the restoration as a biologic seal between the graft particles and the restoration.[44] *(o)* The fully contoured custom healing abutment was adjusted to experience nonocclusal loading only.

support soft tissue healing and deliver some nonocclusal loading to accelerate bone healing.[47,48] When the custom healing abutment was ready for insertion, a PRF clot prepared from the patient's venous blood was skewered over the crown retention screw and the latter screwed into place[45] (Figs 7-7l to 7-7o). After 3 months of healing (Figs 7-7p to 7-7r), implant stability was recorded as ISQ 81, and 1 month later, the definitive restoration was placed (Figs 7-7s and 7-7t). Both clinical and radiographic images of the implant and crown can be seen after 3 years in function in Figs 7-7u and 7-7v.

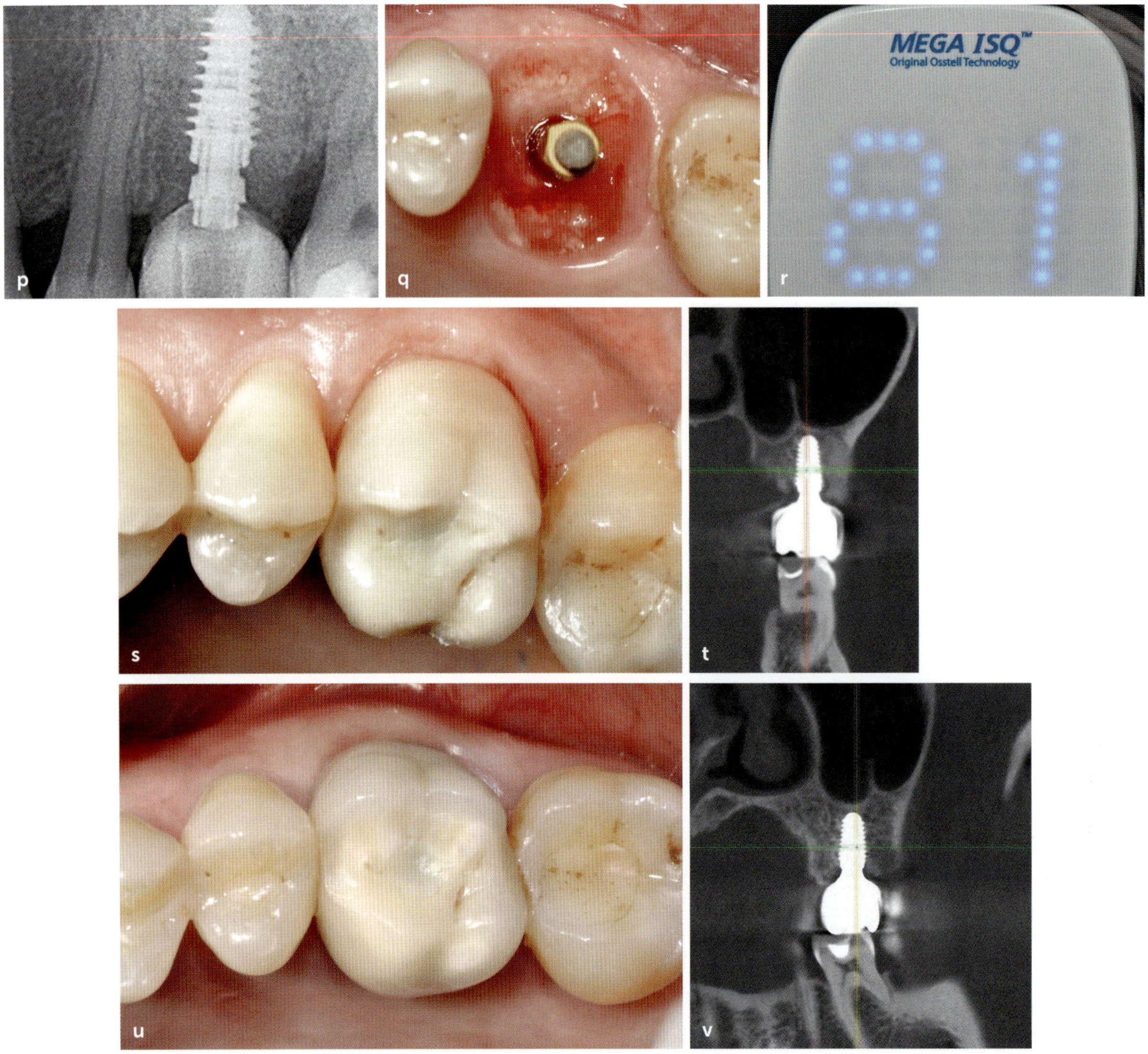

FIG 7-7 *(cont) (p)* The immediate postoperative radiograph shows the healing abutment fully seated and contouring the allograft particles. *(q and r)* After 3 months of healing, implant stability was recorded as ISQ 81, and 1 month later, the definitive restoration was placed. *(s)* The final implant crown was delivered after 4 months of site healing. *(t)* This CBCT image shows the implant at the crown delivery date. *(u)* A clinical photograph of the implant crown after 3 years in function. *(v)* A CBCT scan taken after 3 years in function shows an excellent bony housing and stable crestal bone level.

Case 3: Type B mandibular molar septum

This patient was a 68-year-old man with no significant medical history who presented with nonrestorable recurrent decay under the crown of the mandibular left first molar (Fig 7-8a). The existing crown was easily removed (Fig 7-8b), and the two roots were separated and removed atraumatically (Fig 7-8c). The type B IRS was converted to type A using Densah burs (Fig 7-8d). Following insertion of a 10 × 4.8-mm Straumann Tissue Level implant (Fig 7-8e), any remaining gaps were filled with particulate allograft subsequently covered with a collagen dressing (Collagen Repair Patch, Zimmer Biomet) and insertion of a large-diameter healing abutment (PEEK tissue former,

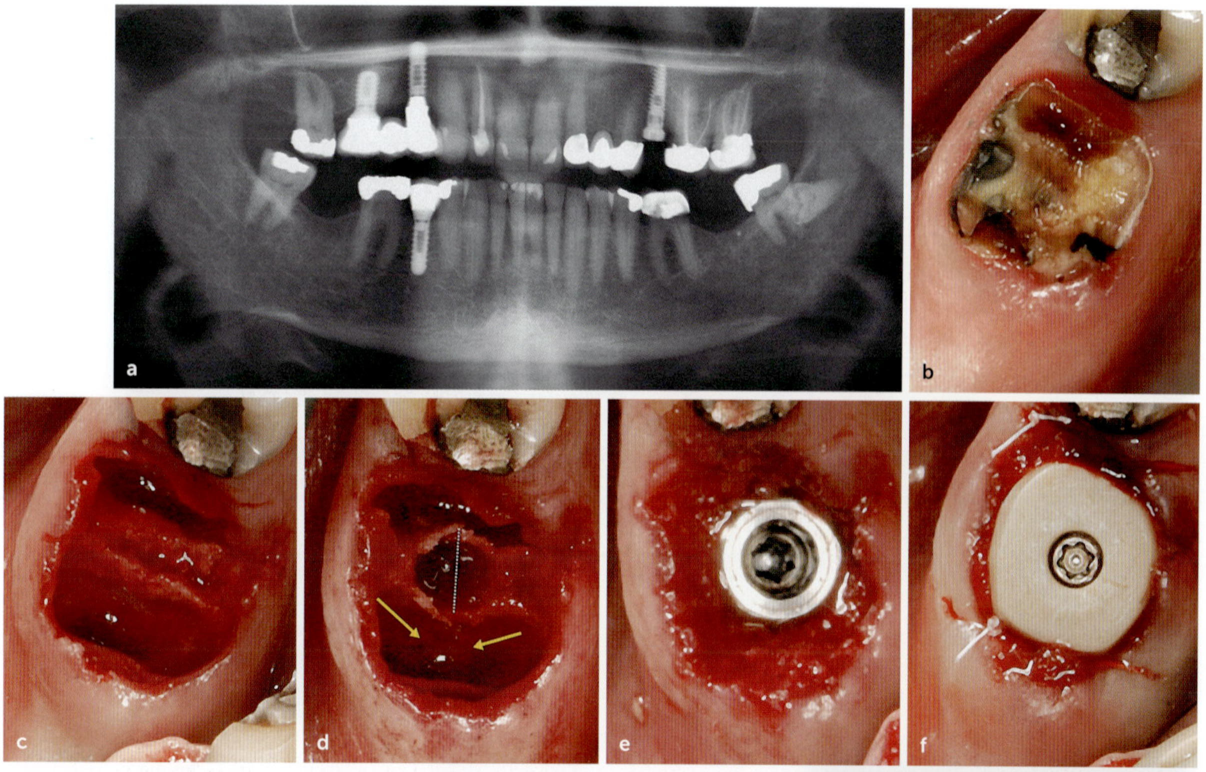

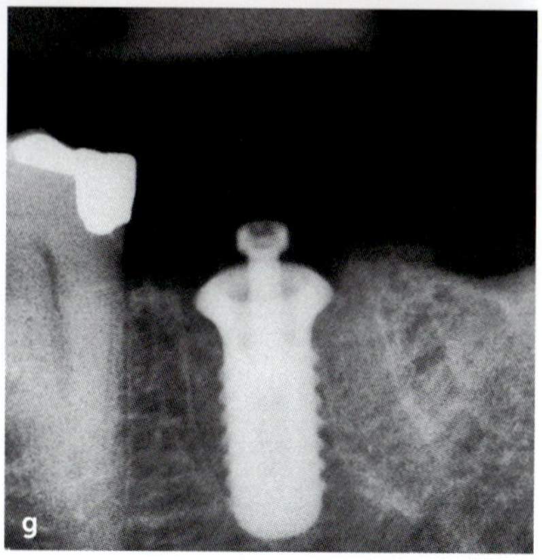

FIG 7-8 *(a)* The preoperative panoramic radiograph confirmed the presence of advanced recurrent decay under the crown of the mandibular left first molar. *(b)* The clinical state of the tooth after crown removal. *(c)* A type B septum (3.5-mm width mesiodistally) was preserved following removal of the two roots. *(d)* The original type B IRS was converted to a type A one (4.5-mm width mesiodistally) using osseodensification with a sequence of burs to a depth of 11.5 mm as follows: A 1.6-mm diameter pilot bur in CW mode; Densah bur VT1525 (2.0) in CCW mode; Densah bur VT1828 (2.3) in CCW mode; Densah bur VT2535 (3.0) in CCW mode; Densah bur VT2838 (3.3) in CCW mode; and Densah bur VT3545 (4.0) in CCW mode. Because of the small increases in Densah burs and osteotomy diameter, the expanding IRS remained intact throughout. *(e)* The chosen implant (10 × 4.8–mm Straumann Tissue Level) was successfully inserted with its coronal aspect completely surrounded with septal bone. *(f)* Following gap grafting with a covering of a resorbable collagen dressing, a large-diameter healing abutment was connected to the implant and two interproximal sutures used to stabilize the papillae. *(g)* The immediate postoperative radiograph.

Straumann; Fig 7-8f) The immediate postoperative radiograph with a connected healing abutment can be seen in Fig 7-8g.

After 3 months of site healing, the healing abutment was replaced with a porcelain-fused-to-metal definitive restoration (Figs 7-8h and 7-8i). Figures 7-8j to 7-8l show the clinical and radiographic status of the implant after 5 years in clinical function.

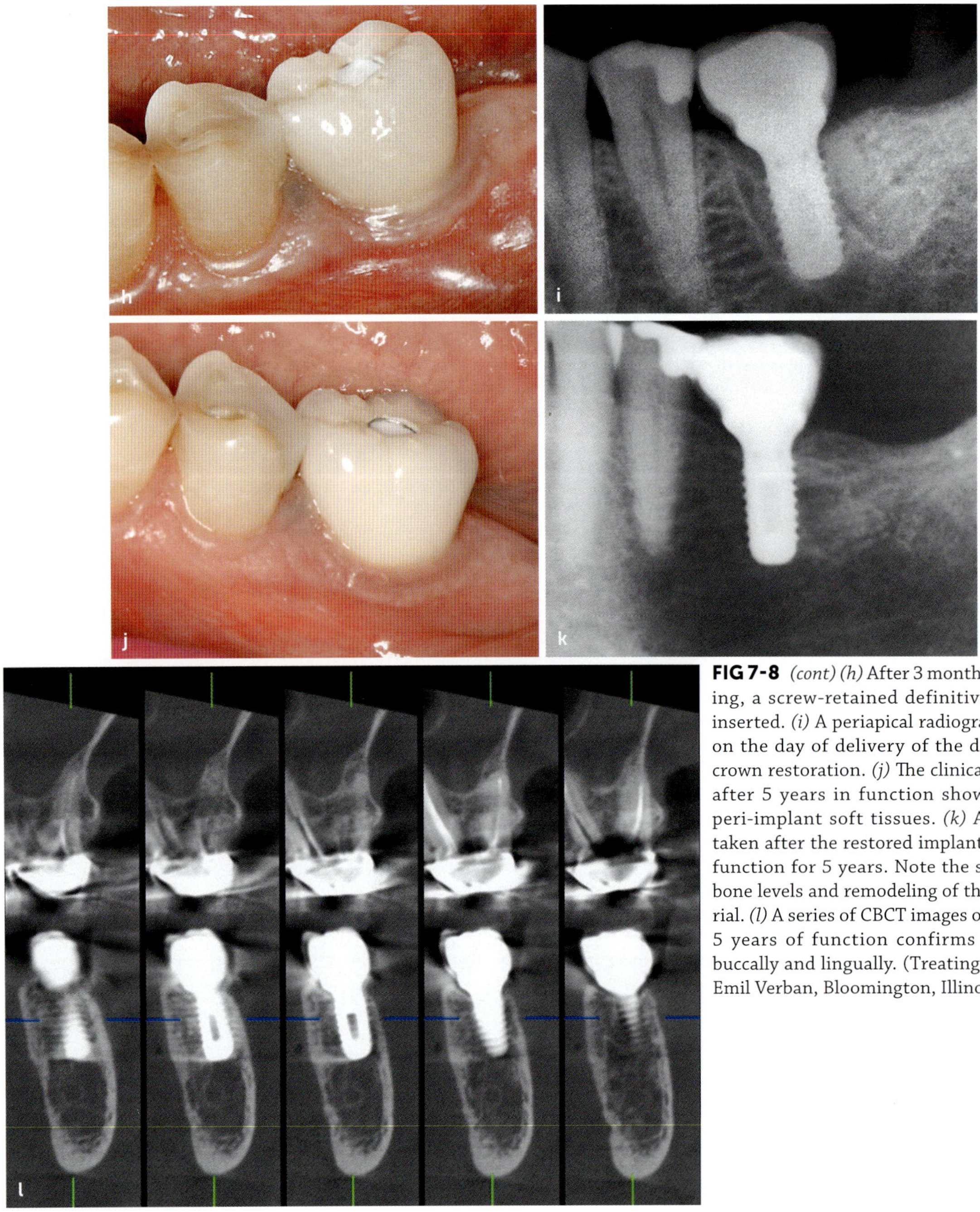

FIG 7-8 *(cont) (h)* After 3 months of site healing, a screw-retained definitive crown was inserted. *(i)* A periapical radiograph obtained on the day of delivery of the definitive full crown restoration. *(j)* The clinical appearance after 5 years in function showing healthy peri-implant soft tissues. *(k)* A radiograph taken after the restored implant had been in function for 5 years. Note the stable crestal bone levels and remodeling of the graft material. *(l)* A series of CBCT images obtained after 5 years of function confirms stable bone buccally and lingually. (Treating clinician: Dr Emil Verban, Bloomington, Illinois.)

Case 4: Maxillary type A septum management, including simultaneous minor sinus floor elevation

The final case is that of an IMI treatment in a healthy patient who presented with a hopeless maxillary right first molar due to a fracture and periapical lesion (Figs 7-9a and 7-9b). The treatment planned was to extract the tooth without raising a flap and develop the osteotomy in the remaining type A IRS along with a simultaneous indirect/transcrestal sinus elevation using osseodensification burs and an established protocol.

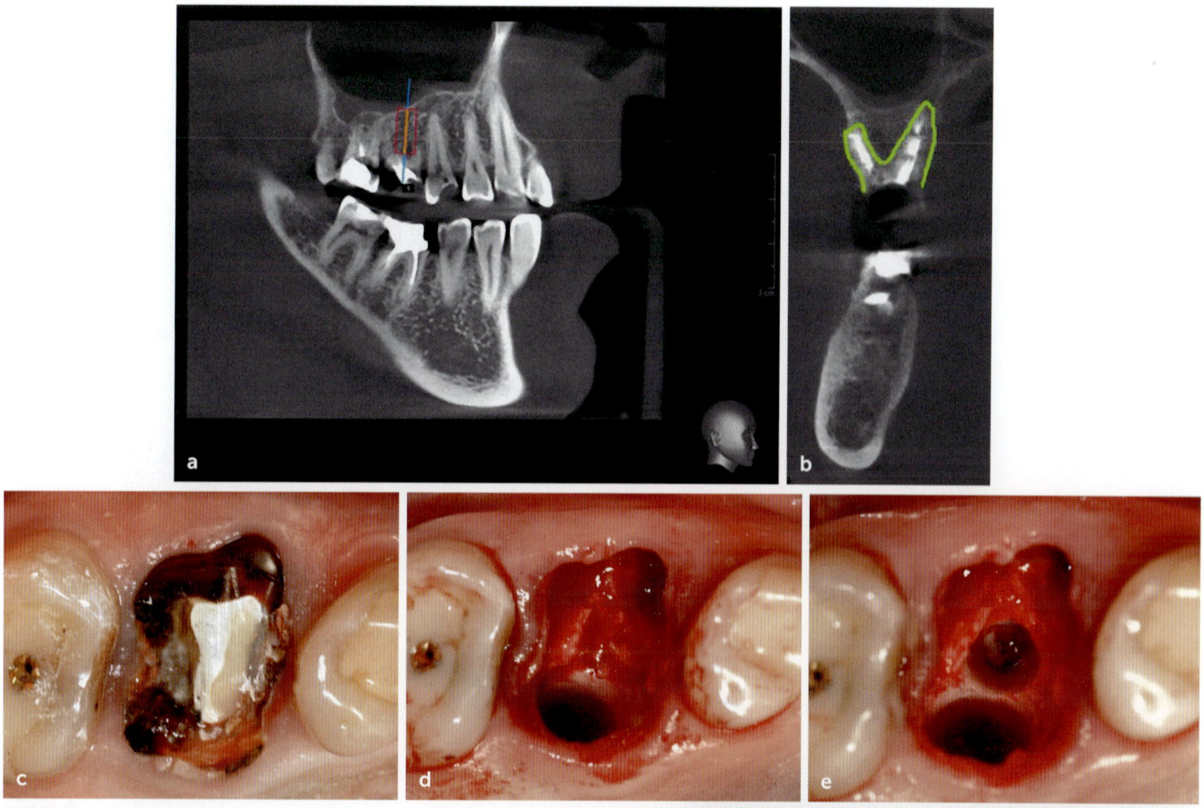

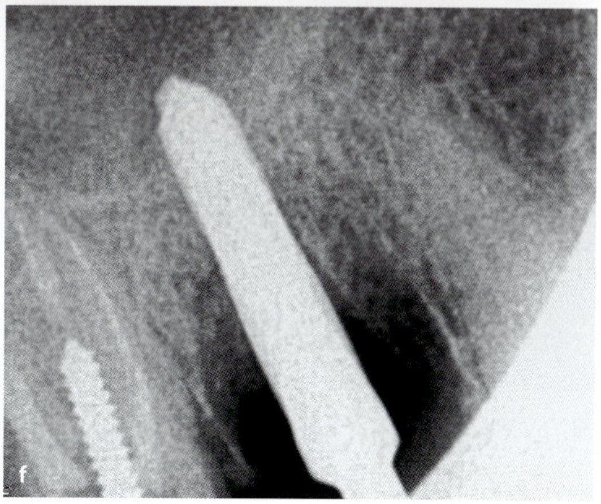

FIG 7-9 *(a)* The patient's maxillary right first molar was deemed hopeless, and plans were made to place a 10 × 5-mm IMI along with simultaneous localized indirect sinus floor elevation. *(b)* The pretreatment CBCT scan showed the presence of a type A septum with good width and 7 mm of crestal bone height below the sinus floor. *(c)* The maxillary right first molar required extraction. *(d)* Following flapless, atraumatic extraction of the three roots, a large type A septum was retained. The septum had a minimum diameter of 5 mm. *(e)* The final osteotomy was completely contained within the septal bone. Note the sinus membrane with autograft. *(f)* Because a 5-mm-diameter implant was planned, the final drilling was done by bur VT3848, leaving the osteotomy slightly undersized. The sinus floor was intentionally breached with bur VT2535 (3.0) used in CCW mode to a total depth of 10 mm. This radiograph shows the depth of penetration of the final bur VT3848 (4.3) extending 3 mm into the sinus domain. Autogenous bone shavings have been pushed apically by the CCW action of the burs, elevating the sinus floor by approximately 3 mm.

The chosen implant (NeoBiotech IS II Active) was 10 × 5 mm. The CBCT scan indicated that in order to place a 10 × 5–mm implant, approximately 3 mm of sinus floor elevation would be needed, and the plan was to accomplish this using the densification burs. The tooth presented as shown in Fig 7-9c. Following sectioning, the tooth roots were removed separately and atraumatically with preservation of the type A septum (Fig 7-9d). Site preparation began using a pilot bur in cutting mode to a depth of approximately 6 mm, ie, about 1 mm short of the sinus floor. Next, the Densah bur VT1525 (2.0) was used in CCW mode to a depth of 7 mm. At this point, the Densah bur VT2535 (3.0) was used in CCW mode to cut through the sinus floor to a final depth of 10 mm. Following this, the Densah burs VT3545 (4.0) and VT3848 (4.3) were used in CCW mode to the same depth (10 mm), and the completed osteotomy remained contained entirely within septal bone (Figs 7-9e and 7-9f).

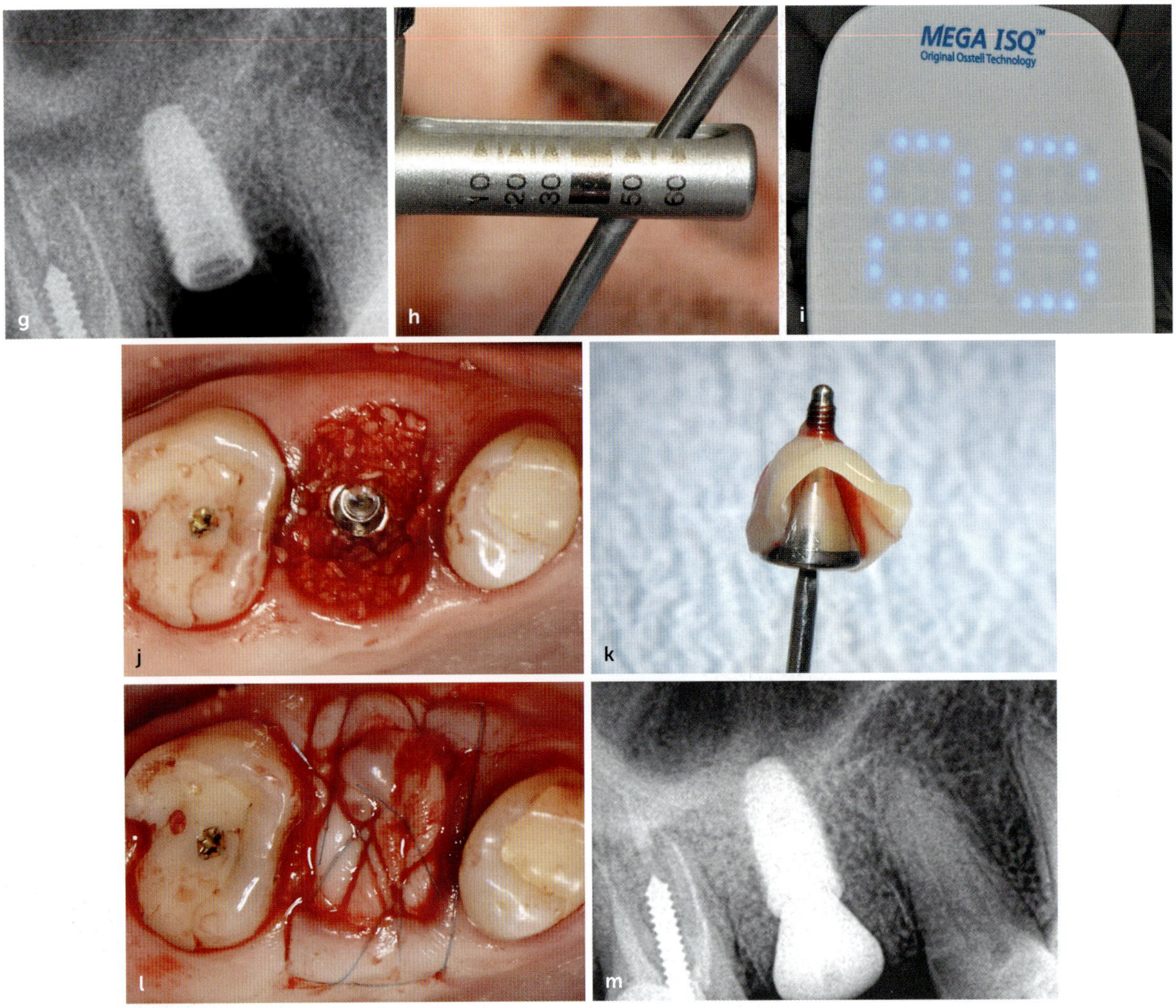

FIG 7-9 *(cont) (g)* A 10 × 5–mm implant was placed with 3 mm of its apex extending into the sinus domain, but surrounded by autogenous bone pushed upward by the osseodensification burs used in CCW mode. *(h and i)* A torquing force of 50 Ncm and ISQ value of 86 were required to fully seat the NeoBiotech IS II Active implant. *(j)* The peri-implant gaps were filled with particulate allograft material to be covered by a PRF clot. *(k)* An autogenous PRF clot was skewered over the low-profile wide healing abutment screw before the screw was connected to the implant. *(l)* Once the healing abutment was fully seated, a second autologous fibrin clot secured with sutures was used to cover and seal the surgical site. *(m)* The immediate postoperative radiograph confirmed that a significant amount of autogenous bone had been pushed upward, lifting the sinus membrane and surrounding the 2 to 3 mm of implant apex protruding beyond the original sinus floor.

Following implant insertion (Fig 7-9g), which required a torquing force of 50 Ncm and ISQ value of 86 (Figs 7-9h and 7-9i), the peri-implant gaps were filled with particulate allograft (Fig 7-9j). An autologous PRF clot was skewered over the screw of the expanded healing cap (Fig 7-9k), which was then connected to the implant. Finally, a second fibrin clot was placed over the site and secured with sutures (Fig 7-9l). An immediate postoperative radiograph confirmed that the implant apex protruded up to 3 mm into the sinus, but the apex was separated from the sinus space by a dome of compacted autogenous bone shavings driven upward by the osseodensification procedure (Fig 7-9m).

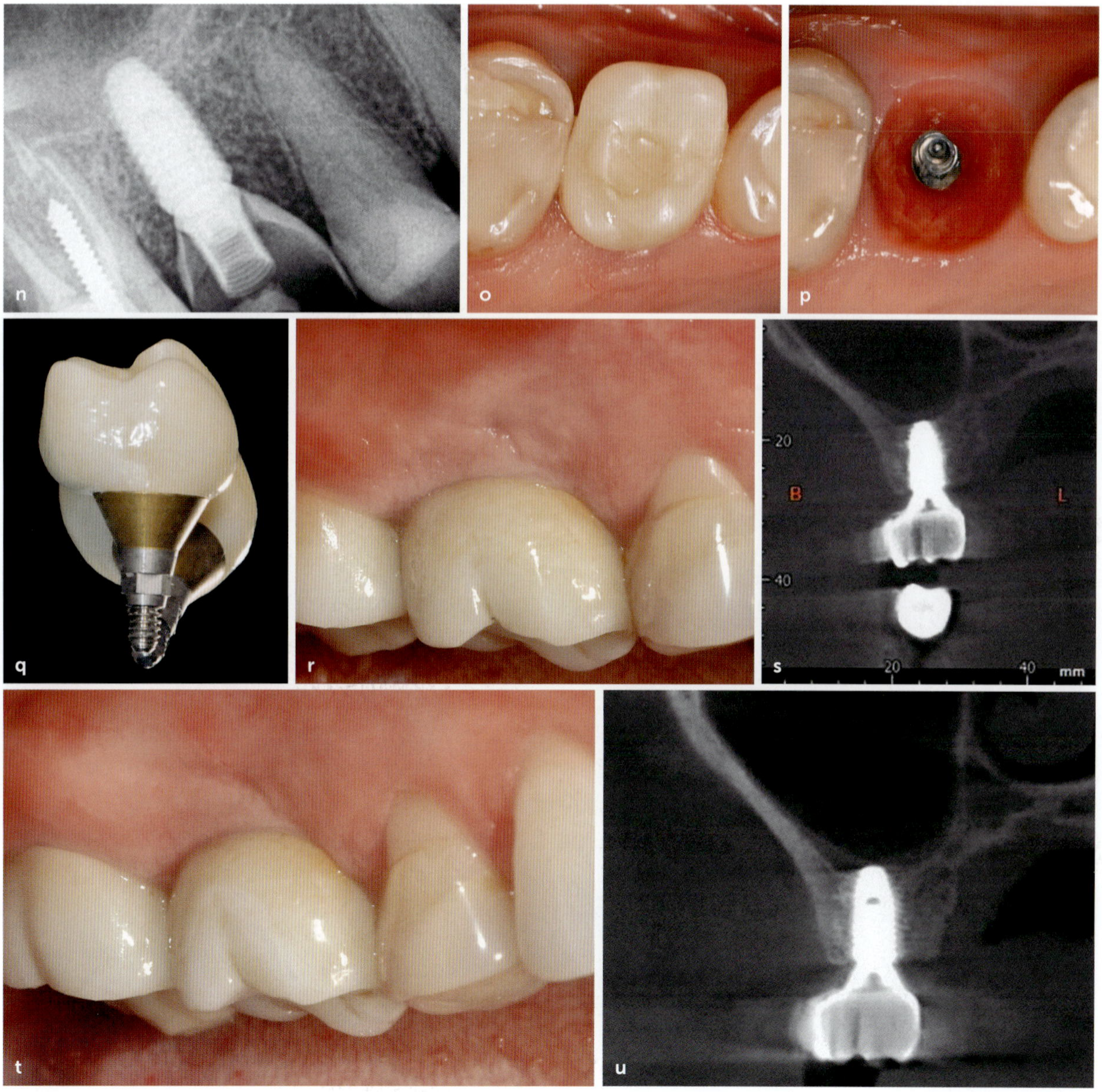

FIG 7-9 *(cont) (n)* A radiograph at 3 months shows the chairside custom provisional restoration meant to guide soft tissue healing in preparation for the definitive crown fabrication.[49] *(o)* The provisional restoration in position. *(p)* One month later, impressions were taken for the definitive restoration. *(q)* The definitive restoration was a porcelain-fused-to-metal screw-retained crown. *(r)* The definitive restoration at insertion. *(s)* A CBCT image taken at the time of crown insertion showing expansive bone supporting the implant. *(t)* The clinical condition of the definitive restoration after 30 months in function. *(u)* A CBCT scan obtained of the restored implant after 30 months in function. Note that significant new bone has formed around the implant apex.

After 3 months of site healing, the healing abutment was replaced with a chairside custom provisional crown to help shape the soft tissues prior to fabricating the definitive restoration (Figs 7-9n and 7-9o).[49] One month later (Fig 7-9p), the site was ready for an impression to be taken for the definitive crown (Figs 7-9q to 7-9s). The clinical status of the restoration after 30 months in function is shown is Fig 7-9t. Finally, the radiographic image after 30 months shows that new bone has formed around the implant apex (Fig 7-9u).

Conclusion

While the placement of IMIs is a difficult procedure, it is our contention that osseodensification is of benefit in expanding IRS bone to be able to position molar implants optimally while ensuring initial implant stability. Specific osseodensification protocols to use with most currently available endosseous dental implant devices have been developed and published. Osseodensification permits the plastic deformation of trabecular bone around molars in either jaw using outward strains and bone compaction. As a result, the osteotomy bony walls become denser due to the compaction-autografting and display an elastic "spring-back" effect, in both instances contributing to increased initial implant stability. Further, this lateral and apical compaction-grafting facilitates adequate molar septum expansion and crestal sinus grafting.

Acknowledgment

All images in this chapter are courtesy of Versah and used with permission.

KEY POINTS

- Sites with a thick gingival biotype are preferred, along with flapless surgery.
- Atraumatic tooth removal is crucial, meaning that the crown should first be removed with a high-speed handpiece, exposing the furcation and separating the tooth roots.
- Tooth roots should be removed individually before osteotomy preparation.
- Both type A and type B sockets can be used, and osteotomy preparation should be located centrally in the IRS, ie, in optimal prosthetic position.
- After use of a pilot bur in CW mode, further site development should proceed using densification burs in CCW mode with progressive small increases in bur diameter to enhance bone plasticity and not to overstress the osteotomy walls.
- A constant, well-controlled "bouncing" motion of the handpiece/bur and copious saline irrigation should be used within the developing osteotomy.
- In the mandible only, the osteotomy depth should be 1 mm deeper than the intended implant length to accommodate the bone shavings being propelled apically.
- Good initial implant stability is crucial to success.
- If up to 3 mm of transcrestal sinus floor elevation is needed, this can be done using the densification burs without added graft materials. Allograft materials can be added to facilitate additional crestal elevation.
- The decision whether or not to graft peri-implant gaps should be made by the treating clinician, recognizing that its necessity in < 2-mm gaps is presently controversial.
- A large-diameter healing abutment or custom chairside provisional restoration should be used to cover the peri-implant gaps, whether grafted or not.

References

1. Dawson A, Chen S (eds). The SAC Classification in Implant Dentistry. Berlin: Quintessence, 2009.
2. Jemt T, Olsson M, Renouard F, Stenport V, Friberg B. Early implant failures related to individual surgeons: An analysis covering 11,074 operations performed during 28 years. Clin Implant Dent Relat Res 2016;18:861–872.
3. Atieh MA, Payne AG, Duncan WJ, de Silva RK, Cullinan MP. Immediate placement or immediate restoration/loading of single implants for molar tooth replacement: A systematic review and meta-analysis. Int J Oral Maxillofac Implants 2010;25:401–415.
4. Ketabi M, Deporter D, Atenafu EG. A systematic review of outcomes following immediate molar implant placement based on recently published studies. Clin Implant Dent Relat Res 2016; 18:1084–1094.
5. Lang NP, Pun L, Lau KY, Li KY, Wong MC. A systematic review on survival and success rates of implants placed immediately into fresh extraction sockets after at least 1 year. Clin Oral Implants Res 2012;23(suppl 5):39–66.
6. Esposito M, Grusovin MG, Polyzos IP, Felice P, Worthington HV. Interventions for replacing missing teeth: Dental implants in fresh extraction sockets (immediate, immediate-delayed and delayed implants). Cochrane Database Syst Rev 2010:CD005968.
7. Trisi P, Perfetti G, Baldoni E, Berardi D, Colagiovanni M, Scogna G. Implant micromotion is related to peak insertion torque and bone density. Clin Oral Implants Res 2009;20:467–471.
8. Trisi P, Berardini M, Falco A, Podaliri Vulpiani M. Validation of value of actual micromotion as a direct measure of implant micromobility after healing (secondary implant stability). An in vivo histologic and biomechanical study. Clin Oral Implants Res 2016;27:1423–1430.
9. Gehrke SA, da Silva Neto UT, Rossetti PH, Watinaga SE, Giro G, Shibli JA. Stability of implants placed in fresh sockets versus healed alveolar sites: Early findings. Clin Oral Implants Res 2016; 27:577–582.
10. Walker LR, Morris GA, Novotny PJ. Implant insertional torque values predict outcomes. J Oral Maxillofac Surg 2011;69:1344–1349.
11. Atieh MA, Alsabeeha NH, Duncan WJ, et al. Immediate single implant restorations in mandibular molar extraction sockets: A controlled clinical trial. Clin Oral Implants Res 2013;24:484–496.
12. Iacono VJ, Cochran DL. State of the science on implant dentistry: A workshop developed using an evidence-based approach [published correction appears in Int J Oral Maxillofac Implants 2008;23:56]. Int J Oral Maxillofac Implants 2007;(22 suppl): 7–10.
13. Hayacibara RM, Gonçalves CS, Garcez-Filho J, Magro-Filho O, Esper H, Hayacibara MF. The success rate of immediate implant placement of mandibular molars: A clinical and radiographic retrospective evaluation between 2 and 8 years. Clin Oral Implants Res 2013;24:806–811.
14. Crespi R, Capparè P, Gherlone EF. Electrical mallet in implants placed in fresh extraction sockets with simultaneous osteotome sinus floor elevation. Int J Oral Maxillofac Implants 2013;28: 869–874.
15. Acocella A, Bertolai R, Sacco R. Modified insertion technique for immediate implant placement into fresh extraction socket in the first maxillary molar sites: A 3-year prospective study. Implant Dent 2010;19:220–228.
16. Fugazzotto PA. Implant placement at the time of maxillary molar extraction: Treatment protocols and report of results. J Periodontol 2008;79:216–223.
17. Bruschi GB, Crespi R, Capparè P, Bravi F, Bruschi E, Gherlone E. Localized management of sinus floor technique for implant placement in fresh molar sockets. Clin Implant Dent Relat Res 2013;15:243–250.
18. Ahn SH, Park EJ, Kim ES. Reamer-mediated transalveolar sinus floor elevation without osteotome and simultaneous implant placement in the maxillary molar area: Clinical outcomes of 391 implants in 380 patients. Clin Oral Implants Res 2012;23:866–872.
19. Kim JM, Sohn DS, Heo JU, et al. Minimally invasive sinus augmentation using ultrasonic piezoelectric vibration and hydraulic pressure: A multicenter retrospective study. Implant Dent 2012;21:536–542.
20. Hamouda NI, Mourad SI, El-Kenawy MH, Maria OM. Immediate implant placement into fresh extraction socket in the mandibular molar sites: A preliminary study of a modified insertion technique. Clin Implant Dent Relat Res 2015;(17 suppl 1):e107–e116.
21. Kurtzman GM, Luchetti CG, Kitrilakis AE, Ostrowicz DI. Immediate implant placement in maxillary molars using septa dilatation with threaded expanders: 3 years follow-up and use of the technique in complex cases. Int J Oral Implantol Clin Res 2012; 3:138–145.
22. Chen ST, Darby IB, Reynolds EC, Clement JG. Immediate implant placement postextraction without flap elevation. J Periodontol 2009;80:163–172.
23. Huwais S, Meyer EG. A novel osseous densification approach in implant osteotomy preparation to increase biomechanical primary stability, bone mineral density, and bone-to-implant contact. Int J Oral Maxillofac Implants 2017;32:27–36.
24. Slete FB, Olin P, Prasad H. Histomorphometric comparison of 3 osteotomy techniques. Implant Dent 2018;27:424–428.
25. Alifarag AM, Lopez CD, Neiva RF, Tovar N, Witek L, Coelho PG. Atemporal osseointegration: Early biomechanical stability through osseodensification. J Orthop Res 2018;36:2516–2523.
26. Green JR, Nemzek JA, Arnoczky SP, Johnson LL, Balas MS. The effect of bone compaction on early fixation of porous-coated implants. J Arthroplasty 1999;14:91–97.
27. Kold S, Bechtold JE, Ding M, Chareancholvanich K, Rahbek O, Søballe K. Compacted cancellous bone has a spring-back effect. Acta Orthop Scand 2003;74:591–595.
28. Trisi P, Berardini M, Falco A, Podaliri Vulpiani M. New osseodensification implant site preparation method to increase bone density in low-density bone: In vivo evaluation in sheep. Implant Dent 2016;25:24–31.
29. Koutouzis T, Huwais S, Hasan F, Trahan W, Waldrop T, Neiva R. Alveolar ridge expansion by osseodensification-mediated plastic deformation and compaction autografting: A multicenter retrospective study. Implant Dent 2019;28:349–355.
30. Neiva R, Tanello B, Duarte W, Coelho P, Witek L, Silva F. Effects of osseodensification on Astra TX and EV implant systems. Clin Oral Implants Res 2018;29(suppl 17):444.
31. Tanello B, Huwais S, Tawil I, Rosen P, Neiva R. Osseodensification protocols for enhancement of primary and secondary implant stability: A retrospective 5-year follow-up multi-center study. Clin Oral Implants Res 2019;30(suppl 19):414.
32. da Rosa JCM, Pértile de Oliveira Rosa AC, Huwais S. Use of the immediate dentoalveolar restoration technique combined with osseodensification in periodontally compromised extraction sites. Int J Periodontics Restorative Dent 2019;39:527–534.
33. Gaspar J, Esteves T, Gaspar R, Rua J, Mendes JJ. Osseodensification for implant site preparation in the maxilla: A prospective study of 97 implants. Clin Oral Implants Res 2018;29(suppl 17):163.

34. Aly A, Tahaa M, Toradb F, Sleema H. The effect of osseodensification technique on primary stability of dental implants. Egypt J Oral Maxillofac Surg 2019;10:123–128.
35. Huwais S, Mazor Z, Ioannou AL, Gluckman H, Neiva R. A multicenter retrospective clinical study with up-to-5-year follow-up utilizing a method that enhances bone density and allows for transcrestal sinus augmentation through compaction grafting. Int J Oral Maxillofac Implants 2018;33:1305–1311.
36. Kumar BT, Narayan V. Minimally invasive crestal approach sinus floor elevation using Densah burs, and Hydraulic lift utilising putty graft in cartridge delivery. Clin Oral Implants Res 2017; 28(suppl 14):203.
37. Froum S, Casanova L, Byrne S, Cho SC. Risk assessment before extraction for immediate implant placement in the posterior mandible: A computerized tomographic scan study. J Periodontol 2011;82:395–402.
38. Smith RB, Tarnow DP. Classification of molar extraction sites for immediate dental implant placement: Technical note. Int J Oral Maxillofac Implants 2013;28:911–916.
39. Sharma SD, Vidya B, Alexander M, Deshmukh S. Periotome as an aid to atraumatic extraction: A comparative double blind randomized controlled trial. J Maxillofac Oral Surg 2015;14: 611–615.
40. Blus C, Szmukler-Moncler S. Atraumatic tooth extraction and immediate implant placement with Piezosurgery: Evaluation of 40 sites after at least 1 year of loading. Int J Periodontics Restorative Dent 2010;30:355–363.
41. Ragucci GM, Elnayef B, Criado-Cámara E, Del Amo FS, Hernández-Alfaro F. Immediate implant placement in molar extraction sockets: A systematic review and meta-analysis. Int J Implant Dent 2020;6:40.
42. Vandeweghe S, Hattingh A, Wennerberg A, Bruyn HD. Surgical protocol and short-term clinical outcome of immediate placement in molar extraction sockets using a wide body implant. J Oral Maxillofac Res 2011;2:e1.
43. Miron RJ, Zucchelli G, Pikos MA, et al. Use of platelet-rich fibrin in regenerative dentistry: A systematic review. Clin Oral Investig 2017;21:1913–1927.
44. Bleyan S, Gaspar J, Huwais S, et al. Molar septum expansion with osseodensification for immediate implant placement. Retrospective multicenter study with up-to-5-year follow-up, introducing a new molar socket classification. J Funct Biomater 2021;12:66.
45. Sohn DS, Huang B, Kim J, Park I, Park CC. Utilization of autologous concentrated growth factors (CGF) enriched bone graft matrix (sticky bone) and CGF-enriched fibrin membrane in implant dentistry. J Implant Adv Clin Dent 2015;7(10):11–29.
46. Smith RB, Tarnow DP, Sarnachiaro G. Immediate placement of dental implants in molar extraction sockets: An 11-year retrospective analysis. Compend Contin Educ Dent 2019;40:166–170.
47. Sommer M, Zimmermann J, Grize L, Stübinger S. Marginal bone loss one year after implantation: A systematic review of different loading protocols. Int J Oral Maxillofac Surg 2020;49: 121–134.
48. Wazen RM, Currey JA, Guo H, Brunski JB, Helms JA, Nanci A. Micromotion-induced strain fields influence early stages of repair at bone-implant interfaces. Acta Biomater 2013;9:6663–6674.
49. Beretta M, Poli PP, Pieriboni S, et al. Peri-implant soft tissue conditioning by means of customized healing abutment: A randomized controlled clinical trial. Materials (Basel) 2019;12:3041.

8

ULTRA-WIDE IMMEDIATE MOLAR IMPLANTS

Andre Hattingh
Andrew Ackermann

An important consideration in treatment planning for immediate implant placement in molar extraction sockets is whether the site will allow adequate primary stability to be achieved. In this regard, wider-diameter implants may offer an advantage in molar sockets with minimal to no interradicular septum (IRS) bone. Furthermore, wider implants may allow for more favorable emergence profiles for molar crown restorations and reduce the impact of functional stresses at the bone-to-implant interface in the crestal region,[1] particularly if platform switching is employed.[2,3] While most implant manufacturers now provide implants of 5 mm in diameter, one implant manufacturer offers molar-specific implants in "ultra-wide" diameters (ie, up to 9 mm) with a strongly tapered configuration.

The original Brånemark-type endosseous implant with a "wide" (ie, 5 or 5.5 mm) diameter was designed for use as a "rescue" implant to replace those of standard diameter that had failed.[4] However, when these wider-diameter implants were used more generally, the early results were not promising. For example, in a retrospective report from the first Brånemark implant study in North America (the "Toronto Study"), Attard and Zarb[5] reported up to 15-year data that showed a significant negative impact of increased implant diameter. By 5 years in function, standard-diameter Brånemark-type implants had a 95% survival compared to 76% survival for 5-mm-diameter implants. The investigators also reported poor survival of short (ie, 7-mm) implants in the same patient group. Similar poor outcomes with the same wide implant had earlier been published by Eckert et al,[6] with 19% failure in the posterior mandible and 29% in the posterior maxilla. In retrospect, however, these high failure rates with 5-mm-diameter implants, as well as those with short implants reported by Attard and Zarb, were likely due to inexperience and inappropriate surgical techniques.[7] In addition, poor site selection, eg, placing wide implants in alveolar bone of insufficient buccolingual/palatal width to avoid engagement of the

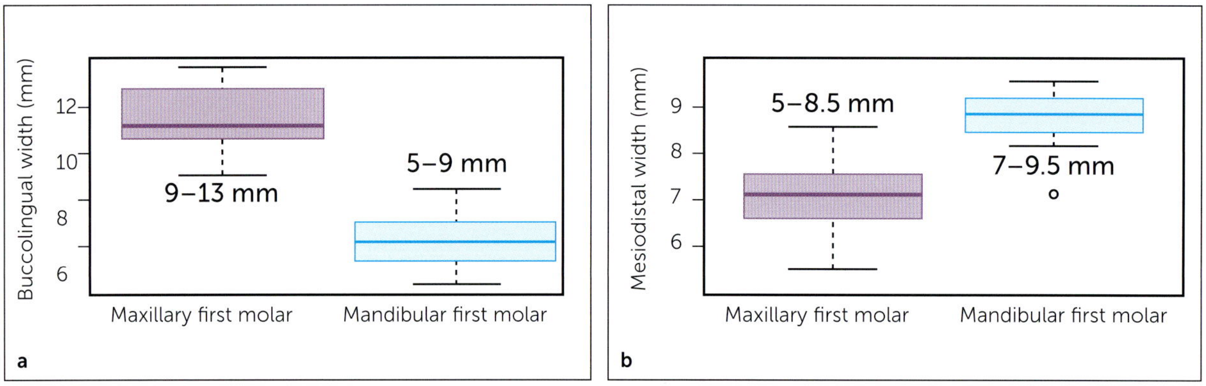

FIG 8-1 Typical buccolingual *(a)* and mesiodistal *(b)* widths of maxillary and mandibular first molars.[11]

buccal bone during implant insertion, likely resulted in further negative consequences during site remodeling.[8] Moderately rough–surfaced[9] (eg, particle-blasted and/or acid-treated) wide-diameter implants led to far better outcomes. For example, Bornstein et al[10] reported that only one such implant of 151 placed in partially edentulous individuals failed (success rate of 99.3%). Adapted drilling protocols also may have played a role here.

The MAX Implant

The original molar-specific ultra-wide-diameter threaded and tapered dental implant was developed in South Africa (MAX implant; Southern Implants) and was intended to be used primarily as an immediate molar implant (IMI). A micro-CT study measured the mesiodistal and buccolingual dimensions of maxillary and mandibular molars at different levels (Fig 8-1).[11] The mesiodistal widths of maxillary first molars typically range from 5.47 to 8.56 mm (mean: 7.05 mm), while their buccopalatal widths have a range of 9.51 to 13.33 mm (mean: 11.58 mm). Mean buccolingual dimensions of mandibular first molars are 7.24 mm, while their mesiodistal widths are around 8.80 mm. These measurements are in agreement with previous references to the cervical dimensions of human molars.[12]

Accordingly, the MAX implant was created with diameters originally ranging from 7 to 9 mm, but it is now also available with a diameter of 6 mm (Fig 8-2). The MAX implant has a sharply tapered body, which has several advantages, including the ability to achieve excellent primary stability, conservation of bone more apically, reduced risk of perforating into a lingual undercut in mandible, and minimizing risk of damaging adjacent tooth roots. The apex also has a benign, rounded shape to reduce the risk of rupturing the sinus membrane should the implant advance beyond the sinus floor during seating. A built-in platform-switch feature is provided to minimize crestal bone loss after restoration and loading. Ultra-wide-diameter implants also will eliminate the risk of implant fracture due to the high biomechanical loads experienced at molar sites, a concern with implants of diameters less than 5 mm used as molar replacments.[13–17] The wider prosthetic platform allows for more natural emergence profiles of molar crowns, thereby markedly reducing the risk of lateral food impaction/entrapment, a reason for patient dissatisfaction with molar implant restorations,[18] and caries risk at adjacent teeth.[19] Because of the considerable increase in surface area with wider bodies, the implant was offered only in lengths of 7, 9, and 11 mm.

Literature review

The first report with this device was that of Vandeweghe et al.[20] Forty-seven implants with diameters of 8 or 9 mm were placed as IMIs in 38 patients and followed for a mean period of 20 months before publication of the results. Implant success was reported as 97.9% with only 0.38 mm (range of 0.50 to 1.95 mm) mean crestal bone loss. A subsequent report[21] disclosed outcomes from a multicenter study in which 93 ultra-wide-diameter implants (59 in the posterior

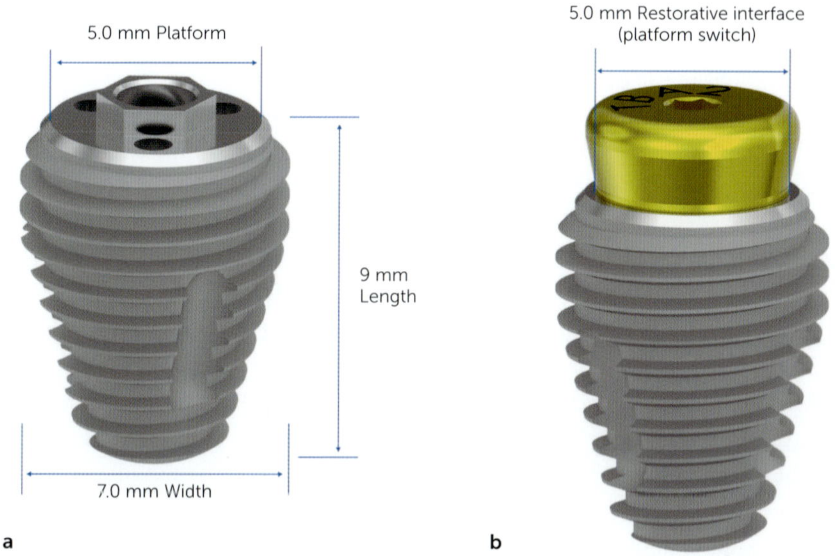

FIG 8-2 *(a)* Sample dimensions of an ultra-wide MAX implant (9 × 7 mm). *(b)* MAX implant (9 × 7 mm) with a healing abutment demonstrating the built-in platform-switch feature.

maxilla and 34 in the posterior mandible) had been placed in 75 patients. Unfortunately, patients were not all treated similarly. Twenty-seven implants were placed immediately into molar extraction sockets, while two were placed in healed sites, and all 29 were loaded immediately. Meanwhile, another 42 implants placed immediately into extraction sockets and 22 placed in mature bone were loaded in a delayed protocol (3 months postimplantation). The mean follow-up was 14 months (range of 6 to 34), by which time four implants (4.3%) had been lost, all before loading. Based on the criteria that crestal bone loss should be less than 1.5 mm at 1 year in function, another four implants were considered failures, giving an overall success rate of 91.4%. Implant survival rates were similar for immediate versus delayed implant placement (both close to 96%), but dropped to 89.7% when they had been immediately loaded.

Atieh et al[22] published less favorable results after using the MAX as an immediate replacement for mandibular molars. In their relatively small study, 24 MAX implants of 8- or 9-mm-diameter were placed either immediately or after extraction site healing, and all were loaded with provisional crowns within 48 hours to be restored with definitive crowns after only 8 weeks of healing. The overall implant success rate for both groups at 1 year was 75%, but lower at 66.7% for the IMIs. The authors mentioned that the coronal threads of the ultra-wide-diameter implants often came into contact with cortical bone of the extraction sockets, a possible indication that there was direct contact between the implant and inner aspect of the buccal wall. Although this had no impact on the reported radiographic bone levels at 1 year, one can only speculate on the negative impact this may have had on buccal wall integrity and long-term implant survival. They also reported removing the IRS as part of osteotomy preparation and did not use a sequenced gradual increase in drill diameter. These actions could have resulted in full obliteration of the extraction socket by the wide implant body, which again could have had detrimental long-term consequences. All the failed implants lost integration within the first 3 months except for two, which failed by the 1-year follow-up. With a sample size of only 24 implants, this easily resulted in a high failure rate. The authors speculated on other reasons for their high failure rate, such as the high degree of taper of the MAX design[23] and the possibility that the excessive torque required to seat the ultra-wide implants in the posterior mandible could have delivered unacceptably high compressive forces on crestal bone with microfractures, delayed bone remodeling, and failed integration.[24] Interestingly, they did not focus on immediate loading as a more likely contributor to the high failure rate. Since the rate of bone remodeling associated with immediately loaded implants is a critical factor, the placement of provisional crowns within 48 hours and definitive restorations at 8 weeks postsurgery may have played a major role in the poor outcome in this study.[25]

In a more recent publication, Checchi et al[26] reported outcomes from a prospective study with 100 patients comparing the use of 6- to 8-mm-diameter (6, 6.5, 7, 7.5, and 8 mm) moderately rough threaded implants as IMIs with 4- or 5-mm-diameter ones placed at healed molar sites treated at the time of extraction with socket preservation grafting using a porcine xenograft covered with resorbable collagen membranes (all implants provided by MegaGen). The latter sites were allowed 4 months of healing before implant placement surgery. The total numbers of implants reported were 54 in the IMI group and 53 in the healed, previously grafted extraction site group. As well as differences in diameter, the two groups had markedly different ranges of implant lengths. For example, 64.8% of the wide-diameter implants were only 5 or 6 mm in length, while 72.8% of the smaller-diameter implants were 8.5 to 13 mm in length. Delayed loading was used in both patient groups. By 1 year, three patients had dropped out from the IMI group versus six from the delayed group. Failure rates at 1 year were 10.6% for the IMIs and 4.6% for the delayed group with grafted sockets. Also, by the end of year 1, patients with IMIs had on average 1.06 mm of crestal bone loss compared to 0.63 mm for the 4- to 5-mm-diameter implants placed at grafted molar sites, the difference being statistically significant ($P < .0001$). The wide implants gave less favorable esthetic outcomes according to the investigators, but this was likely related to the advanced bone loss present at the time of tooth extraction rather than to implant diameter per se. They also resulted in more complications, including loss of buccal bone with soft tissue dehiscences and exposure of implant threads. Clearly, the treatment choices in the IMI group could be considered heroic with only sufficient bone remaining to receive implants of 5- or 6-mm length, and not at all similar to the usual patient for whom one would consider an IMI.

Tallarico et al[27] published a small randomized controlled study using 7-mm-diameter implants (Osstem Implant) either as IMIs or with delayed placement following extraction site preservation grafting. There were 12 patients in each group, and each individual received a single implant, primarily in lengths 8.5 or 10 mm with the majority placed at first molar sites in either arch. Both groups were loaded in the traditional delayed fashion. At the 1-year postloading follow-up, no implants or prostheses had failed, and no complications were encountered. Unlike the patients in Checchi et al's study,[26] none of these patients were smokers, and none had lost so much bone that they could only be managed using 5- or 6-mm-long implants.

Most recently, Hattingh et al[28] presented longer-term outcomes with the MAX implant. The investigators invited all of their patients previously treated with immediate MAX implants to attend for reassessment after they had been in function for 3 years or more. Unfortunately, only 85 out of 230 treated patients (37%) made themselves available for the recall. Thus, 96 implants were available for assessment: 47 in the maxilla and 49 in the mandible. Because so few patients agreed to attend for assessment, no survival data could be estimated, but crestal bone levels in the patients who did attend appeared to be stable.

In a subsequent prospective study, Hattingh et al[29] evaluated 51 consecutively treated MAX implant cases (26 maxilla, 25 mandible), recording an average insertion torque of 116 Ncm. Implant diameters were mostly 7 or 8 mm. A standardized protocol was used with all implants placed at the time of molar removal. Mean crestal bone levels were 1.16 mm apical to the implant-abutment junction after an average period of 23 months, but the actual bone remodeling associated with socket healing resulted in a mean coronal bone gain of 0.15 mm. No gap grafting had been performed in any of the 51 IMI sites. As a result, when changes in alveolar ridge volume were calculated in a parallel study,[30] there were mean midfacial and midpalatal/midlingual horizontal ridge reductions at 1 year of 1.45 mm and 1.16 mm, respectively. This would support the notion that grafting at the time of implant placement may be needed, particularly on the buccal aspect, to fully maintain the preextraction peri-implant ridge anatomy.

Suggested placement protocols

Detailed protocols for using MAX implants as IMIs in the maxilla and mandible have been published by Vandeweghe et al[20] and Hattingh et al[31] but have been somewhat modified by the present authors. Case planning should include the use of CBCT scans to allow assessment of socket anatomy, presence of intact socket walls, amount of IRS bone, proximity of the mandibular canal, presence and extent of any lingual fossae, and of course the thickness of buccal bone plate. Ideally, the buccal bone thickness should be 1.5 mm or greater[32] and have no fenestrations or dehiscences. Should the buccal bone be less than 1.5 mm in thickness, special measures such as guided bone regeneration may needed to avoid its compromise during osteotomy preparation and implant insertion. This risk can also be reduced by using flapless surgery to prevent any negative impacts on the local vascularity.[33] The simplest way to deal with the situation, however, is to select the MAX implant diameter most likely to leave a buccal gap of 1 to 2 mm between the implant perimeter and existing buccal plate.

As has been repeatedly stressed in the literature, atraumatic tooth extraction is crucial for successful outcomes where immediate implant insertion is intended. To achieve this goal, it is best to avoid raising a flap and in particular to make every effort to avoid trauma to the buccal plate. Conventional extraction using forceps is contraindicated, as this could cause unacceptable damage to bone and soft tissues. As described elsewhere in this book, the tooth must first be decoronated and its roots separated at the level of the furcation for subsequent removal individually using periotomes, piezoelectric tips, narrow diamond high-speed burs, and/or narrow-beak root forceps. As a result, the most time-consuming phase of the procedure may be the extraction, even for highly experienced surgeons. While root removal prior to osteotomy preparation for a MAX implant was originally recommended in published protocols,[20,21] many clinicians found it very difficult to stabilize the specialized implant burs in a vacant socket with irregular walls, sometimes resulting in sufficient damage to the remaining bone to preclude immediate implant placement. As a result, the protocols were altered following the approach of Rodrigues-Tizcareño and Bravo-Flores,[34] whereby the roots are removed only after the implant osteotomy has been largely completed.[35]

Protocol for Placing a Maxillary MAX Implant

General guidelines

Molar sockets being considered for IMI placement have been classified by Smith and Tarnow[36] according to the amount of IRS existing between the tooth roots. Type A sockets are those with sufficient bulk of IRS to completely house the crestal portion of a standard-diameter implant. On the other hand, type B sockets may have sufficient IRS to stabilize a standard-diameter IMI but not completely house its crestal aspect, while type C sockets have too little IRS to be able to stabilize an implant at all. Type A sockets are rare and only exist in association with a small percentage of maxillary first molars. If an ultra-wide implant is being considered for a type A site, the molar roots could well be removed before commencing the osteotomy, as the amount of IRS bone will readily stabilize the implant burs during site preparation.

Of utmost importance, however, is that the osteotomy must be initiated slightly toward the mesial of the midpoint of the molar socket so as to not end up too close to the second molar, if present. There are two reasons for the tendency of the drill site to drift to the distal during preparation. First, there is often a septum of dense interdental bone between the second maxillary premolar and the first maxillary molar; second, the palatal root of the first molar is often distopalatally inclined in relation to the center of the socket (Fig 8-3a). These two anatomical aspects should be checked preoperatively (radiographically) so that the important starting point of the osteotomy preparation can be adjusted accordingly. The pilot hole should be started at least 1 to 2 mm mesial to the central point (Fig 8-3b) as a way of compensating for likely distal bur drift. The buccopalatal dimension of maxillary first molar sockets is more forgiving because it is always wider than the mesiodistal dimension. One should therefore keep the buccopalatal starting point central within the IRS and in line with the central fossa line of adjacent teeth (Fig 8-3c).

The reality, however, is that the IRS of some maxillary first molars will be type B or C—or in the case of maxillary second molars, often be missing altogether. In the latter situation (no IRS present), rather than trying to place an ultra-wide implant, the authors suggest that site preservation grafting and delayed implant placement may be the preferred approach. In addition to having type B or C IRS, maxillary molar sites will generally have lower bone density (types III to IV),[37] meaning that the majority will best be handled by cutting off the crown and retaining the tooth roots in situ until the implant osteotomy has

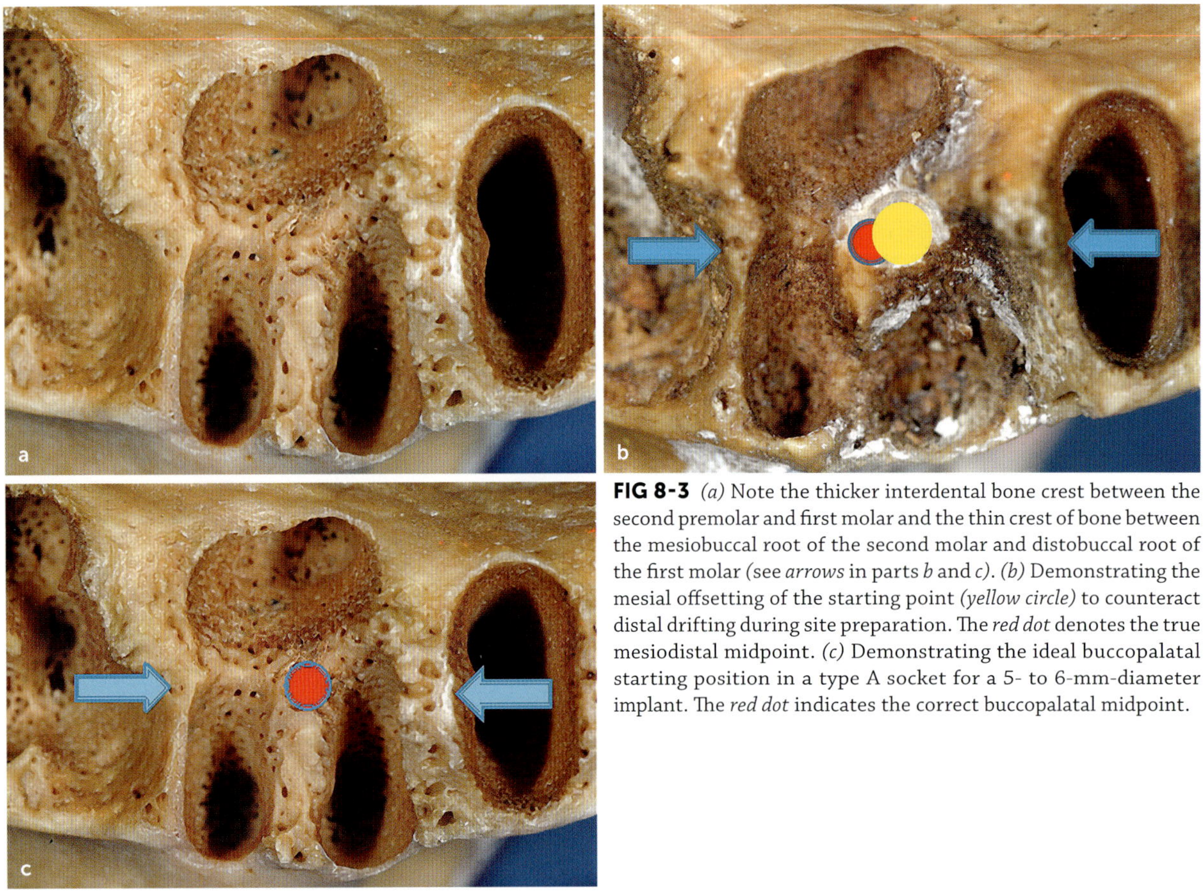

FIG 8-3 *(a)* Note the thicker interdental bone crest between the second premolar and first molar and the thin crest of bone between the mesiobuccal root of the second molar and distobuccal root of the first molar (see *arrows* in parts *b* and *c*). *(b)* Demonstrating the mesial offsetting of the starting point *(yellow circle)* to counteract distal drifting during site preparation. The *red dot* denotes the true mesiodistal midpoint. *(c)* Demonstrating the ideal buccopalatal starting position in a type A socket for a 5- to 6-mm-diameter implant. The *red dot* indicates the correct buccopalatal midpoint.

been largely completed. This will allow the operator to stabilize the implant burs using the roots as guidance and support.

Practical example

An example of a hopeless maxillary right first molar managed with an ultra-wide implant is shown in Fig 8-4. A pretreatment radiograph (see Fig 8-4a) showed the IRS to be type B with sufficient residual bone height to house a 9-mm-long implant without risk of invading the sinus cavity. The molar was carefully mobilized by manipulation with extraction forceps. This facilitates the later removal of the sectioned roots. No attempt was made to remove the tooth using the forceps, and once some mobility was established, the crown was removed with a high-speed handpiece, and the remaining tooth structure was flattened with a large round diamond bur, identifying the pulpal floor and root positions (see Fig 8-4c).

Osteotomy preparation was initiated through the dentin of the pulpal floor using a carbide bur, taking care to locate the entry point slightly mesial to the center of the tooth in order to compensate for any distal drift during site preparation (see Fig 8-4d). Following this, a 3Spade drill (Southern Implants; Figs 8-5 and 8-6) was used at 1,000 to 1,500 rpm with copious irrigation to establish the desired osteotomy depth, drilling through both the tooth structure and underlying bone. Sufficient depth is required to submerge the implant platform 2 mm below the buccal bone crest of the socket. Further pilot drilling with the 2-mm twist drill was used to finalize the desired depth and position of the osteotomy. The intention is to prepare bone slightly beyond the tooth root apices (see Fig 8-5c) if this can be safely accomplished (respecting anatomical structures) to allow for a purchase point for subsequent implant burs and taps, particularly after the roots have been removed. At this stage, a radiograph should be taken with a drill or profile gauge

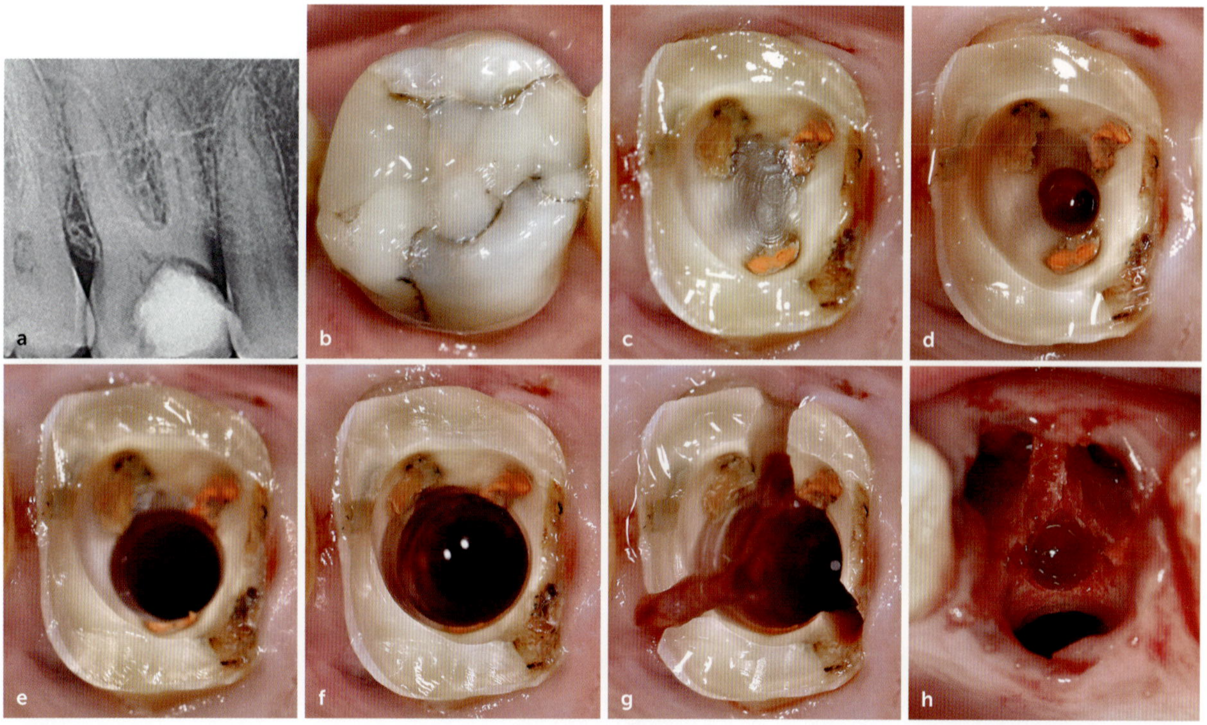

FIG 8-4 *(a and b)* Maxillary right first molar to be removed. *(c)* Flattening of decoronated tooth structure to expose the pulpal floor and identify root positions. *(d)* Initiation of the osteotomy through the pulpal floor, slightly mesial but in line with the central fossa line. *(e)* Widening of the preparation to 4-mm diameter. *(f)* Incremental widening to 5- and then 6-mm diameter. *(g)* Separation of roots. *(h)* Removal of the roots, leaving the primary osteotomy preparation visible. Note: Use of the dedicated MAX tap is recommended at this stage.

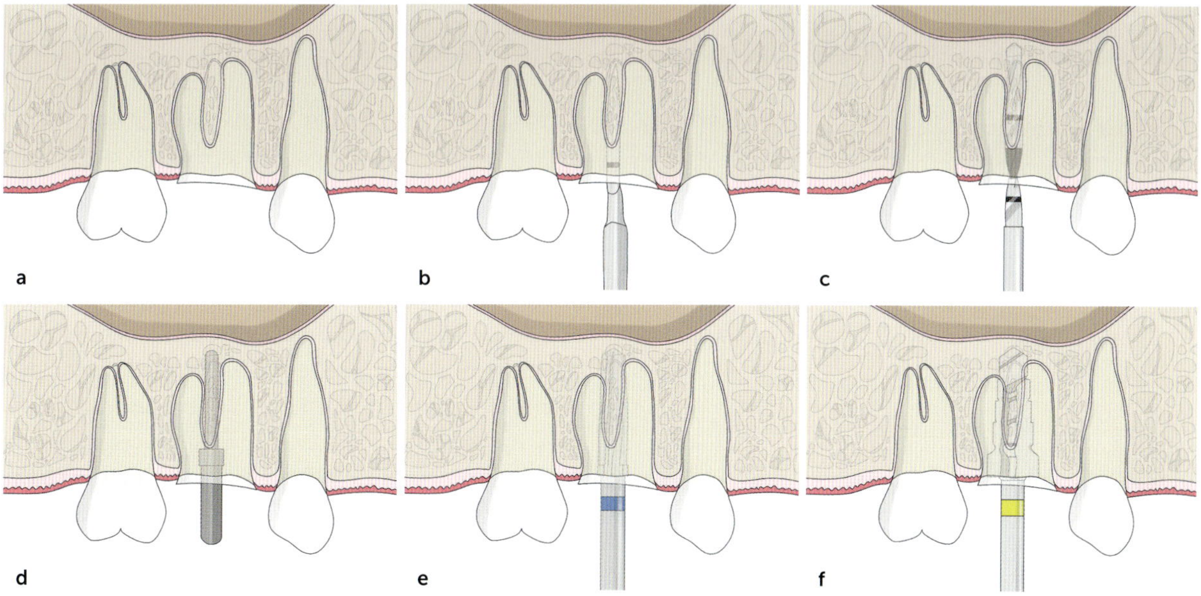

FIG 8-5 *(a)* Maxillary right first molar decoronated at the cervical level. *(b)* Start of the osteotomy through the pulpal floor slightly mesial to but in line with the central fossa line using 3Spade drill. *(c)* Continuation of osteotomy development through the pulpal floor with a 2-mm twist drill. *(d)* Radiographic depth and position check with a 2-mm-diameter profile gauge. *(e)* Incremental widening of preparation using 3.3-mm- followed by 4-mm-diameter tapered drill. *(f)* Further widening of preparation using 5-mm-diameter tapered drill.

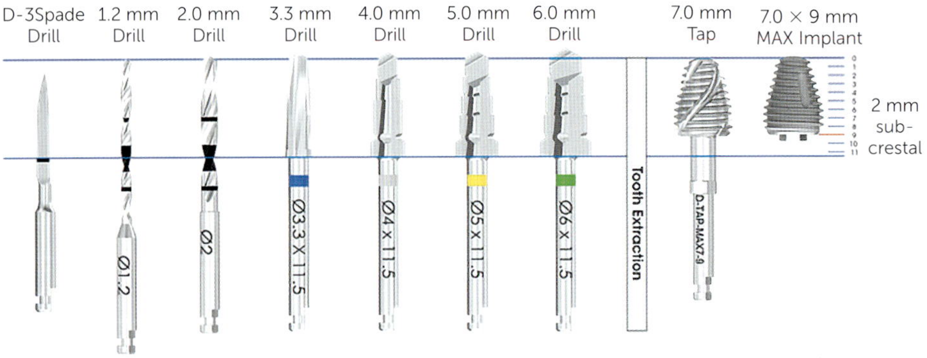

FIG 8-6 The drill sequence to prepare a 9-mm-length × 7-mm-diameter MAX implant in the maxilla.

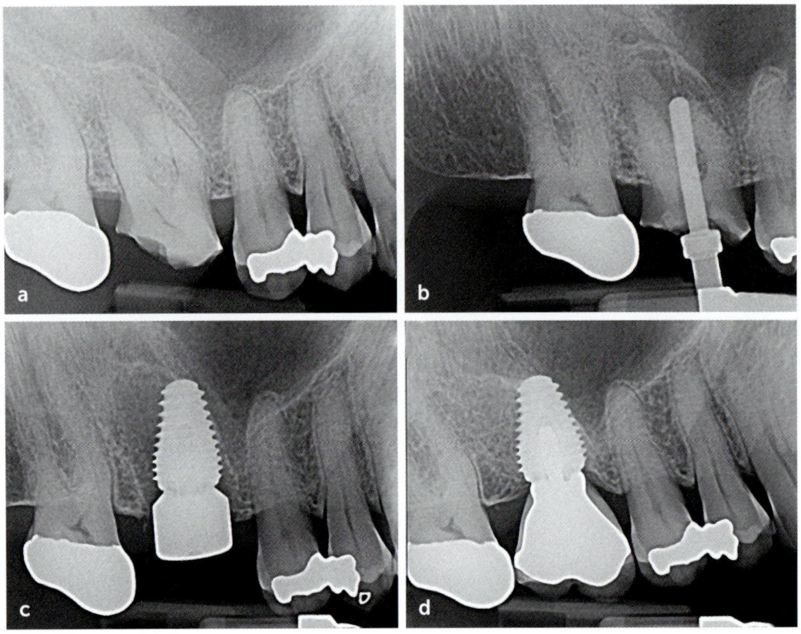

FIG 8-7 *(a)* A maxillary right first molar to be removed. *(b)* A radiograph for depth check with profile gauge in position. *(c)* A MAX 9 × 7–mm implant in position with a wide-diameter healing abutment added. *(d)* The 1-year follow-up showing full maturation of supporting bone around the implant.

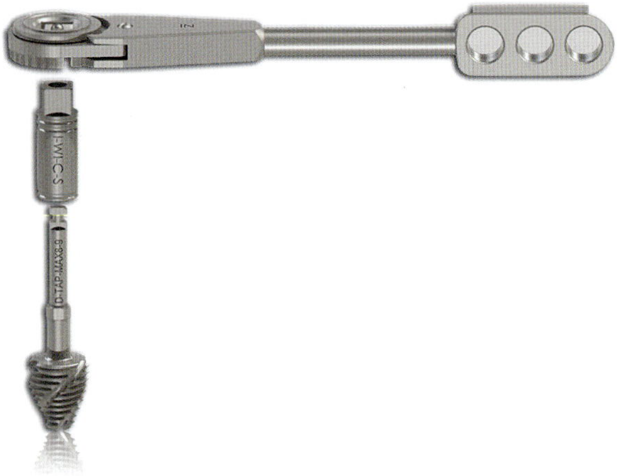

FIG 8-8 A sample tap device for the MAX implant includes spiral flutes to increase cutting efficiency. The hex drive on the tap shaft in addition to the latch connection allows high insertion torque to be applied. Each implant model has a dedicated tap (matching length and diameter) that should always be used in finishing the osteotomy regardless of bone density. If the appropriate tap is stable and fully seated in the osteotomy, the corresponding implant can then be predictably inserted.

in situ to confirm the osteotomy depth developed thus far (Fig 8-7). After radiographic confirmation, the osteotomy can be continued using the sequence of instruments depicted in Fig 8-6 at 800 rpm and ending with the 6-mm-diameter implant bur. Depth of preparation as well as mesiodistal and buccopalatal positioning should be controlled throughout. At this point, the root remnants can be sectioned to allow their individual removal (see Fig 8-4g) by careful elevation toward the center of the prepared osteotomy.

Once the root remnants have been removed, the appropriate implant diameter can be determined, keeping in mind that it should be the smallest diameter that will allow adequate stability. Most commonly, the diameter needed in the maxilla will be either 7 or 8 mm. Regardless, the next step is to use the dedicated 6-mm-diameter tap of appropriate length (Figs 8-8 and 8-9). The tap is first introduced using a handpiece

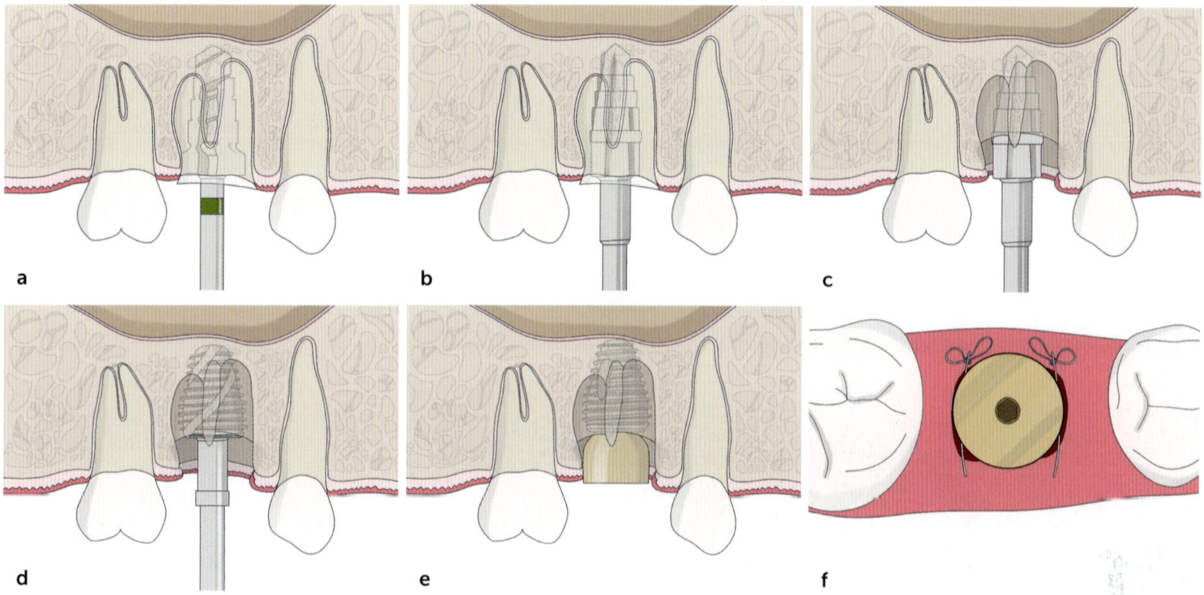

FIG 8-9 *(a)* Drilling is complete after the use of the 6-mm-diameter drill. *(b)* A 6-mm-diameter tap then is used after tooth removal. *(c)* A 7-mm-diameter tap follows the 6-mm tap. *(d)* The selected implant can then be placed to full depth. *(e)* A wide healing abutment is connected to the implant. *(f)* The soft tissues can be secured around the healing abutment with sutures.

FIG 8-10 *(a)* At full seating, the implant platform must be 2 mm subcrestal to the lowest point of the buccal socket wall. *(b)* There should be at least a 2-mm gap between the implant shoulder and the buccal bone crest.

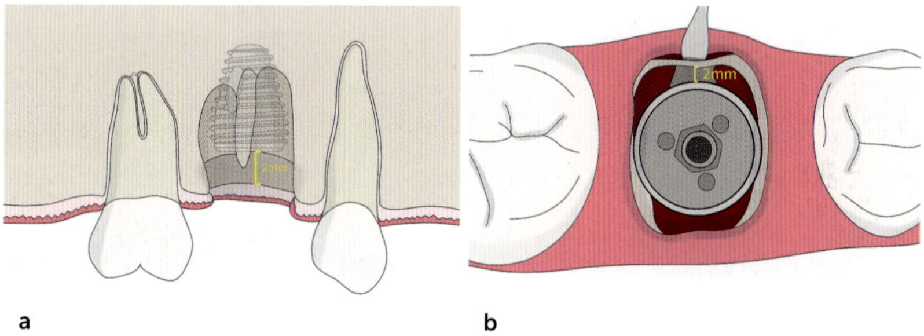

set to high torque (eg, 50 Ncm) and low speed (15 to 20 rpm).

Since the last drill diameter used is 6 mm (see Fig 8-9a), a 6-mm-diameter tap of appropriate length is used next (see Fig 8-9b), followed by the 7-mm-diameter tap (see Fig 8-9c). This sequential tapping technique provides greater control and stability of preparation than using burs, while also providing lateral compression and expansion of the osteotomy site to help increase the primary stability of the implant. The aim should be for the 7-mm-diameter tap to achieve adequate stability at the correct depth of insertion. A radiograph then should be taken to check the depth of placement relative to the sinus floor. If the 7-mm-diameter tap does not achieve adequate stability, then the corresponding 8-mm-diameter tap should be used. In the example shown, it was determined that the appropriate implant would be one of 7-mm diameter and 9-mm length, and this was inserted using a high-torque (50-Ncm) handpiece at 15 to 20 rpm, followed by use of the manual surgical wrench. At full seating, the implant platform must be 2 mm subcrestal to the lowest point of the buccal socket wall (Figs 8-10 and 8-11).

Another radiograph can be taken to verify that the implant has been fully and safely seated without penetrating significantly beyond the cortical sinus floor and with adequate interproximal bone mesially and distally (see Fig 8-7c). Establishing proper insertion depth with the prosthetic platform 2 mm apical to the buccal bone crest may result in some interference from the mesial or distal interproximal bone when

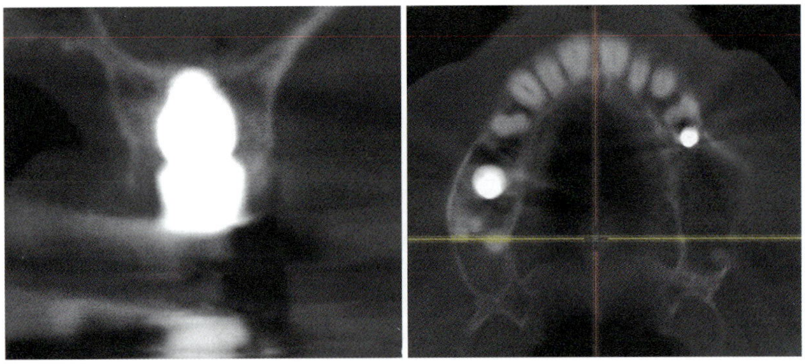

FIG 8-11 This immediate postoperative CBCT of a MAX 9 × 7–mm implant demonstrates the relationship between the implant shoulder and the lowest point of the buccal bone crest. The implant shoulder is 2 mm apical and 2 mm palatal to the buccal bone crest.

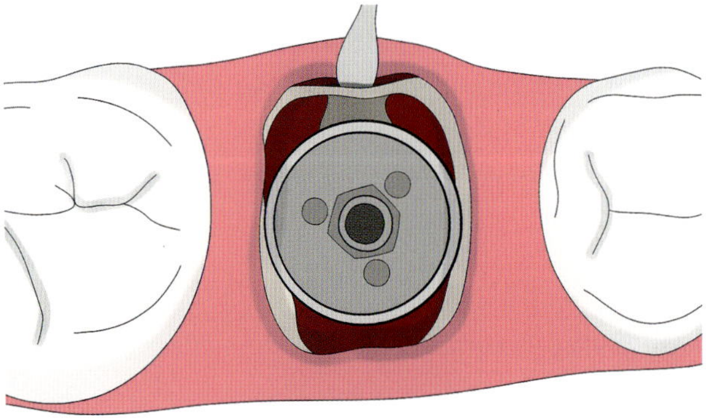

FIG 8-12 Blood will fill the residual socket voids, and these blood clots should be protected with a wide-diameter stock or custom healing abutment.

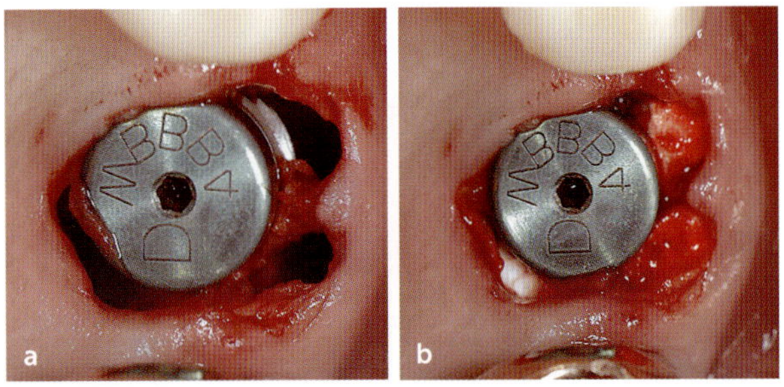

FIG 8-13 *(a)* Voids visible around healing abutment. *(b)* Voids closed at abutment level using only collagen sponge.

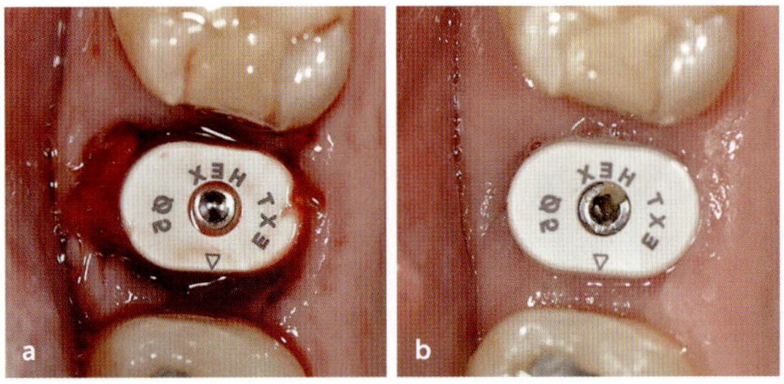

FIG 8-14 *(a)* A PEEK abutment in place with collagen to close the remaining void on the buccal aspect. *(b)* Healing after 2 weeks, showing the voids fully closed.

trying to seat a healing abutment. This may necessitate the use of a bone mill. Residual peri-implant gaps will generally be present after implant placement and can be allowed to fill spontaneously with blood clots (Fig 8-12).

While the operator may elect to graft these gaps with allograft material or with platelet-rich fibrin clots prepared from the patient's blood, the authors often prefer to use only absorbent collagen sponge material (Hemocollagene, Septodont) to protect the blood clots in the socket gaps after connecting a healing abutment to the implant. The collagen is placed only at an abutment level and is not pushed into the voids (Fig 8-13).

The healing abutment chosen should be the largest diameter possible in order to further protect the blood-filled gaps and provide support for the peri-implant soft tissues once these have been stabilized with sutures. One can also use an oval-shaped PEEK (polyetheretherketone) healing abutment (Fig 8-14), which is easily adjustable and can greatly assist in sheltering the peri-implant voids. Soft tissue adaptation should then be completed using a minimum of two interrupted sutures, one through the mesial papilla and one through the distal. The authors also recommend an additional horizontal mattress suture for soft tissue support around the healing abutment

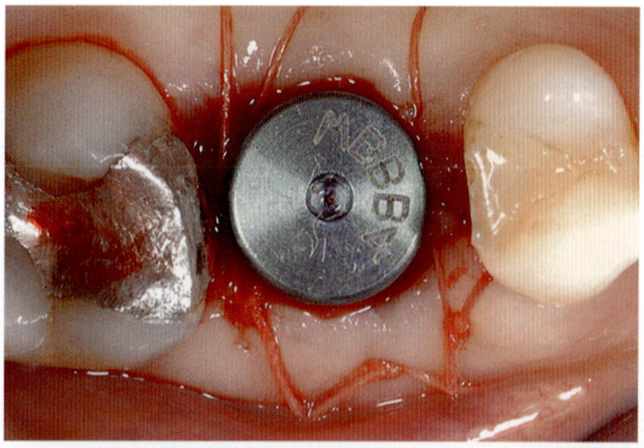

FIG 8-15 Suturing around the healing abutment greatly assists with void management and soft tissue adaptation. Two sling sutures are combined with a horizontal mattress suture to adapt the soft tissue lightly against the healing abutment.

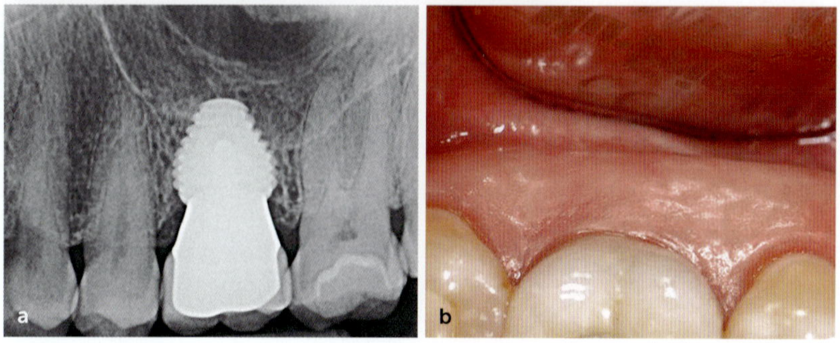

FIG 8-16 *(a and b)* Follow-up of a MAX implant demonstrating good maintenance of interproximal bone and buccal tissue dimensions after 9 years despite the short implant length.

(Fig 8-15). Figure 8-16 shows an example of a well-executed ultra-wide-diameter implant after many years in function.

Protocol for Placing a Mandibular MAX Implant

Placing an ultra-wide implant immediately into a mandibular molar socket offers its own challenges because the surrounding bone is likely to be dense. Again, most mandibular molars will have types B or C IRS,[36] and therefore, delaying tooth extraction until after the osteotomy has been largely prepared is the current preferred approach. Once the tooth has been decoronated, the entry point for the osteotomy should be established with a high-speed handpiece and large round bur. This starting point should be off-center toward the lingual by at least 2 mm (Fig 8-17). The entry point through the pulp floor can be performed with a carbide bur.

Site drilling should begin using a 2-mm-diameter twist drill at 2,000 rpm under copious sterile saline irrigation and should aim to establish a purchase point in bone apically for stabilization of subsequent burs. The osteotomy must be incrementally enlarged and likely will require use of the full sequence of burs (ie, 2-mm-diameter twist followed by tapered implant burs with diameters of 3.3, 4.0, 5.0, and 6.0 mm) and lengths appropriate for the site (Fig 8-18). Verification of preparation depth relative to the infra-alveolar canal should be done intermittently with radiographs (Fig 8-19). The root remnants are removed after use of the 6-mm-diameter drill. Unlike the situation in the maxilla, it is often necessary for the diameter of bur coinciding with the planned implant (6-, 7-, 8-, or 9-mm diameter) to be employed before finishing the site with the implant-specific tap, as described previously.

As in the maxilla, every attempt should be made to use the narrowest MAX implant that will achieve adequate primary stability. Most frequently in the mandible, this will be one of 7-mm diameter. If the 7-mm-diameter tap is unstable in the osteotomy, the 8-mm-diameter one should be used—provided that there is enough buccolingual dimension to allow for the placement of an 8-mm-diameter implant without risking direct contact with the buccal socket wall. Further use of MAX drills in the site preparation should only be considered as a last resort, should the use of taps prove not possible due to the density of the mandibular bone.

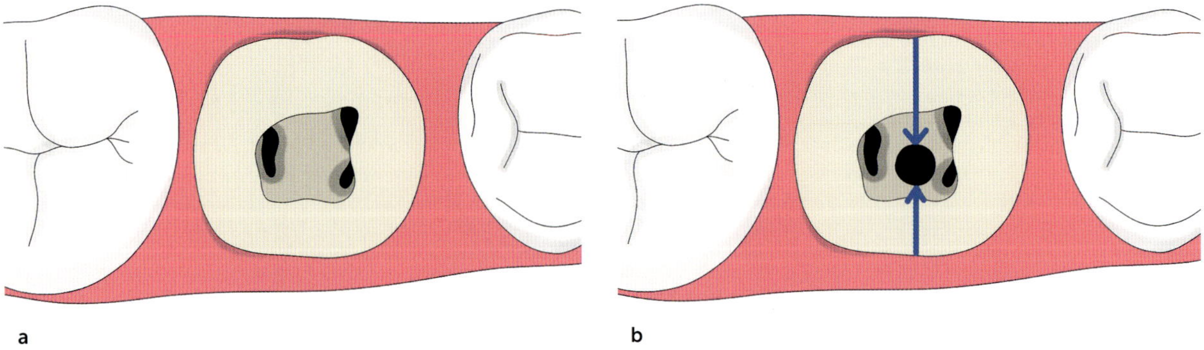

FIG 8-17 *(a)* Mandibular molars are first decoronated to expose the pulpal floor and confirm root positions. *(b)* The starting point of the osteotomy in a mandibular molar should be offset lingually relative to the central fossa line.

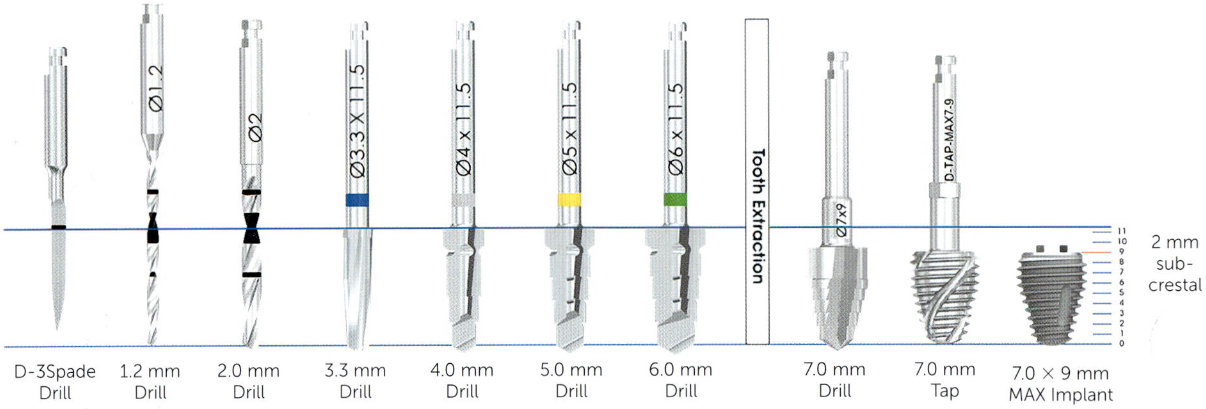

FIG 8-18 This image shows the full sequence of burs that would be needed to complete the osteotomy for a 9-mm-long × 7-mm-diameter MAX implant in the mandible.

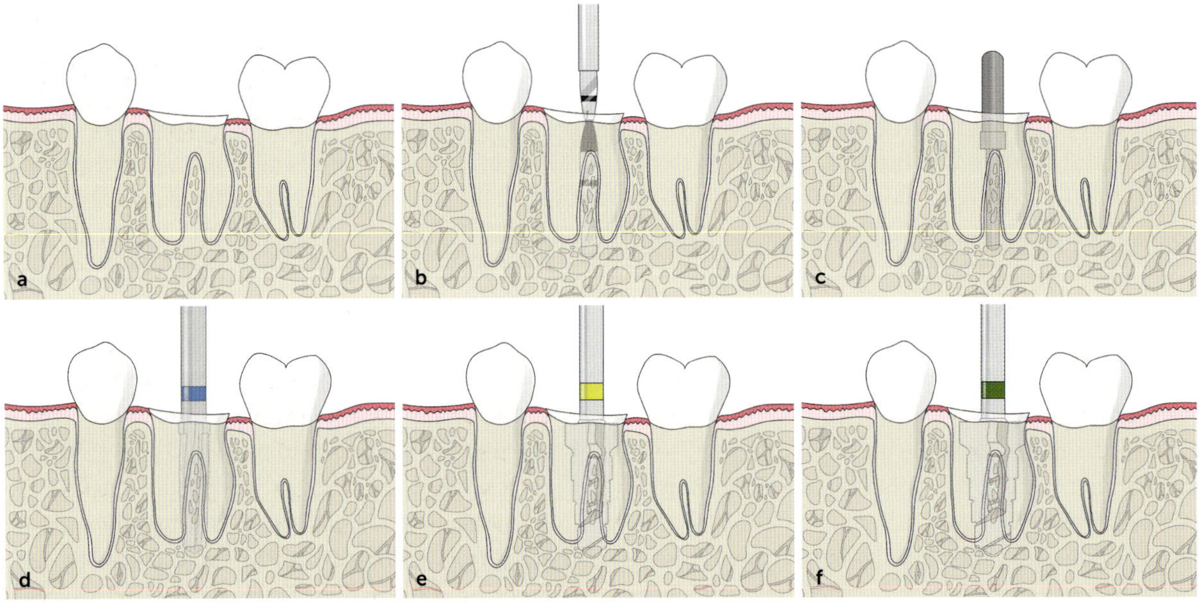

FIG 8-19 *(a)* A mandibular molar is decoronated at the cervical level. *(b)* Initiation of osteotomy preparation is through the pulpal floor using a 2-mm twist drill. *(c)* A radiographic depth and position check is performed with a 2-mm-diameter profile gauge. *(d to f)* Incremental widening of preparation using a 3.3-mm-diameter tapered drill followed by the corresponding 4-, 5-, and 6-mm tapered drills.

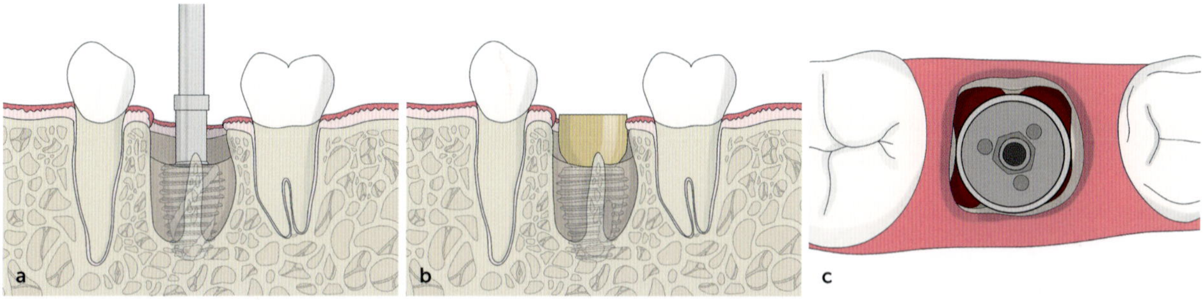

FIG 8-20 *(a)* Taps are used to finalize osteotomy preparation. *(b)* The implant is placed 2 mm apical to the buccal bone crest, and a wide healing abutment is added. *(c)* The implant shoulder must be seated at least 2 mm away from the buccal cortical plate.

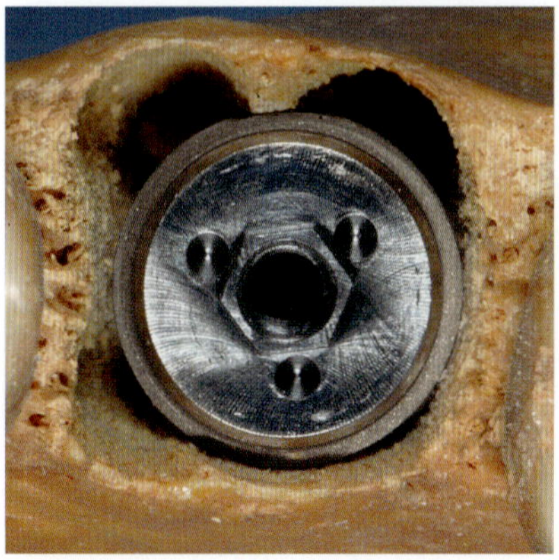

FIG 8-21 Simulation of a MAX implant insertion demonstrating the desired relationships between implant and socket walls. The implant shoulder is 2 mm away from the buccal bone crest, making contact only with the remaining buccal strut of the IRS, but not with the buccal bone plate itself.

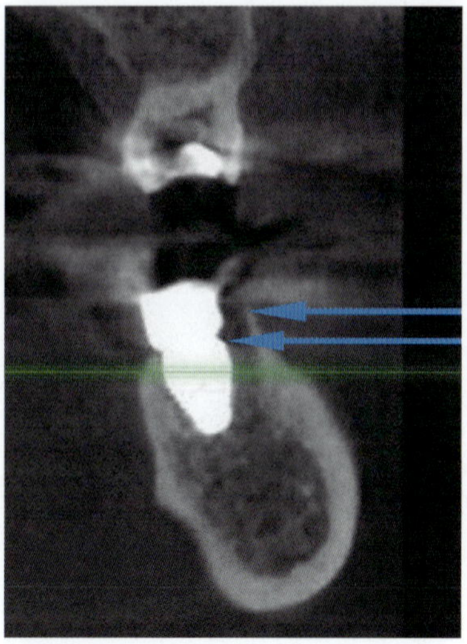

FIG 8-22 An immediate postoperative CBCT of a MAX implant demonstrating the relationship between the implant and the surrounding socket dimensions. The implant shoulder is 2 mm apical and 2 mm lingual to the buccal bone crest.

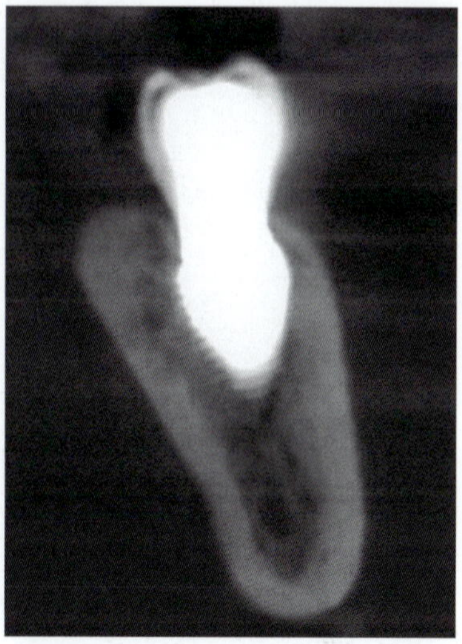

FIG 8-23 Follow-up CBCT of a MAX implant demonstrating the relationship between the implant and the surrounding socket walls after 8 years.

As in the maxilla, the depth of implant insertion must be extended to at least 2 mm apical to the existing buccal crest of bone to compensate for the inevitable postimplantation crestal bone remodeling and ensure optimal emergence for the final implant restoration (Fig 8-20). In preparing mandibular MAX osteotomies, due care must be given to the planning and execution of the osteotomy depth to avoid injury to the mandibular nerve. In addition to engaging apical bone (where there is a safe distance of at least 2 mm between the root apices and the nerve canal), the implant should rely on contact with the buccal and lingual buttresses of the IRS (Fig 8-21). It is very important that implant engagement of the buccal bone plate be avoided. Indeed, as discussed already, residual gaps of at least 1 to 2 mm should always be sought between implant perimeter and buccal bone plate (Figs 8-22 and 8-23). The marked taper of the implant allows preservation of and contact with the more apical remains of the IRS bone. A bone mill may be required to allow insertion of a wide healing abutment and ensure a favorable emergence profile for the final implant crown.

During implant seating, particularly in the mandible, it is not uncommon for MAX implants to require insertion torques as high as 70 to 100 Ncm. If higher torque than this is needed, it will be necessary to back out the implant and refine the osteotomy again with the aid of the implant-specific tap.

Conclusion

Ultra-wide threaded dental implants used as IMIs offer certain prosthetic advantages, such as optimizing emergence profiles and moderation of force transfer to crestal bone. However, they require intact socket walls and generally must be stabilized by the remaining buttresses of IRS, with care to avoid contact with the buccal bone wall by leaving large buccal gaps.

KEY POINTS

- The pretreatment CBCT scan should indicate adequate buccolingual/palatal ridge width to allow implant placement while still leaving a gap of at least 1 to 2 mm buccally.
- The pretreatment CBCT scan ideally will confirm an intact buccal bone thickness of 1.5 mm or more.
- Sites with a thick gingival biotype are preferred.
- Flapless surgery should be performed.
- Atraumatic tooth removal is crucial.
- In most instances, tooth roots should not be removed before osteotomy preparation.
- Osteotomy preparation should be begun through the pulpal floor and into the IRS bone.
- In low-density maxillary bone, a dedicated tap should be used for final preparation of the osteotomy walls using a handpiece (15 to 20 rpm) initially and followed by manual wrenching.
- The smallest-diameter implant that will achieve adequate primary implant stability should be chosen.
- Higher torque values than those required for placing standard-diameter implants will be needed, particularly in the mandible.
- In the maxilla, some transcrestal sinus floor elevation may be needed, and can be achieved by using osteotomes with or without added graft material.
- Placement of the implant subcrestal to the buccal bone crest by at least 2 mm is essential to allow for buccal bone remodeling and gingival recession while avoiding exposure of implant threads.
- Buccally, the implant should contact only the buccal IRS buttress while leaving gaps of at least 1- to 2-mm width between the implant and buccal plate of bone.

References

1. Himmlová L, Dostálová T, Kácovský A, Konvicková S. Influence of implant length and diameter on stress distribution: A finite element analysis. J Prosthet Dent 2004;91:20–25.
2. Lazzara RJ, Porter SS. Platform switching: A new concept in implant dentistry for controlling postrestorative crestal bone levels. Int J Periodontics Restorative Dent 2006;26:9–17.
3. Tabata LF, Rocha EP, Barão VA, Assunção WG. Platform switching: Biomechanical evaluation using three-dimensional finite element analysis. Int J Oral Maxillofac Implants 2011;26:482–491.
4. Langer B, Langer L, Herrmann I, Jorneus L. The wide fixture: A solution for special bone situations and a rescue for the compromised implant. Part 1. Int J Oral Maxillofac Implants 1993;8:400–408.

5. Attard NJ, Zarb GA. Implant prosthodontic management of partially edentulous patients missing posterior teeth: The Toronto experience. J Prosthet Dent 2003;89:352–359.
6. Eckert SE, Meraw SJ, Weaver AL, Lohse CM. Early experience with Wide-Platform Mk II implants. Part I: Implant survival. Part II: Evaluation of risk factors involving implant survival. Int J Oral Maxillofac Implants 2001;16:208–216.
7. Ivanoff CJ, Gröndahl K, Sennerby L, Bergström C, Lekholm U. Influence of variations in implant diameters: A 3- to 5-year retrospective clinical report. Int J Oral Maxillofac Implants 1999; 14:173–180.
8. Shin SW, Bryant SR, Zarb GA. A retrospective study on the treatment outcome of wide-bodied implants. Int J Prosthodont 2004;17:52–58.
9. Albrektsson T, Wennerberg A. Oral implant surfaces: Part 1—Review focusing on topographic and chemical properties of different surfaces and in vivo responses to them. Int J Prosthodont 2004;17:536–543.
10. Bornstein MM, Harnisch H, Lussi A, Buser D. Clinical performance of wide-body implants with a sandblasted and acid-etched (SLA) surface: Results of a 3-year follow-up study in a referral clinic. Int J Oral Maxillofac Implants 2007;22:631–638.
11. Theye CEG, Hattingh A, Cracknell TJ, Oettlé AC, Steyn M, Vandeweghe S. Dento-alveolar measurements and histomorphometric parameters of maxillary and mandibular first molars, using micro-CT. Clin Implant Dent Relat Res 2018;20:550–561.
12. Scheid RC, Weiss G. Woelfel's Dental Anatomy, ed 8. Philadelphia: Lippincott Williams & Wilkins, 2012.
13. Brånemark PI, Hansson BO, Adell R, et al. Osseointegrated implants in the treatment of the edentulous jaw. Experience from a 10-year period. Scand J Plast Reconstr Surg Suppl 1977;16:1–132.
14. Velásquez-Plata D, Lutonsky J, Oshida Y, Jones R. A close-up look at an implant fracture: A case report. Int J Periodontics Restorative Dent 2002;22:483–491.
15. Chrcanovic BR, Kisch J, Albrektsson T, Wennerberg A. Factors influencing the fracture of dental implants. Clin Implant Dent Relat Res 2018;20:58–67.
16. Tagger Green N, Machtei EE, Horwitz J, Peled M. Fracture of dental implants: Literature review and report of a case. Implant Dent 2002;11:137–143.
17. Hattori Y, Satoh C, Kunieda T, Endoh R, Hisamatsu H, Watanabe M. Bite forces and their resultants during forceful intercuspal clenching in humans. J Biomech 2009;42:1533–1538.
18. Vandeweghe S, De Bruyn H. A within-implant comparison to evaluate the concept of platform switching: A randomised controlled trial. Eur J Oral Implantol 2012;5:253–262.
19. Smith RB, Rawdin SB, Kagan V. Influence of implant-tooth proximity on incidence of caries in teeth adjacent to implants in molar sites: A retrospective radiographic analysis of 300 consecutive implants. Compend Contin Educ Dent 2020;41:e1–e5.
20. Vandeweghe S, Hattingh A, Wennerberg A, Bruyn HD. Surgical protocol and short-term clinical outcome of immediate placement in molar extraction sockets using a wide body implant. J Oral Maxillofac Res 2011;2:e1.
21. Vandeweghe S, Ackermann A, Bronner J, Hattingh A, Tschakaloff A, De Bruyn H. A retrospective, multicenter study on a novo wide-body implant for posterior regions. Clin Implant Dent Relat Res 2012;14:281–292.
22. Atieh MA, Alsabeeha NH, Duncan WJ, et al. Immediate single implant restorations in mandibular molar extraction sockets: A controlled clinical trial. Clin Oral Implants Res 2013;24:484–496.
23. Atieh MA, Shahmiri RA. Evaluation of optimal taper of immediately loaded wide-diameter implants: A finite element analysis. J Oral Implantol 2013;39:123–132.
24. Atieh MA, Alsabeeha NH, Payne AG, Schwass DR, Duncan WJ. Insertion torque of immediate wide-diameter implants: A finite element analysis. Quintessence Int 2012;43:e115–e126.
25. Raghavendra S, Wood MC, Taylor TD. Early wound healing around endosseous implants: A review of the literature. Int J Oral Maxillofac Implants 2005;20:425–431.
26. Checchi V, Felice P, Zucchelli G, et al. Wide diameter immediate post-extractive implants vs delayed placement of normal-diameter implants in preserved sockets in the molar region: 1-year post-loading outcome of a randomised controlled trial. Eur J Oral Implantol 2017;10:263–278.
27. Tallarico M, Xhanari E, Pisano M, Gatti F, Meloni SM. Molar replacement with 7 mm-wide diameter implants: To place the implant immediately or to wait 4 months after socket preservation? 1 year after loading results from a randomised controlled trial. Eur J Oral Implantol 2017;10:169–178.
28. Hattingh A, De Bruyn H, Vandeweghe S. A retrospective study on ultra-wide diameter dental implants for immediate molar replacement. Clin Implant Dent Relat Res 2019;21:879–887.
29. Hattingh A, Hommez G, De Bruyn H, Huyghe M, Vandeweghe S. A prospective study on ultra-wide diameter dental implants for immediate molar replacement. Clin Implant Dent Relat Res 2018;20:1009–1015.
30. Hattingh A, De Bruyn H, Van Weehaeghe M, Hommez G, Vandeweghe S. Contour changes following immediate placement of ultra-wide implants in molar extraction sockets without bone grafting. J Clin Med 2020;9:2504.
31. Hattingh AC, De Bruyn H, Ackermann A, Vandeweghe S. Immediate placement of ultrawide-diameter implants in molar sockets: Description of a recommended technique. Int J Periodontics Restorative Dent 2018;38:17–23.
32. Monje A, Chappuis V, Monje F, et al. The critical peri-implant buccal bone wall thickness revisited: An experimental study in the beagle dog. Int J Oral Maxillofac Implants 2019;34:1328–1336.
33. Merheb J, Vercruyssen M, Coucke W, Beckers L, Teughels W, Quirynen M. The fate of buccal bone around dental implants. A 12-month postloading follow-up study. Clin Oral Implants Res 2017;28:103–108.
34. Rodriguez-Tizcareño MH, Bravo-Flores C. Anatomically guided implant site preparation technique at molar sites. Implant Dent 2009;18:393–401.
35. Rebele SF, Zuhr O, Hürzeler MB. Pre-extractive interradicular implant bed preparation: Case presentations of a novel approach to immediate implant placement at multirooted molar sites. Int J Periodontics Restorative Dent 2013;33:89–96.
36. Smith RB, Tarnow DP. Classification of molar extraction sites for immediate dental implant placement: Technical note. Int J Oral Maxillofac Implants 2013;28:911–916.
37. Lekholm U, Zarb G. Patient selection and preparation. In: Branemark P-I, Zarb G, Albrektsson T (eds). Tissue-Integrated Prostheses: Osseointegration in Clinical Dentistry. Chicago: Quintessence, 1985:199–209.

9

PRESS-FIT IMMEDIATE MOLAR IMPLANTS

Miguel Simancas-Pallares
Mauro Marincola
Shadi Daher

General Concepts with PRF Implants

Unlike the majority of endosseous threaded dental implant designs, which are torqued to depth using a handpiece and/or manual torque wrench, plateau root form (PRF) implants have moderately rough–surfaced horizontal fins or plateaus (Fig 9-1) and are designed to be press-fitted into precisely prepared osteotomies.[1] Given this major difference in concept, the first part of this chapter aims to describe the macro geometry and biomechanics of the PRF implant as well as its pattern of initial bone healing. A major advantage with the design is that it is intended for use in short lengths (≤ 8 mm) only, although generally in wider-than-standard implant diameters.[2–4] We will present clinical evidence supporting the use of short PRF implants for molar replacement, as well as suggest clinical protocols for their immediate placement at molar sites in both maxilla and mandible. A review of possible surgical complications, and available clinical approaches to address them, is also included.

Molars frequently require extraction due to advanced caries, periodontal disease, and untreatable fractures often associated with parafunctional habits. Their loss may diminish oral health–related quality of life, affecting proper mastication of food, stability of adjacent teeth, changes in orofacial appearance, loss in occlusal vertical dimension, and orofacial muscle and temporomandibular joint dysfunction or pain. Therefore, it is important to minimize the time that a patient is without teeth, and this has led to the concept and use of the immediate molar implant (IMI).

Historically, immediate placement of dental implants began with the replacement of nonmolar teeth, and numerous reports have documented high survival and success rates.[5,6] More recently, the use of IMIs has proved feasible, again showing excellent survival rates.[7,8] Careful case planning and the choice of a suitable implant design are, however, crucial factors in determining positive

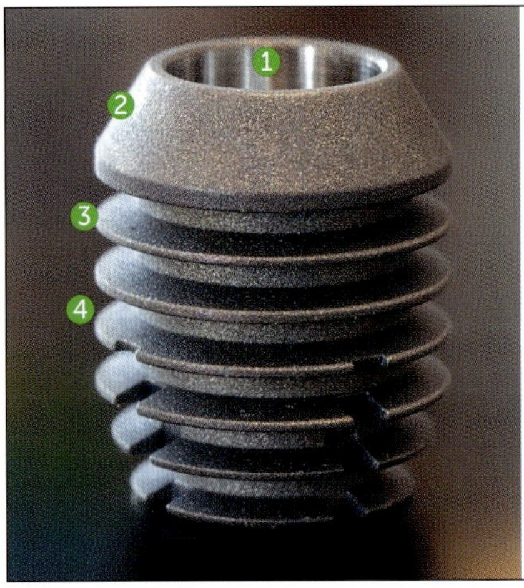

1. Implant well to allow connection of the implant body with prosthetic components.
2. A sloping shoulder allows substantial new crestal bone formation following grafting of the associated initial peri-implant gaps.
3. The tips of implant "plateaus" along the implant body allow for an initial tight press-fit with the osteotomy walls.
4. The interplateau spaces act as healing chambers for initial woven bone formation.

FIG 9-1 The Bicon implant design and some of its macro geometric features.

outcomes. Using a large collection of CBCT records, Demircan and Çankaya[9] determined that socket dimensions in the maxillary first molar area are often appropriate for immediate placement of wide-diameter (> 5 mm) IMIs, but that the maximum possible implant length usable in this location can often be no longer than ~ 8 mm due to the risk of sinus perforation (see also chapter 2). In the past, such short implant lengths were considered inappropriate, but more recent data have shown this not to be the case provided that certain precautions are exercised.[10,11] Crucial to successful outcomes with IMIs is adequate initial implant stability, ie, mechanical stability, which relies heavily on implant size and design.[12] Without good initial implant stability, adequate osseointegration (bone-to-implant surface contact) is unlikely to occur. Therefore, the success of IMIs will be highly dependent on implant geometry and surface topography, the preferred topography being a moderately rough surface[13] such as one created by particle blasting and/or acid etching. This will promote differentiation and proliferation of osteoblasts and upregulation of transcription factors responsible for the expression of bone matrix formation genes.[14] Once initial integration has been achieved, implant geometry then must permit favorable distribution of the considerable strains experienced in molar regions at the bone-to-implant interfaces under conditions of compression, tension, and shear loading.

Most currently available endosseous dental implant systems have a root shape and threaded design (SRF or screw root form) to confer benefits in biomechanical fixation during their insertion stage.[15] Since the groundbreaking publication on the osseointegration of titanium SRF implants,[16] SRF implants have become the most accepted designs. However, PRF implants (also called "finned" or "serrated" implants) have also been in clinical use for decades. Geometrically, the differences between PRF and SRF dental implants are essentially that PRF implants have a series of separate circumferential fins spaced along the long axis of the bone-interfacing portion of the fixture[17] (see Fig 9-1). Another difference is that SRF implants were—until recently—promoted for use in long lengths, while PRF implants were designed for use in short lengths from the outset.

The early healing with moderately rough SRF implants has been well described.[14] Immediately after implant insertion, platelet activation in the forming blood clot leads to directed osteogenic cell migration toward the textured implant surface, direction being given by blood clot fibrin fibrils anchored to the implant surface. Integration then begins with the formation of a mineralized interfacial matrix, comparable to the cement line seen in natural bone, followed by de novo bone formation via contact osteogenesis,[14] ie, directly onto the implant surface.

Lemons[18] provided histologic evidence of the bone healing patterns around PRF and SRF implants explanted from human subjects and concluded that they differed considerably. Unlike SRF implants, PRF implants make initial contact with the outer osteotomy walls only at the tips of their plateaus. Immediately thereafter, the spaces between the plateaus (termed "healing chambers") fill with blood clots followed by vascular ingrowth, differentiation of osteoblasts, and formation of callus-like or woven bone, ie, by intramembranous bone formation.[19] By 3 months postimplantation, overall integration of both SRF and PRF implants appears to be comparable. With time, the intramembranous bone formed in the healing chambers associated with PRF implants slowly becomes converted to lamellar bone, which continues to remodel after the implants go into function.[15,17] Coelho et al[12] conducted a histomorphologic study of PRF implants retrieved from humans after 8 to 13 years in function and reported the average bone-to-implant plateau contact (BIC) to be 62%. Other studies focused on the mechanical properties (elastic modulus and hardness) of bone surrounding PRF implants after up to 24 years of clinical function. Both elastic modulus and hardness increased up to the fifth year of function, after which they remained stable.[20] PRF implants also showed a progressive increase in BIC and bone area fraction occupancy levels,[21] demonstrating effective ongoing bone remodeling in response to implant loading.

Even though PRF implants clearly have been shown to develop adequate integration with bone, they have in the past been criticized because of their perceived low primary stability, essentially because they exhibit a less intimate relationship with the osteotomy walls when compared with SRF implants. This argument extends to their use in immediate implantation, given that extraction socket dimensions are generally greater, in both width and height, than available PRF implant dimensions. The essential point here, however, is that rigid primary stability is not an indispensable prerequisite during initial healing. In fact, it is this very feature that provides the main advantage in using PRF implants in the more challenging socket conditions encountered with immediate implant placement at molar sites. Rather than relying on high primary stability to allow integration, PRF implants are purposefully submerged up to 3 mm subcrestally to allow undisturbed healing and osseointegration. Unlike the situation with SRF implants, there is no need to record initial stability of PRF implants.

Following the onset of PRF implant function, load transfer is again different from that which occurs with SRF implants. Thus, occlusal forces have been predicted from finite element analysis studies[22] to be dissipated by the bone formed between PRF implant plateaus rather than by the inner and outer diameter regions of threads as occurs with SRF implants.[19] The same study indicated that PRF implants will be unlikely to suffer overload or failure with moderate levels of occlusal loads, ie, up to 300 Ncm. However, with extreme occlusal loading (> 1,000 Ncm), as may occur with parafunctional habits like bruxism, like most implant designs, PRF implants may suffer biologic failure, ie, excessive bone loss.

PRF implants are suitable for IMI usage because their initial placement subcrestally allows undisturbed healing and fill of the sometimes large peri-implant gaps with new bone. They also are suitable for use in short lengths, an important feature since they need to be placed up to 3 mm subcrestally to allow successful integration. Lengths as short as 6 mm help to ensure that vital structures such as the mandibular neurovascular canal or maxillary sinus are not compromised during implant placement. Interestingly, other evidence shows that short implants are superior to longer ones in mechanotransductive qualities, minimizing crestal bone loss.[23]

Immediate Molar Implantation

While no published data on outcomes with PRF implants used as IMIs have been reported to date, a recent systematic literature review with meta-analysis compared the survival rate of SRF implants inserted into fresh extraction versus healed (delayed implant placement) sockets.[24] Results indicated that after (on average) 30 months of follow-up, the overall survival rate of delayed implants was higher (98.4%) than that for immediate implants (95.2%; $P < .005$). However, there were no differences in radiologic or clinical parameters with surviving implants, such as marginal bone loss (slightly higher for immediate implants), implant stability after 30 months (slightly higher for delayed implants), or pocket probing depth (equal for both implants). The study had combined outcomes with both anterior and posterior teeth, and most likely immediate implant survival rates will vary according to tooth position in the jaw, with IMI survival possibly being lower. Nevertheless, numerous other studies have verified that IMIs can be a predictable albeit challenging treatment approach.[25-27] For example, a recent report from Amato and Polara[28] showed that after a mean follow-up of 3 years, an overall cumulative success rate of 99% was found (98.1% in the mandible and 100% in the maxilla). Another literature review and meta-analysis[29] showed no difference in the survival rates between immediate and delayed molar implants (98% for both), and no difference between the maxilla (98%) and mandible (99%). Combined average bone loss after at least 1 year was 0.57 mm. It seems clear then that there is little practical downside in choosing to place IMIs if conditions are favorable.

Specific to PRF short implants, Lombardo et al[30] reported 3-year outcomes with 139 implants placed in the posterior maxillae of 65 patients. Implant lengths used included 93 short (6 or 8 mm) and 46 ultra-short (5 mm) PRF implants. Standard protocol was respected, including subcrestal insertion and submerged healing. Afterward, all implants were restored with single crowns. Although the implants had not been placed immediately after tooth extraction, the cumulative survival rates at 3 years were highly favorable at 97.9% for short and 95.1% for ultra-short implants.

Consider the scenario that a clinician treats 100 patients with dental implants in the molar area (one implant per patient), and that the choice is whether to do immediate or delayed placement. Based on the findings of current data like that of the first literature review referenced above, if the clinician chooses the delayed option, after 30 months in function, 98 out of 100 implants will have survived. On the other hand, if they choose the immediate implant approach, then 95 out of 100 implants will have survived. Does this difference in survival rate appear clinically significant? As long as the patient is adequately informed, might that small difference (3%) in survival rate be offset by positive factors such as avoiding the need, time, cost, and morbidity associated with socket preservation grafting and a second surgical procedure to place the implant? What follows then are suggested clinical protocols for the use of PRF implants as IMIs. We will not present general aspects such as patient selection and presurgical assessment (clinical and/or radiologic; see chapters 1 and 2), but rather focus on the surgical steps needed for successful treatment outcomes with PRF designs.

Suggested Clinical Protocols Using PRF Implants as IMIs

Maxillary placement

After initiating osteotomy site development for a PRF implant using a pilot drill, site development is continued not with surgical burs, but rather with an incremental series of increasing-diameter reamers used at very low speed (50 rpm) and without saline irrigation. These reamers have flutes that create a parallel-walled socket while collecting bone shaved from the osteotomy walls for later use in grafting (Fig 9-2). If the residual subantral bone height in the maxillary IMI site is approximately 8 mm, a 6-mm PRF implant can be placed 2 mm subcrestally without affecting the sinus. If, however, the residual bone height is less than 8 mm, the same implant can be placed along with a minor indirect sinus floor elevation using a modified approach after Summers[31] or others.[32] More specifically, sinus floor upfracture is delayed until the final-diameter reamer chosen for the site has been used. At that point, a 3.5-mm-diameter hand reamer can be used to breach the sinus floor, followed by the addition of an appropriate graft material if need be before implant placement.

The preoperative radiographic status of a sample molar requiring extraction is shown in Fig 9-3. Evidence of deep tooth decay extending into the furcation was seen at the maxillary first molar. It was estimated that there was approximately 8 mm of bone height in the interradicular septum (IRS) area. The placement of an IMI was planned, and the patient was given a loading dose (2 g) of amoxicillin 1 hour prior to the surgery. A local anesthetic with low-dose (2%) vasoconstrictor was chosen to ensure that a small quantity of blood could be easily collected from the osteotomy in a sterile syringe and set aside for later use. Atraumatic tooth extraction was performed using periotomes to sever but preserve as much periodontal ligament tissue attached to the socket walls as possible in an attempt to capture the ligament's potential in new bone formation.[33] Fine straight luxation elevators can also be used, but care must be exercised to avoid root or crown fractures. Once the tooth had been adequately luxated, it was sectioned through its furcation area using a carbide bur to allow separation of the roots for individual removal. Thereaf-

1. Handpiece attaching head
2. Extending arm that connects the attaching head with the reamer body
3. Flute wherein bone is harvested during the reaming process
4. Tapered, noncutting reamer tip
5. Reamer length indicator for 6 mm
6. Reamer length indicator for 8 mm
7. Reamer length indicator for 11 mm
8. Reamer length indicator for 14 mm

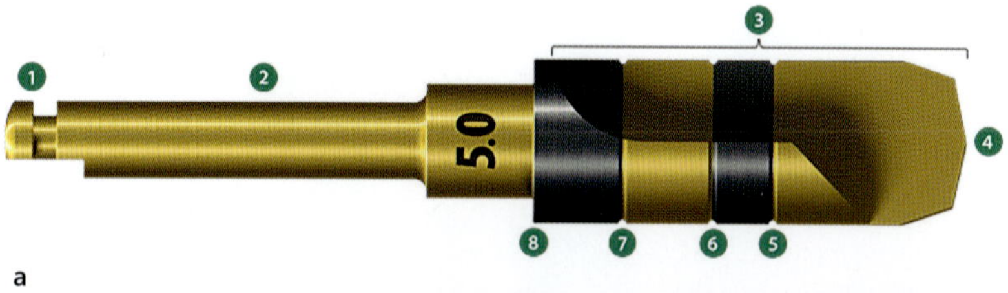

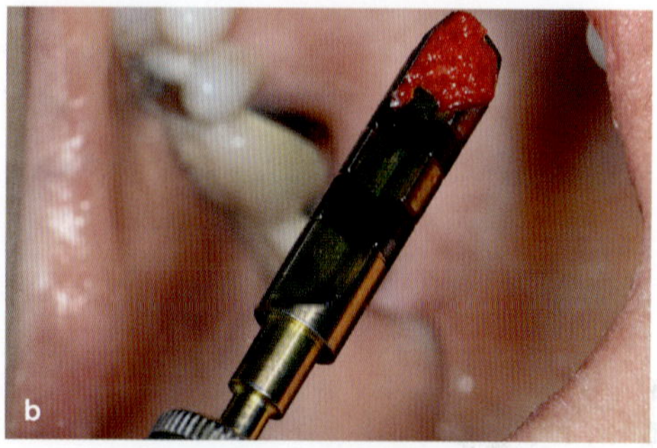

FIG 9-2 *(a)* A 5.0-mm-diameter Bicon standard latch reamer and its components. *(b)* Latch reamers are used at slow speeds without coolant to allow the collection of autogenous bone from the osteotomy walls. In this example, the flute was used to collect bone up to the 6-mm length indicator.

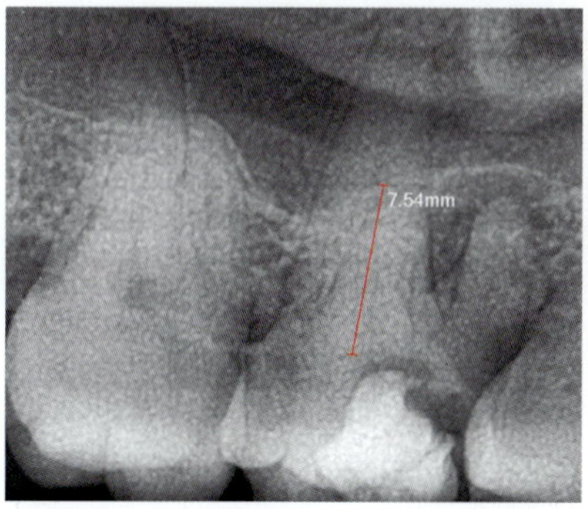

FIG 9-3 A preoperative radiograph was used to estimate approximately 7.5 mm of bone height at the planned maxillary first molar osteotomy site. The prognosis of the tooth was classified as hopeless.

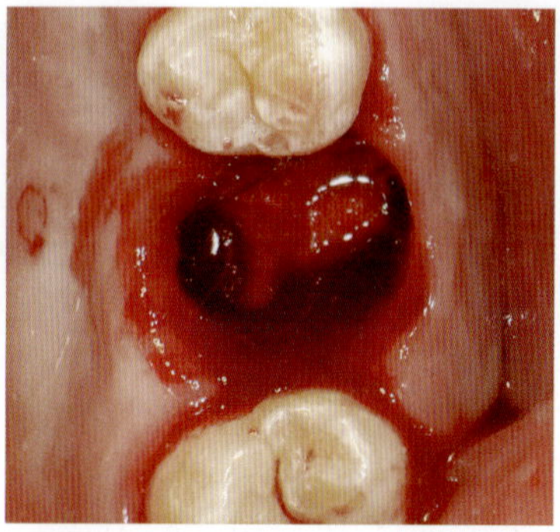

FIG 9-4 Alveolar cavity (socket) after extraction. Notice the thick type A septum.[34]

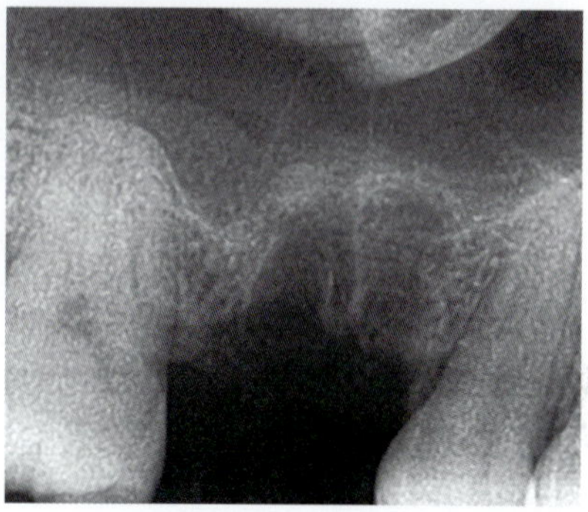

FIG 9-5 Periapical radiograph after extraction. Notice the proximity to the sinus floor. This appears to be an ideal site to place a short implant.

ter, careful inspection of the socket walls and their integrity was performed using a curette. The same instrument was used to gently yet thoroughly remove any pathologic soft tissue remnants from the socket apex. Socket walls were intact, and a substantial bone septum remained[34] (Fig 9-4). While the root apices had extended into the sinus domain, no sinus perforation was detected (Fig 9-5).

Should a minor defect such as a fenestration be discovered in any of the socket walls, it may be possible to repair it while proceeding with implant placement. On the other hand, if a major bone defect exists, the clinician must determine whether immediate implant placement is still appropriate or whether guided bone regeneration (GBR) with delayed implant placement is more appropriate. If it is concluded that an IMI is still the preferred approach, it is important first to obtain a radiologic measure of the remaining bone height (distance from the most apical portion of the socket to the floor of the sinus). This measurement enables the clinician to determine whether there is enough native bone height to accommodate the implant, or whether a controlled entry into the maxillary sinus will be required. In the case demonstrated, the remaining bone height was ~ 7.5 mm.

Site preparation began in the center of the remaining IRS using a pilot drill in a 20:1 handpiece rotating at 1,100 rpm and cooled with external saline irriga-

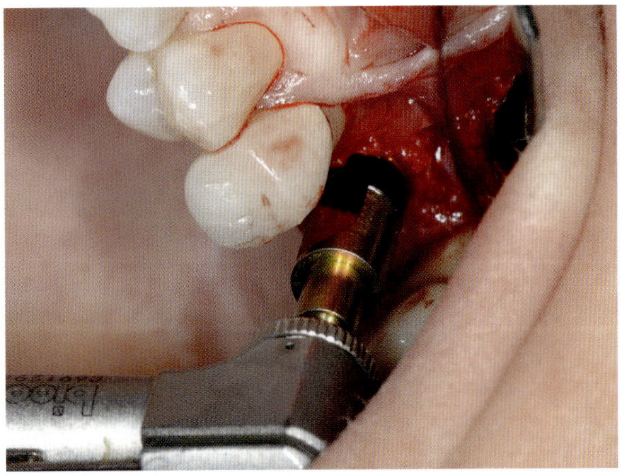

FIG 9-6 After pilot drill use, latch reamers are used to widen the osteotomy. Slow speeds (~ 50 rpm) are used without saline irrigation to allow collection of autogenous bone from the osteotomy walls (see Fig 9-2b).

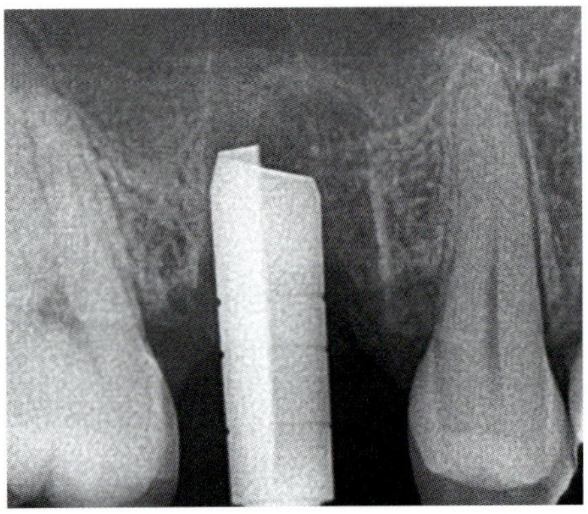

FIG 9-7 Radiograph of a 5-mm-diameter reamer, the last one of a series establishing the final width of the osteotomy.

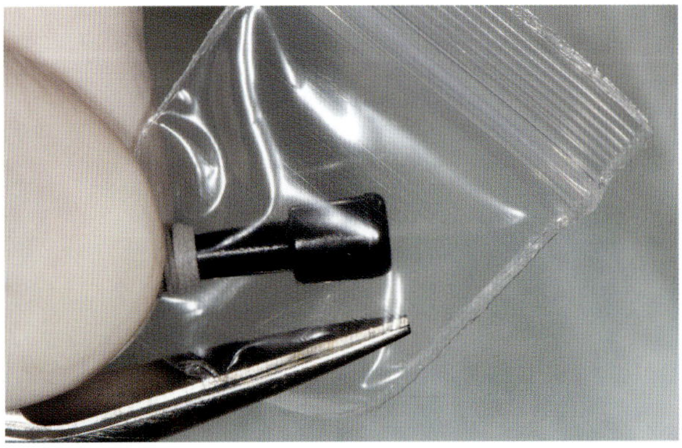

FIG 9-8 The PRF implant is received with a black plastic healing plug inserted into its well.

tion. A 6-mm-long implant was planned for the site, and since it needed to be placed 2 mm subcrestally, the final depth of the osteotomy was planned for 8 mm. However, initial drilling depth was stopped at 6 mm, at which point a new periapical radiograph was obtained with a paralleling pin in position in the osteotomy to assess the proximity of the implant tip to the sinus floor as well as the implant's overall spatial orientation. Thereafter, the pilot drilling was finished to the planned depth (8 mm).

Once the pilot osteotomy was completed, reamers were used to widen it (Fig 9-6). It is important to realize that these reamers do not have a cutting tip; their cutting blades are located on their lateral surfaces (see Fig 9-2). They are specifically designed to widen the osteotomy without deepening it, thereby minimizing risk of damage to vital structures—in this case the sinus membrane. The reamers are used in the 20:1 high-torque handpiece, but with speeds as low as 50 rpm, meaning that external coolant is no longer necessary. During use, bone will collect in the flutes of the reamers and can be saved for later grafting, either alone or mixed with a xenograft or even a synthetic graft material (eg, SynthoGraft, Bicon), to fill any peri-implant gaps. Hand reamers with only one cutting edge and a cutting tip also are available. These can be helpful in expanding the septum as well as enabling the clinician to limit cutting to a specific aspect of the osteotomy when it is advantageous to do so.

Once the reamer corresponding to the chosen implant diameter has been used (Fig 9-7), the implant can be inserted. The implant is received with a black healing plug in place (Fig 9-8), and this must be removed to allow the implant to be mounted on the implant inserter for its delivery into the socket (Fig 9-9). Seating is achieved with a gentle turning motion of the inserter device, after which the inserter can be disconnected. Then, a seating tip with a width consistent with that of the implant inner well is mounted on a

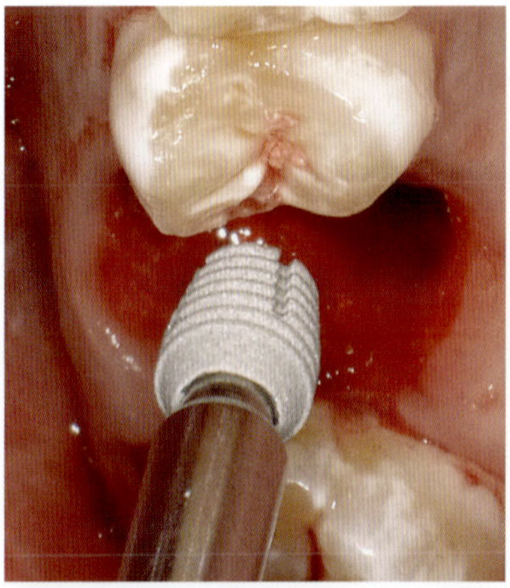

FIG 9-9 The 6-mm-length × 5-mm-width PRF implant (Bicon) was inserted into the prepared osteotomy using an implant inserter device.

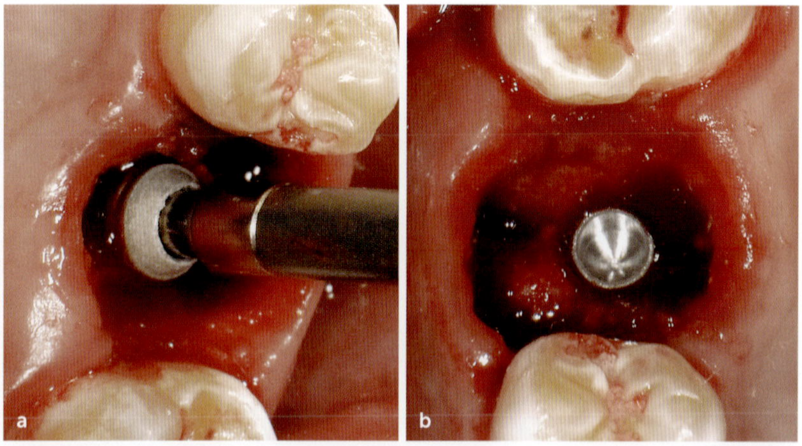

FIG 9-10 *(a)* The final seating of this press-fit implant was achieved with a seating tip screwed onto a straight handle, and a surgical mallet was used to tap the implant into its final position in the osteotomy. *(b)* The implant located inside the expanded septum. Notice the implant well without threads and its diameter (3 mm) as compared with the 5-mm width of the implant body. This is an example of platform switching.

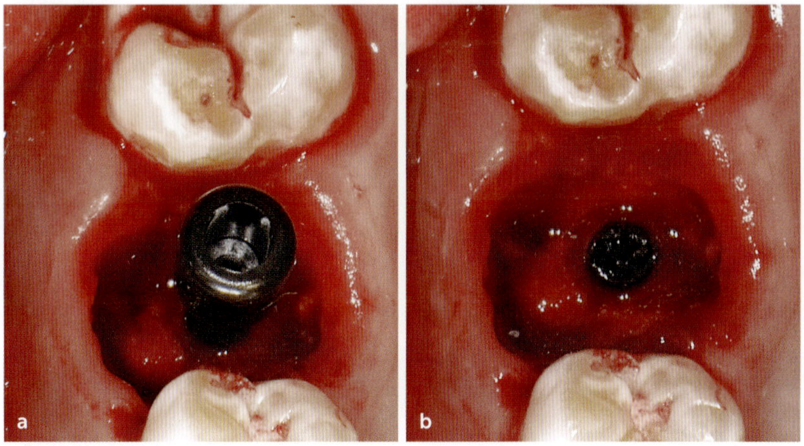

FIG 9-11 *(a)* The polytetrafluoroethylene (PTFE) healing plug was reinserted into the implant well. The plug can also be used to help confirm the proper prosthetic positioning of the implant. *(b)* The healing plug was cut at crestal level. It protects the implant well during the bone healing. Notice how the implant is subcrestally placed and not visible at the crest.

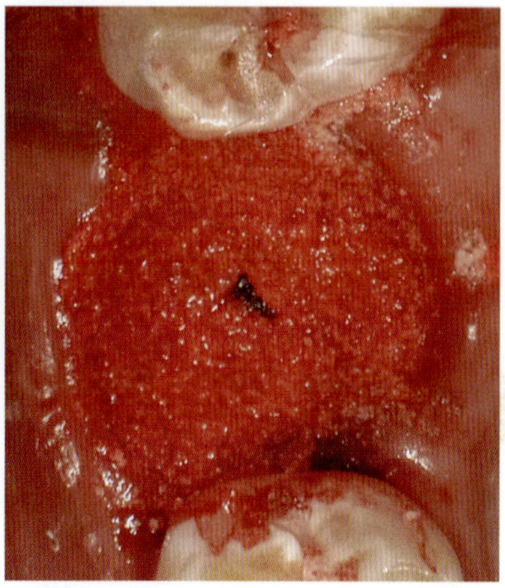

FIG 9-12 The grafting material completely filled the socket and covered the implant.

straight handle, positioned into the implant well, and tapped with a surgical mallet to fully seat the implant (Fig 9-10). Next, the black healing plug is reinserted into the implant well and shortened with a plug cutter to the level of the surrounding crestal bone (Fig 9-11).

To fill the remaining peri-implant gaps, the autogenous bone collected with the reamers was mixed with alloplast particles and the patient's blood for delivery using a syringe (Fig 9-12). The graft was protected by covering it with a collagen plug (Fig 9-13), and the flap margins were stabilized with sutures, making no attempt at primary closure (Fig 9-14). A final periapical radiograph showed the implant to be well-positioned without breaching of the sinus floor (Fig 9-15). The implant was restored after 6 months of site healing using an Integrated Abutment Crown (IAC; Bicon), a screwless and cementless restorative technique whereby a zirconium silicate microceramic crown is formed directly onto a Bicon abutment, forming a one-piece abutment–crown unit[1,35] (Fig 9-16a). A radiograph taken after 1 year in function is shown in Fig 9-16b, while the most recent one at 5 years is seen in Fig 9-16c.

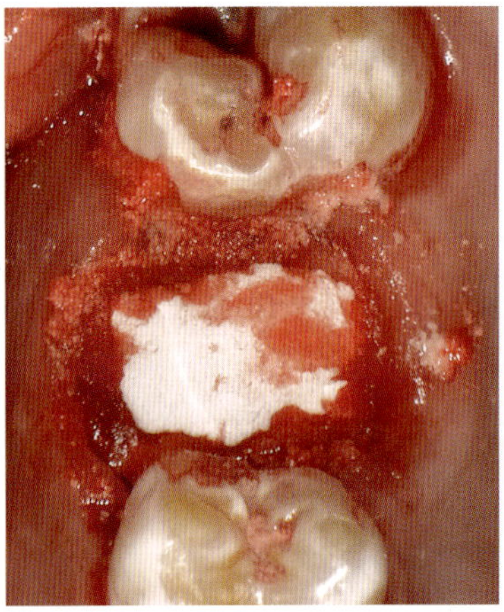

FIG 9-13 A double layer of collagen plugs was placed over the graft and tucked underneath the soft tissue margin to keep it in place.

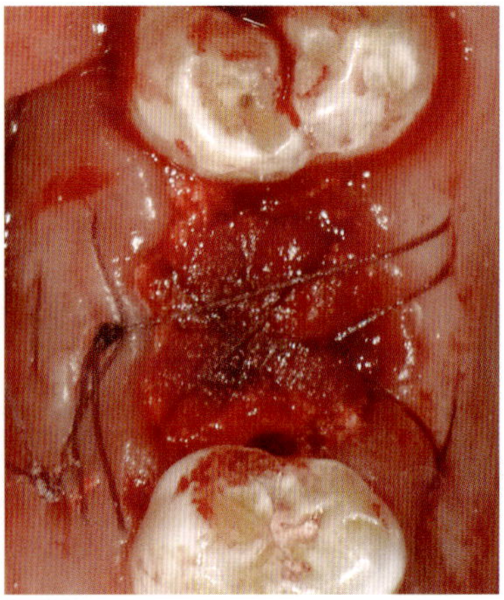

FIG 9-14 Horizontal cross mattress sutures and single sutures were placed to maintain the plugs in position.

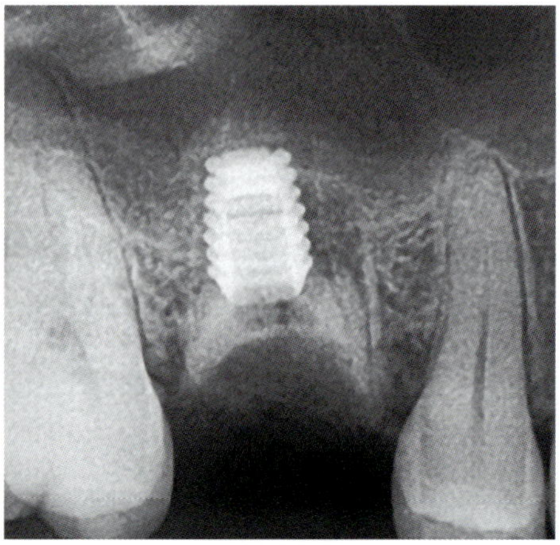

FIG 9-15 A postoperative radiograph was taken after surgery and confirmed the implant's proximity to the sinus floor. This demonstrates another advantage of short implants—avoiding unnecessary sinus elevation surgery.

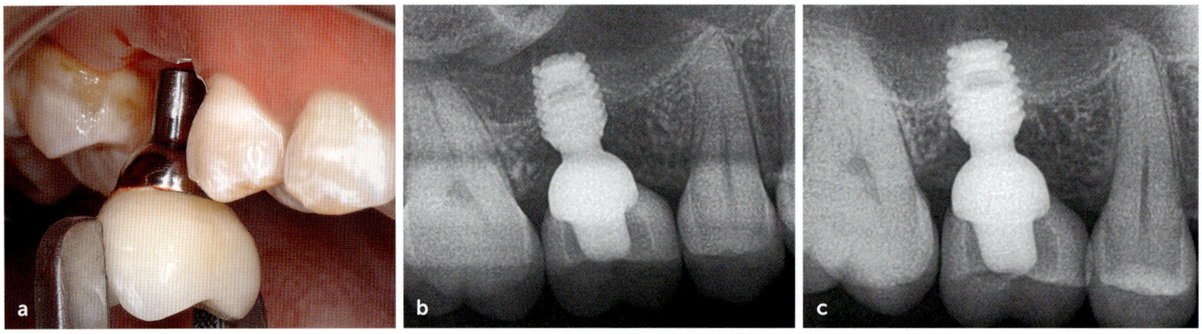

FIG 9-16 *(a)* The implant was restored after 6 months of site healing using an IAC. *(b)* This radiograph taken at the recall visit at 1 year in function shows bone growth over the sloped implant shoulder and around the ball-shaped prosthetic abutment, the latter also allowing for an effective platform switch at the interface between implant neck and abutment. *(c)* The most recent recall radiograph after 5 years in function.

Mandibular placement

The protocol for immediate mandibular molar PRF implant placement is similar to that for maxillary implant placement with only minor variances. Ideally, a substantial IRS (type B) will remain after atraumatic tooth removal.[34] If not, the clinician may opt to use the better of the mesial or distal root sockets, as shown in the case presented here. The patient shown required extraction of a mandibular left first molar, as it was nonrestorable and had endodontic complications (Fig 9-17).

The radiograph showed some loss of the IRS bone, making its use for positioning of an IMI questionable. Therefore, rather than opting for socket preservation and delayed implant placement, it was decided to use the distal root socket to receive the implant. The rationale here was as follows:

- The septum was minimal and not centrally located.
- The bone between the second premolar and first molar generally has less buccolingual ridge width than that between the two molars.
- The surface area of the distal root of a mandibular first molar is generally smaller than that of its mesial counterpart and therefore more appropriate for a press-fit implant design.

FIG 9-17 *(a)* Radiograph of compromised mandibular left molar with deficient endodontic treatment and apparent furcation involvement. *(b)* Clinical view of the tooth after crown removal.

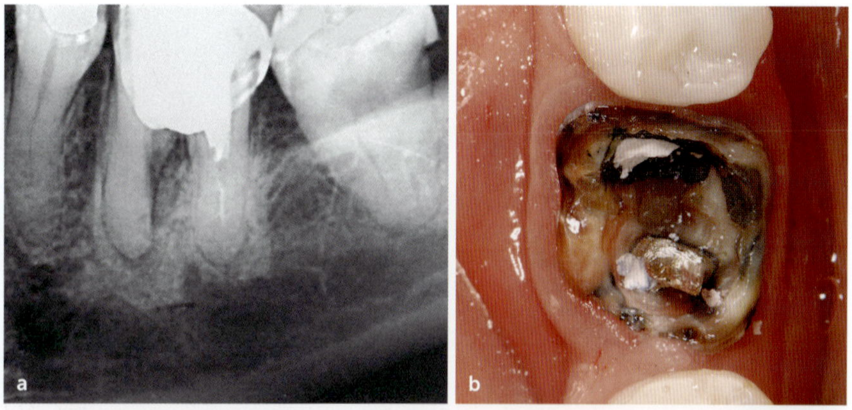

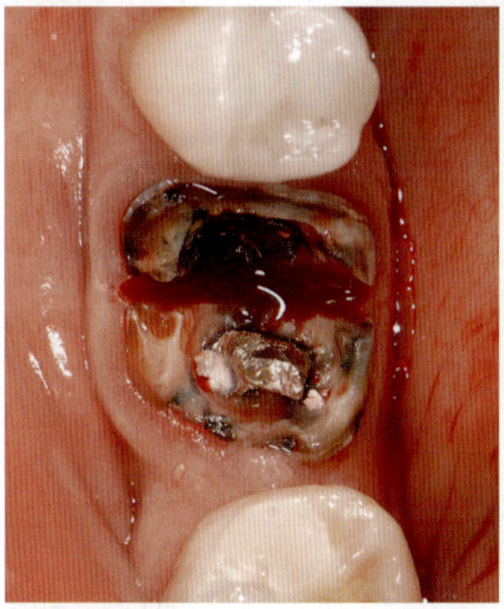

FIG 9-18 Root separation with tungsten carbide surgical burs after severing the periodontal ligament and carrying out gentle luxation using periotomes. This is followed by removing each of the now-mobile roots while preserving the socket integrity.

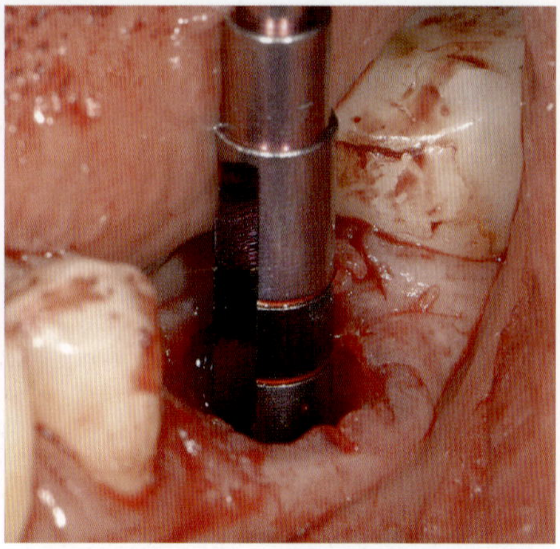

FIG 9-19 Special low-speed latch reamers are used after the pilot drilling to achieve the planned diameter of the osteotomy. The reamer diameters increase in a sequence of 0.5 mm per drill.

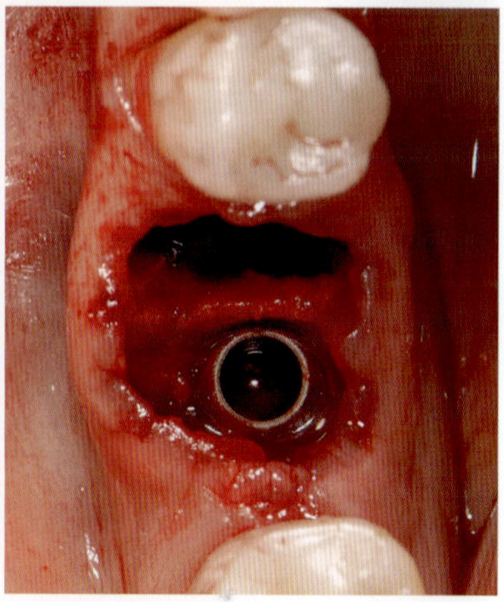

FIG 9-20 Implant seated inside the distal root socket. Notice the expansion of the thin septum toward the mesial.

The tooth was sectioned to allow removal of the two roots separately (Fig 9-18). A 6-mm-long × 5-mm-diameter PRF implant was selected. There was no need to use a pilot drill, and the site was prepared only with reamers, ending with the one corresponding with the planned implant diameter (Fig 9-19). Before implant placement, some of the usual collected and prepared graft material was inserted into the apical part of the implant osteotomy.

Thereafter, the implant was inserted and tapped into place, ensuring a tight initial press-fit with the socket walls (Fig 9-20). The black healing plug was inserted and trimmed to the level of the crestal bone (Fig 9-21a). All peri-implant gaps were filled with the usual graft mixture, as was the mesial root socket in the hope of minimizing loss in alveolar ridge width here (Fig 9-21b). Finally, the graft was protected with a collagen plug and the flap margins secured with sutures (Fig 9-21c). The immediate postoperative radiograph is depicted in Fig 9-21d. The implant integrated successfully and is shown radiographically and clinically in Fig 9-22 after 1 year in function.

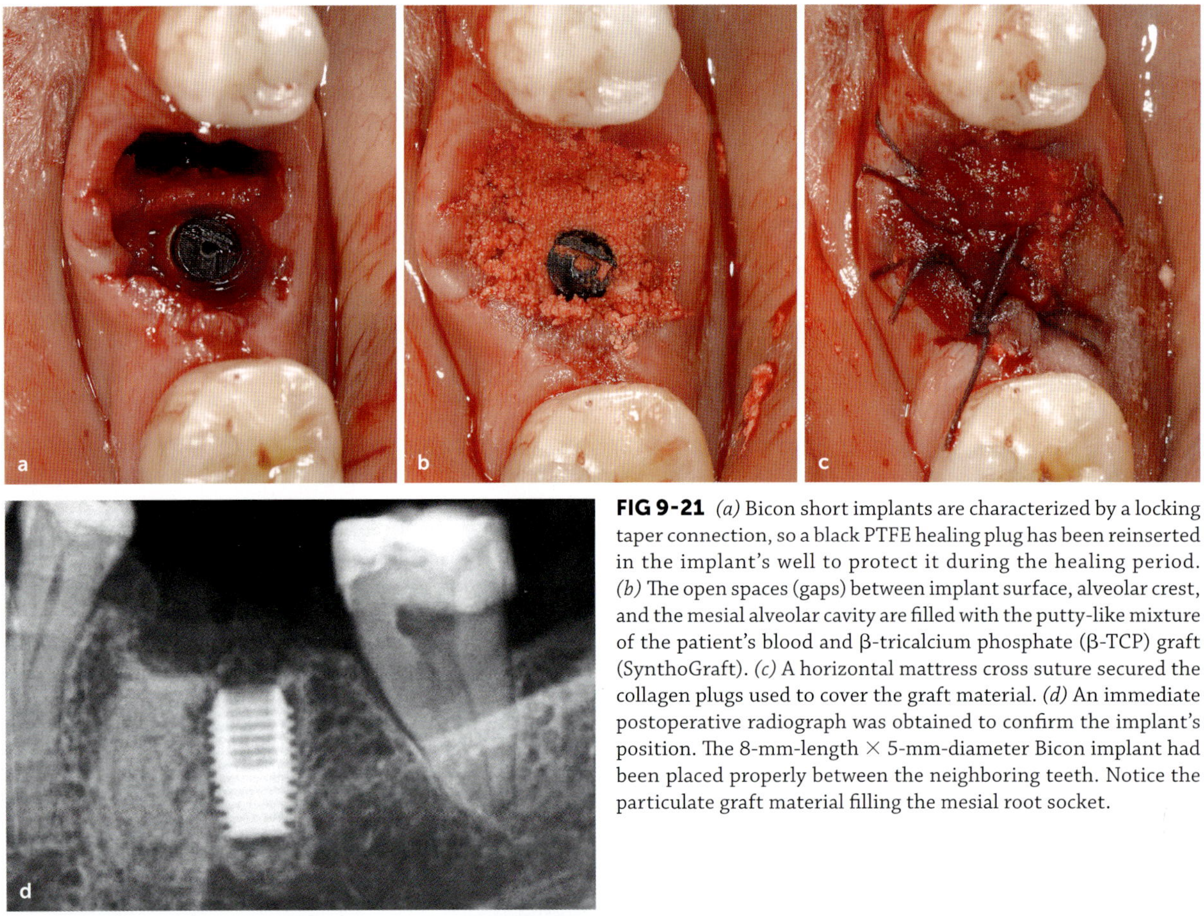

FIG 9-21 *(a)* Bicon short implants are characterized by a locking taper connection, so a black PTFE healing plug has been reinserted in the implant's well to protect it during the healing period. *(b)* The open spaces (gaps) between implant surface, alveolar crest, and the mesial alveolar cavity are filled with the putty-like mixture of the patient's blood and β-tricalcium phosphate (β-TCP) graft (SynthoGraft). *(c)* A horizontal mattress cross suture secured the collagen plugs used to cover the graft material. *(d)* An immediate postoperative radiograph was obtained to confirm the implant's position. The 8-mm-length × 5-mm-diameter Bicon implant had been placed properly between the neighboring teeth. Notice the particulate graft material filling the mesial root socket.

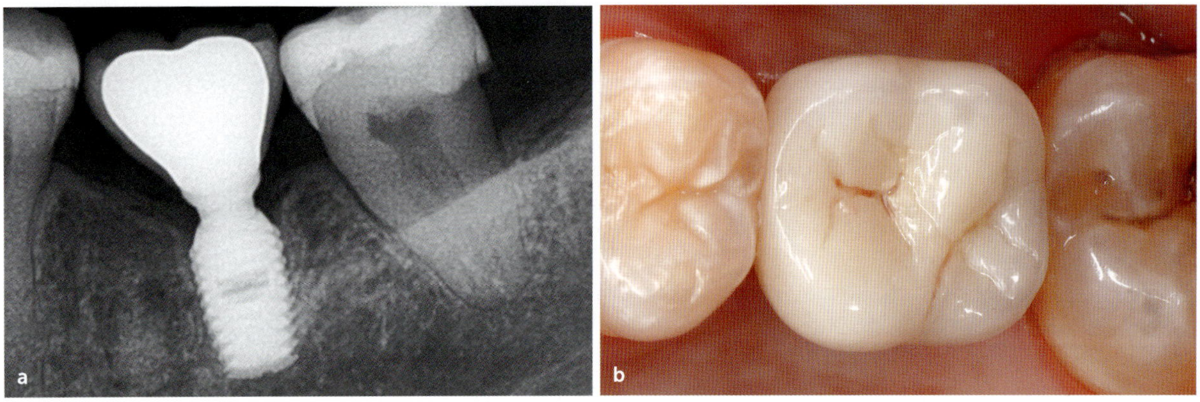

FIG 9-22 *(a)* A radiograph obtained after 1 year showing stable crestal bone. *(b)* The clinical image.

Management of Complications

Relatively few potential complications may occur during placement of PRF implants as IMIs or during their postoperative period. It is clear that there are advantages for the patient, the most evident being fewer surgical procedures and shorter treatment time.[36] Very few press-fit PRF implants will fail to become osseointegrated because they are forcibly seated into precise osteotomies and intentionally submerged subcrestally to allow undisturbed initial healing. The temporary healing plug ensures that the top of the implant will not become completely covered in bone and difficult to locate later. One key issue is that all four extraction socket walls must be intact, and ideally a substantial furcal septum will be present to allow positioning of the IMI in the ideal location for its prosthetic restoration. As with all dental implants, however, complications may occur in cigarette smokers or patients with poorly managed chronic severe periodontitis, both of which can increase the risk of early implant site infection (see also chapter 1).

One complication common with the placement of IMIs in either jaw is the fracture of one or more socket walls during tooth extraction or subsequent osteotomy preparation with the latch reamers. On careful inspection of the severity of the fracture, this complication may change the course of treatment. In some circumstances, such as a large fracture requiring replacement of an entire socket wall or more, the implant placement will have to be delayed for 2 or 3 months, and instead the socket should be grafted using a GBR approach.[37] However, if the socket damage is minor, it may be possible to repair it and continue with the IMI.

In patients with a U-shaped mandible[38] (see also chapter 2), there is often the possibility of perforating the lingual cortical plate in the mandible, particularly in second molar sites, resulting in perforation of the lingual cortex and the risk of hemorrhage or infection of the submandibular spaces. However, this serious risk is most unlikely when 6-mm-long PRF implants are being used.

Laceration of the inferior alveolar nerve is another possible complication during IMI placement in the mandible. In some instances, nerve damage may even arise simply because the distance from the implant apex to the inferior alveolar canal is too small (< 2 mm). Again, this is more likely to occur at second molar than at first molar sites.[38] The risk here can be minimized by examining preoperative CBCT scans, and if need be, by placing the implant in one of the two molar root sockets as shown in the example depicted earlier. Another precautionary move can be to avoid block anesthesia, relying instead on infiltration anesthesia only, delivered both buccally and lingually.

Complications exclusive to the maxilla include sinus floor perforation with or without implant displacement into the sinus. In the case of sinus perforation, the extent of the perforation needs to be assessed. Minor perforations can generally be sealed with a collagen plug[39] or better still with an autologous fibrin clot prepared from the patient's blood,[40,41] (see also chapters 1 and 4) and the IMI procedure completed. Autologous fibrin clots can also be used to seal larger perforations,[42] but implant placement will most likely need to be delayed here. In rare instances, an implant—particularly a short implant—can inadvertently slip into the sinus through an apical sinus floor perforation and may lead to sinusitis.[43] If symptoms do arise and the decision is made to remove the implant, this can be done with a lateral open window sinus procedure[44] or even using transnasal endoscopy.[45]

Conclusion

Immediate placement of PRF implants in molar sites is a feasible and relatively simple treatment provided that established protocols, including subcrestal placement, are followed. High initial stability is not a prerequisite as the implant's subcrestal seating by at least 2 mm will ensure that no early micromovements of the implant will impair its osseointegration. The ability to use short lengths with the PRF design helps to avoid complications that might otherwise arise with the use of longer implants.

KEY POINTS

- PRF implants are appropriate for use in short lengths.
- Placement in the IRS is ideal.
- Osteotomies are developed at low speed (50 rpm) without saline irrigation using side-cutting reamers.
- Autogenous bone is collected during site development and later used to fill peri-implant gaps.
- Implants are intentionally overseated by up to 3 mm to allow undisturbed initial integration.

References

1. Urdaneta RA, Marincola M, Weed M, Chuang SK. A screwless and cementless technique for the restoration of single-tooth implants: A retrospective cohort study. J Prosthodont 2008;17:562–571.
2. Renouard F, Nisand D. Impact of implant length and diameter on survival rates. Clin Oral Implants Res 2006;17(suppl 2):35–51.
3. Urdaneta RA, Daher S, Leary J, Emanuel KM, Chuang SK. The survival of ultrashort locking-taper implants. Int J Oral Maxillofac Implants 2012;27:644–654.
4. Gentile MA, Chuang SK, Dodson TB. Survival estimates and risk factors for failure with 6 × 5.7-mm implants. Int J Oral Maxillofac Implants 2005;20:930–937.
5. Arora H, Khzam N, Roberts D, Bruce WL, Ivanovski S. Immediate implant placement and restoration in the anterior maxilla: Tissue dimensional changes after 2-5 year follow up. Clin Implant Dent Relat Res 2017;19:694–702.
6. Marincola M, Lombardo G, Pighi J, et al. The immediate aesthetic and functional restoration of maxillary incisors compromised by periodontitis using short implants with single crown restorations: A minimally invasive approach and five-year follow-up. Case Rep Dent 2015;2015:716380.
7. Malchiodi L, Balzani L, Cucchi A, Ghensi P, Nocini PF. Primary and secondary stability of implants in postextraction and healed sites: A randomized controlled clinical trial. Int J Oral Maxillofac Implants 2016;31:1435–1443.
8. Checchi V, Felice P, Zucchelli G, et al. Wide diameter immediate post-extractive implants vs delayed placement of normal-diameter implants in preserved sockets in the molar region: 1-year post-loading outcome of a randomised controlled trial. Eur J Oral Implantol 2017;10:263–278.
9. Demircan S, Çankaya AB. Is immediate implant placement possible in the maxillary molar area? An anatomical study. Quintessence Int 2016;47:853–859.
10. Deporter D. Short dental implants: What works and what doesn't? A literature interpretation. Int J Periodontics Restorative Dent 2013;33:457–464.
11. Deporter D (ed). Short and Ultra-Short Implants. Chicago: Quintessence, 2018.
12. Coelho P, Marin C, Granato R, Suzuki M. Histomorphologic analysis of 30 plateau root form implants retrieved after 8 to 13 years in function. A human retrieval study. J Biomed Mater Res Part B Appl Biomater 2009;91:975–979.
13. Albrektsson T, Wennerberg A. Oral implant surfaces: Part 1—Review focusing on topographic and chemical properties of different surfaces and in vivo responses to them. Int J Prosthodont 2004;17:536–543.
14. Davies JE. Understanding peri-implant endosseous healing. J Dent Educ 2003;67:932–949.
15. Coelho PG, Suzuki M, Guimaraes MV, et al. Early bone healing around different implant bulk designs and surgical techniques: A study in dogs. Clin Implant Dent Relat Res 2010;12:202–208.
16. Adell R, Lekholm U, Rockler B, Brånemark PI. A 15-year study of osseointegrated implants in the treatment of the edentulous jaw. Int J Oral Surg 1981;10:387–416.
17. Leonard G, Coelho P, Polyzois I, Stassen L, Claffey N. A study of the bone healing kinetics of plateau versus screw root design titanium dental implants. Clin Oral Implants Res 2009;20:232–239.
18. Lemons JE. Biomaterials, biomechanics, tissue healing, and immediate-function dental implants. J Oral Implantol 2004;30:318–324.
19. Lemons JE. Dental implant retrieval analyses. Int J Oral Implantol 1988;5:41–45.
20. Baldassarri M, Bonfante E, Suzuki M, et al. Mechanical properties of human bone surrounding plateau root form implants retrieved after 0.3-24 years of function. J Biomed Mater Res B Appl Biomater 2012;100:2015–2021.
21. Gil LF, Suzuki M, Janal MN, et al. Progressive plateau root form dental implant osseointegration: A human retrieval study. J Biomed Mater Res B Appl Biomater 2015;103:1328–1332.
22. Bozkaya D, Muftu S, Muftu A. Evaluation of load transfer characteristics of five different implants in compact bone at different load levels by finite elements analysis. J Prosthet Dent 2004;92:523–530.
23. Chou HY, Romanos G, Müftü A, Müftü S. Peri-implant bone remodeling around an extraction socket: Predictions of bone maintenance by finite element method. Int J Oral Maxillofac Implants 2012;27:e39–e48.

24. Mello CC, Lemos CAA, Verri FR, Dos Santos DM, Goiato MC, Pellizzer EP. Immediate implant placement into fresh extraction sockets versus delayed implants into healed sockets: A systematic review and meta-analysis. Int J Oral Maxillofac Surg 2017; 46:1162–1177.
25. Jiansheng H, Dongying X, Xianfeng W, Baoyi X, Qiong L, Jincai Z. Clinical evaluation of short and wide-diameter implants immediately placed into extraction sockets of posterior areas: A 2-year retrospective study. J Oral Implantol 2012;38:729–737.
26. Annibali S, Bignozzi I, Iacovazzi L, La Monaca G, Cristalli MP. Immediate, early, and late implant placement in first-molar sites: A retrospective case series. Int J Oral Maxillofac Implants 2011;26:1108–1122.
27. Vandeweghe S, Ackermann A, Bronner J, Hattingh A, Tschakaloff A, De Bruyn H. A retrospective, multicenter study on a novo wide-body implant for posterior regions. Clin Implant Dent Relat Res 2012;14:281–292.
28. Amato F, Polara G. Immediate implant placement in single-tooth molar extraction sockets: A 1- to 6-year retrospective clinical study. Int J Periodontics Restorative Dent 2018;38:495–501.
29. Ketabi M, Deporter D, Atenafu EG. A systematic review of outcomes following immediate molar implant placement based on recently published studies. Clin Implant Dent Relat Res 2016; 18:1084–1094.
30. Lombardo G, Pighi J, Marincola M, Corrocher G, Simancas-Pallares M, Nocini PF. Cumulative success rate of short and ultrashort implants supporting single crowns in the posterior maxilla: A 3-year retrospective study. Int J Dent 2017; 2017:8434281.
31. Summers RB. The osteotome technique: Part 3—Less invasive methods of elevating the sinus floor. Compendium 1994;15: 698–710.
32. Sohn DS, Heo JU, Kwak DH, et al. Bone regeneration in the maxillary sinus using an autologous fibrin-rich block with concentrated growth factors alone. Implant Dent 2011;20:389–395.
33. Weiss A, Stern A, Dym H. Technological advances in extraction techniques and outpatient oral surgery. Dent Clin North Am 2011;55:501–513.
34. Smith RB, Tarnow DP. Classification of molar extraction sites for immediate dental implant placement: Technical note. Int J Oral Maxillofac Implants 2013;28:911–916.
35. Urdaneta RA, Marincola M. The integrated abutment crown, a screwless and cementless restoration for single-tooth implants: A report on a new technique. J Prosthodont 2007;16:311–318.
36. Urban T, Kostopoulos L, Wenzel A. Immediate implant placement in molar regions: Risk factors for early failure. Clin Oral Implants Res 2012;23:220–227.
37. Gher ME, Quintero G, Assad D, Monaco E, Richardson AC. Bone grafting and guided bone regeneration for immediate dental implants in humans. J Periodontol 1994;65:881–891.
38. Lin MH, Mau LP, Cochran DL, Shieh YS, Huang PH, Huang RY. Risk assessment of inferior alveolar nerve injury for immediate implant placement in the posterior mandible: A virtual implant placement study. J Dent 2014;42:263–270.
39. Doobrow JH, Leite RS, Hirsch HZ. Concomitant oroantral communication repair and immediate implant placement: A five-year case report. Implant Dent 2008;17:176–181.
40. Kim JM, Sohn DS, Bae MS, Moon JW, Lee JH, Park IS. Flapless transcrestal sinus augmentation using hydrodynamic piezoelectric internal sinus elevation with autologous concentrated growth factors alone. Implant Dent 2014;23:168–174.
41. Diss A, Dohan DM, Mouhyi J, Mahler P. Osteotome sinus floor elevation using Choukroun's platelet-rich fibrin as grafting material: A 1-year prospective pilot study with microthreaded implants. Oral Surg Oral Med Oral Pathol Oral Radiol Endod 2008;105:572–579.
42. Gülşen U, Şentürk MF, Mehdiyev İ. Flap-free treatment of an oroantral communication with platelet-rich fibrin. Br J Oral Maxillofac Surg 2016;54:702–703.
43. Conforte JJ, Ponzoni D. Sinusitis due to the presence of a dental implant inside the maxillary sinus. J Craniofac Surg 2018;29: e591.
44. Iida S, Tanaka N, Kogo M, Matsuya T. Migration of a dental implant into the maxillary sinus. A case report. Int J Oral Maxillofac Surg 2000;29:358–359.
45. Kitamura A. Removal of a migrated dental implant from a maxillary sinus by transnasal endoscopy. Br J Oral Maxillofac Surg 2007;45:410–411.

10

GUIDED SURGERY FOR PLACING IMMEDIATE MOLAR IMPLANTS

Ehsan Birang
Jaffer Kermalli
Mohammad Ketabi
Vahid Esfahanian
Nasim Farkhani

Inserting implants on the day of tooth extraction (immediate placement) or in the first few weeks (4 to 8) of soft tissue healing (early placement) is appealing to patients because it shortens treatment time and possibly treatment costs compared with late placement (> 6 months' healing). Systematic literature reviews on the topic of immediate replacement of failed molars using dental implants have suggested this treatment modality to be viable and predictable[1,2] (see also chapter 1). However, immediate molar implant (IMI) placement is recognized as a difficult procedure, and it generally needs be performed by highly skilled and experienced surgeons.[3] There are technical challenges such as avoiding bur chatter, controlling the final implant position, achieving adequate implant stability, and maintaining and/or manipulating adequate soft tissue for appropriate site closure.[4] Based considerably on in vitro testing in models,[5] it has been argued that these difficulties might be reduced by employing the techniques of guided implant surgery after merging CBCT DICOM (digital imaging and communication in medicine) files with intraoral jaw scans using commercially available computer software programs.[6,7] The tooth in question can be virtually eliminated from these preoperative software files to determine the ideal position of the future implant and design a corresponding surgical guide to assist with accurate osteotomy site drilling. This chapter will briefly explain the general principles of guided implant surgery, particularly with regard to IMIs.

As originally described by Brånemark and coworkers,[8] endosseous dental implants, like all oral surgical procedures, were done freehand, and therefore depended heavily on the surgeon's judgement, experience, operative skills, and ability to deal with unexpected and stressful intraoperative complications.[9] More and more, however, despite the added training and possible equipment expenditures required, digital techniques employing computer software and hardware are becoming more mainstream, with the goal of minimizing human errors in terms of implant position, angle, and depth.[10]

Guided computer-assisted implant surgery (CAIS) relies heavily on CBCT images, which allow lower doses of radiation exposure for the patient than standard multislice computed tomography (CT) imaging.[11] Combined with intraoral clinical optical scanning, these images can be used with implant planning computer software to predict the most appropriate implant position and subsequently allow the creation of a corresponding surgical drill guide using 3D printing or laboratory CAD/CAM technology. As a result, the implant can be placed in a prosthetically driven and optimal position for the circumstances encountered. Given the growing popularity of CAIS, many manufacturers now offer computer software programs for sale. Commonly used systems include Simplant Pro (Dentsply Sirona), coDiagnostiX (Dental Wings, Straumann), and NobelGuide (Nobel Biocare).

It should be pointed out that meta-analysis of published data indicates that while CAIS is superior to freehand implant surgery in terms of safety and postoperative morbidity, implant success with CAIS is more or less the same.[12] Furthermore, CAIS involves numerous steps, including fabrication of an optional (depending on the number of teeth remaining and length of edentulous span) radiographic stent to be used by the oral radiologist in obtaining the CBCT images; management of the DICOM files from the CBCT, including their importation into a software program; integration with an intraoral or laboratory scan of the patient's mouth with the CBCT files; and accurate fabrication of a surgical guide without distortion (ie, CAD/CAM milled or 3D-printed) and its use during surgery. One or more of these steps could potentially introduce errors in the final implant positioning.

Advantages of CAIS

The major advantages of digital implant planning software include the following:

- The possibility of planning treatment before tooth extraction
- The ability to discuss in detail the planned prosthetic treatment with the intended restorative dentist and lab technicians
- The ability to show the planned end result to the patient before undertaking it
- Greater accuracy in placing the implant in the preplanned desired location

Accuracy is defined in terms of deviations from the planned osteotomy entry point and apex as well as angle deviation of the implant's long axis and deviation in osteotomy depth (Fig 10-1). The tooth can be virtually extracted to allow a more reliable visual evaluation of its socket, including the presence and amount of interradicular septum (IRS) bone and the condition of its four bony walls. Ideally, IMIs should be placed in the socket's IRS, but if this bone is narrower than ideal (ie, type B and particularly type C of Smith and Tarnow's classification[13]), surgical drill chatter and drift may result in unfavorable final implant positioning. Fortunately, however, these problems can be reduced (although not totally eliminated) using digital implant placement software, as all drilling procedures will be directed by a computer-generated surgical guide prepared beforehand.

Other advantages of CAIS compared with the conventional freehand technique are greater ease in performing implant placement using a flapless and sutureless or a minimally raised flap approach, better final soft tissue profiles, and better collaboration and coordination between the radiologist, surgeon, restorative dentist or prosthodontist, and dental technician in treatment planning (eg, achieving prosthetically driven implant placement). Compared with well-executed CAIS, freehand implant placement can be much less accurate[14–17] (Fig 10-2). Lower postoperative morbidity for the patient also is a beneficial consideration.

CAIS can be used routinely for implant placement surgery but is most useful in the following situations:

- In sites previously augmented using guided bone regeneration where the option to use a flapless technique (eg, using only a small incision or the removal of a plug of keratinized tissue using a soft tissue punch) would reduce the risk of postsurgical bone loss

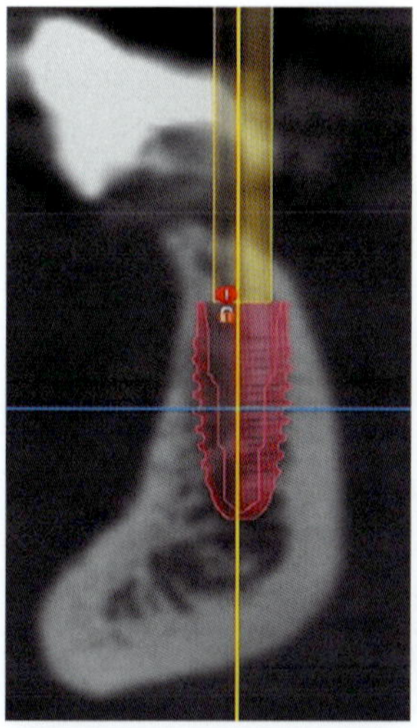

FIG 10-1 Using CAIS, ideal implant positioning and angulation can be achieved.

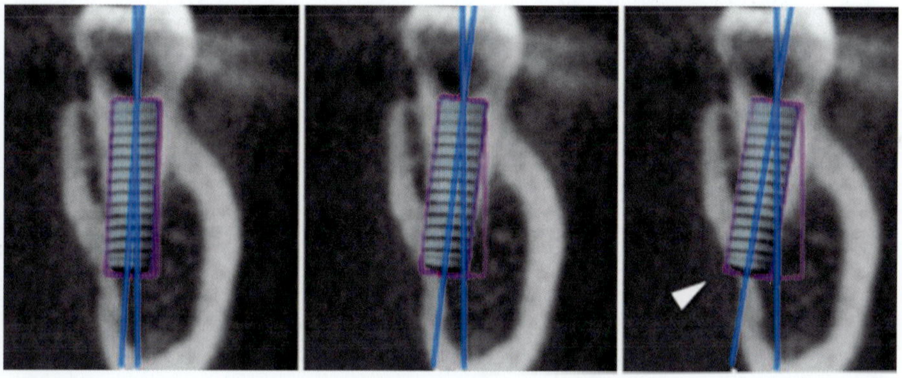

FIG 10-2 Freehand implant placement comes with the risk of improper implant positioning.

- In situations where two or more implants are planned and their parallelism is crucial to ensure ideal esthetics and straightforward use of screw-retained prostheses
- To ensure that osteotomies avoid damage to the maxillary sinus, adjacent teeth, inferior alveolar canal, major vessels, or the nasal cavity
- In simplifying the placement of IMIs, particularly where the socket is type B or C[13]

Limitations of CAIS

There are some practical limitations with CAIS. In their systematic literature review, Jung et al[18] noted that unexpected intraoperative complications can occur, including inadequate interocclusal space to allow CAIS (ie, to accommodate the surgical guide), insufficient primary stability following implant insertion, and possible unexpected need for additional grafting procedures. The quality of the CBCT images is highly important and can be inaccurate, for example, if there is scatter from metal artifacts or if the patient moves during the CBCT examination. As well, using only a small-field CBCT scan may not provide sufficient anatomical landmarks to merge accurately with the intraoral clinical scan. As a result, a larger field scan with some unavoidable increased radiation exposure may be required.

Also, once the surgical guide has been fabricated, its use will not allow any modification from the predetermined implant position during surgery. Any local tissue changes (eg, new soft tissue inflammation/swelling or unexpected loss of one or more of the guide's original abutment teeth) between the time of ordering the surgical guide and actual implant installation can alter the fit of the final prosthesis. Guide dislocation or fracture also can occur during surgery if the guide cannot be adequately stabilized. The best stabilization for these guides can be achieved for CAIS placement of implants in single-tooth gaps.[19] Also, CAIS surgical guides must be prepared to conform to the instrumentation of the implant system intended for use, and changing the implant system being used during surgery is generally not an option. There are also some philosophical hurdles for experienced practitioners in accepting the cost, extra education, time, and learning curves needed to master CAIS technology. An experienced surgeon usually can predictably place an implant freehand with acceptable speed and accuracy, often without a CBCT. The increased costs of a CBCT scan, the surgical guide software, fabrication of the guide, and guided implant-specific surgical instrumentation may be an impairment while not necessarily yielding a significantly different treatment outcome.

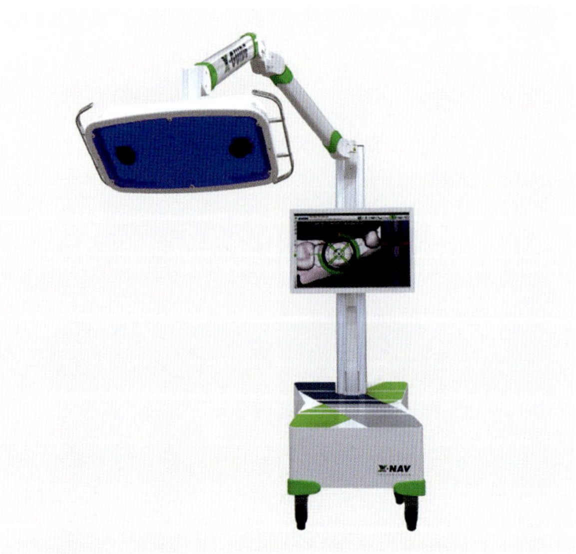

FIG 10-3 An example of a commercially available dynamic, image-guided navigation system.

Types of CAIS

Static and dynamic

There are two general types of CAIS: static and dynamic navigation.[14] The choice of which to use is for the clinician to decide—with the exception of fully edentulous arches, which generally require the static method. *Static navigation* refers to the use of the aforementioned rigid surgical templates/guides and coordinated instrumentation to guide osteotomy site drilling and implant placement according to the pretreatment planning. There are three types of static guides:

1. Nonlimiting, where only the first pilot drill is guided while the other drilling is freehand
2. Semilimiting, where the entire drilling sequence is done using the guide but not during actual implant insertion
3. Fully limiting, where the whole procedure (drilling and implant insertion) is done with the surgical guide in place

The guides can be made by a laboratory using CAD/CAM technology or created in office via 3D printing. The resulting stent or stents (in the past, some clinicians preferred to prepare multiple stents, one for each bur in the sequence needed to finalize the osteotomy) will have a metal guide tube or sleeve located at each intended implant site and meant to direct the burs in creating the osteotomies. This method can result in accurate space management and depth control in drilling as well as apical deviation and angulation errors of less than 5 degrees from the pretreatment plan, all errors being significantly smaller than those using freehand methods. The main disadvantage here, however, is the inability to change the presurgical planned implant position intraoperatively.

Dynamic CAIS systems use visual imaging tools on a computer monitor instead of rigid intraoral stents and allow the surgeon to alter the surgical implant positioning in real time using anatomical information available from the preoperative CBCT scan and displayed at chairside on the monitor.[20] Computerized navigation systems (eg, IGI, Image Navigation; Navident, ClaroNav) are optically based, using infrared cameras to detect and track the intraoperative position of specially designed contra-angle dental surgical handpieces equipped with LEDs that signal their real-time positions to the camera (Fig 10-3). The surgeon can see an icon of the drill bit on the monitor in a 3D relationship to the patient's previously scanned local anatomy. In a patient who has difficulty with mouth opening or requires an implant at a second molar site with limited access, dynamic navigation allows the surgeon to place the implant by monitoring the navigation screen without direct visualization in the patient's mouth. However, a prolonged learning curve in developing proficiency for both the surgeon and assistant may be an issue. The costs of purchasing the necessary equipment also can be a deterrent, making static CAIS systems more practical in private dental practices.[21] A training period is required before use on patients, and the learning curve can be steep.[22] Most experts comment that further clinical investigations are needed to assess the true benefits of this approach, including time consumption analysis in comparison to other methods. Dynamic navigation systems involve considerable financial outlay, and while they generally produce better outcomes than freehand implant surgery, they may not offer better outcomes than static fully-guided CAIS techniques.

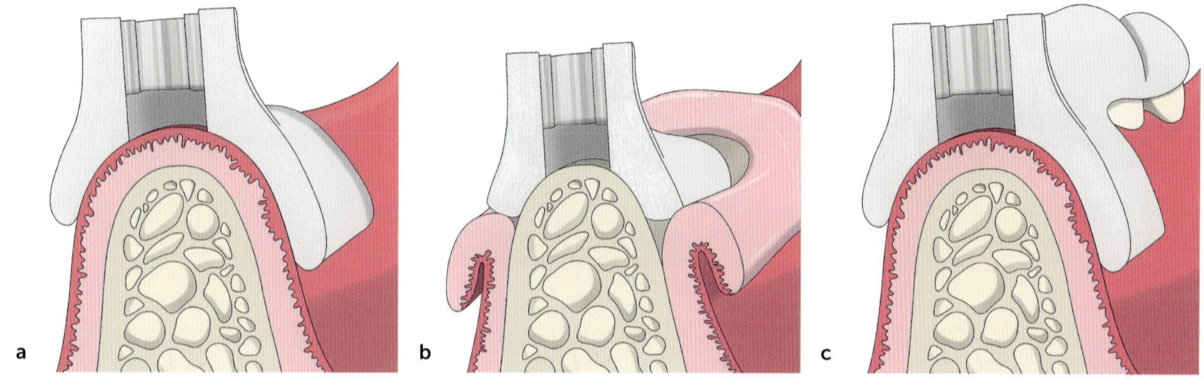

FIG 10-4 Surgical guides can be variously supported as shown. *(a)* Mucosa-supported. *(b)* Bone-supported. *(c)* Tooth- and mucosa-supported. (Illustration provided by Dr Ryan Noh, University of Toronto.)

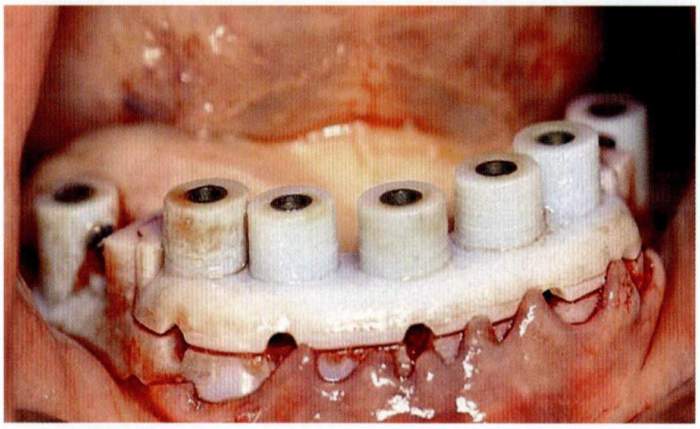

FIG 10-5 An example of a mandibular full-arch, bone-supported static closed CAIS surgical guide. Burs must be frequently removed and reinserted to minimize the risk of elevated temperatures damaging bone.

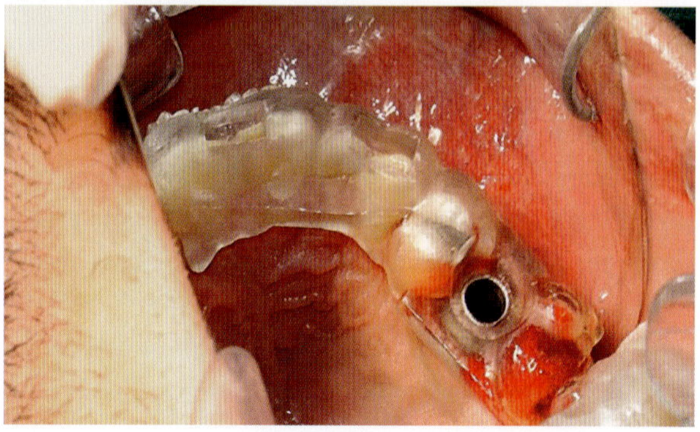

FIG 10-6 An example of a closed half-arch, tooth-supported guide being used to insert a maxillary first molar IMI.

Guide support type

Static navigation currently is the more commonly used approach and can be further classified according to type of guide support being planned. Support for the guide can be mucosal only, directly onto bone, and/or tooth-supported (Fig 10-4). Mucosal support is ideal for full-arch edentulous cases where alveolar ridge anatomy and the quality and quantity of soft tissues are suitable for a flapless surgical procedure. Mucosal support offers greater accuracy than osseous support with fully edentulous interventions,[23] and less risk of surgically created bacteremia.[24] The main drawback when using mucosal support, however, is that it is not possible to include hard tissue augmentation following implant placement should this turn out to be required. In order to make this augmentation feasible with full-arch cases, guide support needs to be planned using bone, may require using special mini implants for guide stabilization,[25] will require longer in-chair treatment times, and will result in increased postoperative morbidity because of the need to raise flaps (Fig 10-5). In partially edentulous patients such as those requiring one or two IMIs, CAIS guides can also be prepared with the support of the patient's remaining teeth in the same jaw segment or arch[26] (Fig 10-6).

Closed and open guides

Static CAIS guides can also be designed as closed or open. Closed guides cover the entire surgical field and do not allow visibility of the underlying bone or soft tissues during the bone drilling sequence and implant placement. They are more restrictive than open guides and may not allow sufficient cooling fluid to come in direct contact with drills during bone preparation, thereby increasing the risk of elevated bone tempera-

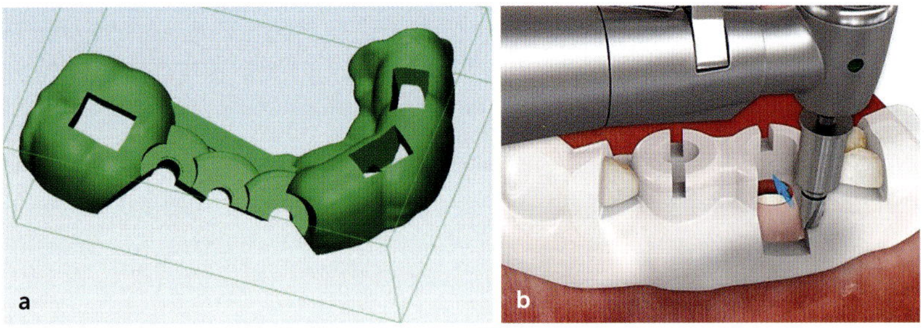

FIG 10-7 *(a and b)* Examples of open guides that allow the operator some visual control, access to sites affected by limited mouth opening, and avoidance of overheating.

tures and compromised healing. As a result, some authors have suggested the use of precooled irrigation fluid with closed guides[27] and that the drills be frequently removed and reinserted during site preparation.[28] Open CAIS guides have accesses located on their sides at each planned implant site, allowing direct visual monitoring of the tissues during osteotomy preparation (Fig 10-7). Some presurgical errors in planning or guided system inaccuracies discovered during drilling can be overcome with this added direct visual monitoring. For example, hard or soft tissue defects can be detected and corrected. Open guides also allow better cooling of drills during bone preparation. One disadvantage may be increased risk of errors in implant positioning, as an open guide provides less restrictive drilling, allowing the burs to drift buccally.

Fully or half-guided

Finally, static guides can be used for fully guided or half-guided implant placement.[29] In both approaches, CBCT exploration, 3D planning, and prosthetic analysis are used before preparing a surgical guide. The only difference is that, with the fully guided approach, the usual metal guiding tubes or sleeves for each drill are included, whereas with the half-guided approach, the metal tubing is omitted or a sleeve for only the first drill is included so that osteotomy preparation is manually controlled by the surgeon. At least one group concluded that the accuracy of half-guided implant surgery is comparable to that of the fully guided method. Drill-to-sleeve tolerance is also an issue with the fully guided technique because if the bur-to-sleeve gap is too large, bur drift is possible, while if it is too small, friction with the formation of metal debris may be a problem. By the same token, this tolerance needs to be intimate enough to avoid bur tilting or rocking within the guide.

Researchers have used randomized clinical trials to compare fully guided static CAIS to freehand implant placement without the use of templates. For example, Arisan et al[30] assessed errors in interproximal emergence, insufficient interimplant distance, and improper parallelism using freehand versus fully guided CAIS. Each of 54 patients presented with at least one fully edentulous arch and were seeking its restoration with an implant-supported fixed prosthesis. Patients were allocated to have either fully guided or freehand implant surgery. In total, 353 implants were placed in the 54 patients. Either mucosal- or bone-supported guides were chosen as required for the 21 patients enrolled in the CAIS group. The probability of errors in implant positioning with freehand placement was significantly higher than with fully guided surgery (88% with freehand vs 6% with fully guided placement using a single guide with all of the implant burs needed for implant placement). However, CAIS-positioned implants more often ended up more lingually or buccally positioned compared with those placed freehand. In another study, Farley et al[31] compared implant placement using fully guided surgical templates compared with conventional guides prepared without computer input. Two implants were placed bilaterally by the same surgeon in 10 patients. CAIS-directed implants were placed on one side of each patient's mouth using flapless surgery, while flaps were raised on the contralateral side to allow conventional guides to be employed. Implants placed with computer-generated guides generally were placed closer to their planned positions, although the differences from those placed using conventional guides were mostly not statistically significant.

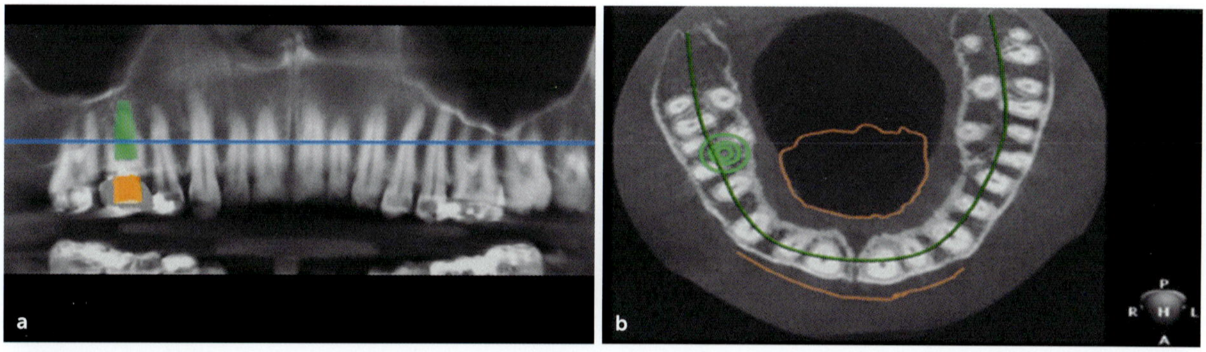

FIG 10-8 *(a and b)* CBCT images are prepared in DICOM format in preparation for IMI placement at the maxillary right first molar site.

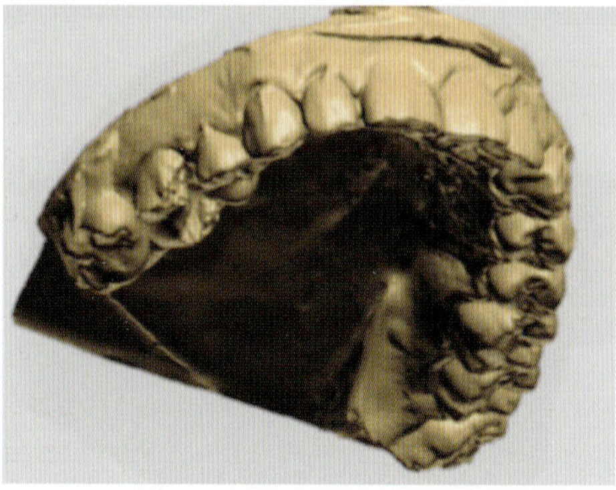

FIG 10-9 An optical scan of the patient's jaw can be done intraorally or from a model using a 3D laboratory scanning machine.

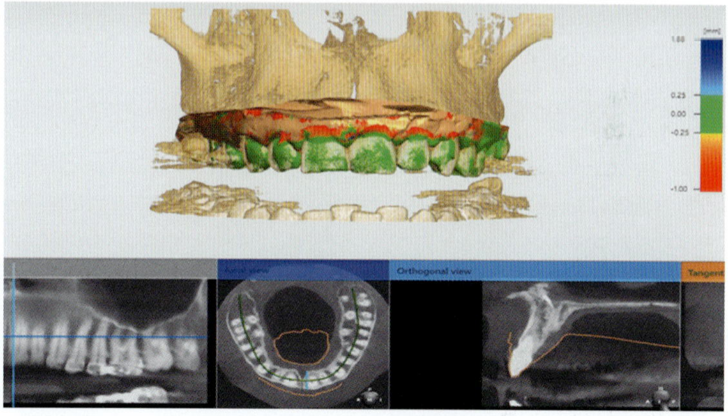

FIG 10-10 Super-impositioning of DICOM (CBCT) and STL (scanned) files for measurement and analysis of soft and hard tissues.

CAIS for IMIs

CBCT scan

Should a molar appear to be a candidate for IMI treatment, the first step is to obtain a high-quality 3D CBCT scan of the site. This will allow an initial assessment of the bone quality and quantity, the molar socket anatomy and overall configuration of the surrounding alveolus, any root proximity to vital anatomical structures, the dimensions of the IRS, possible bony dehiscences and/or fenestrations, and the presence of any periradicular infection. The CBCT file needs to be prepared in DICOM format (Fig 10-8) and uploaded to the planning software program being used.

Jaw scanning

Optical scanning of the jaw involved is also required (Fig 10-9) and can be done either directly in the patient's mouth using an intraoral scanner (eg, CEREC Omnicam, Dentsply Sirona; Virtuo Vivo, Straumann) or indirectly from casts using scanners in the dental laboratory. The scanning must include both hard and soft tissues and be prepared in stereolithography (STL) file format, making it suitable for 3D printing. Thereafter, the DICOM file of the CBCT scan and the STL file of the intraoral or laboratory scan are merged (Fig 10-10). This will then allow evaluation of the available bone, the soft and hard tissue relationships, 3D planning of implant positioning, determination of ideal size and position of the fixture, and likelihood of any grafting procedures being required at the time of implant placement surgery.

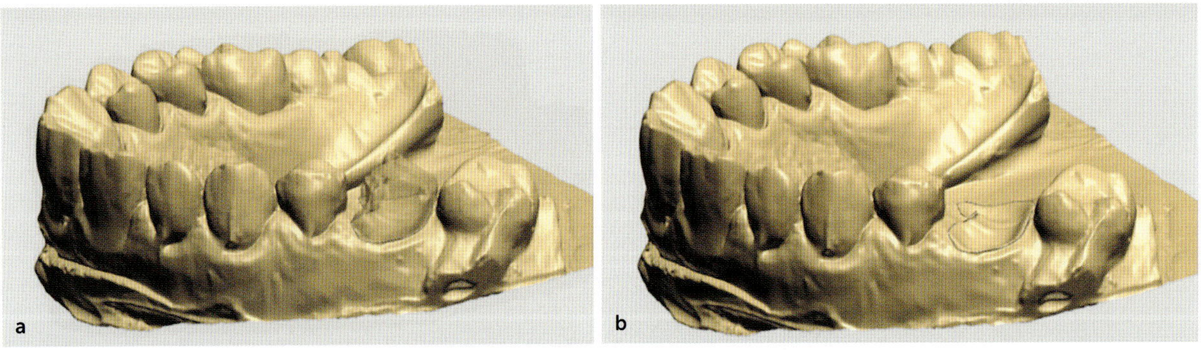

FIG 10-11 *(a and b)* The scanned image of the condemned tooth can be removed virtually as part of the planning process.

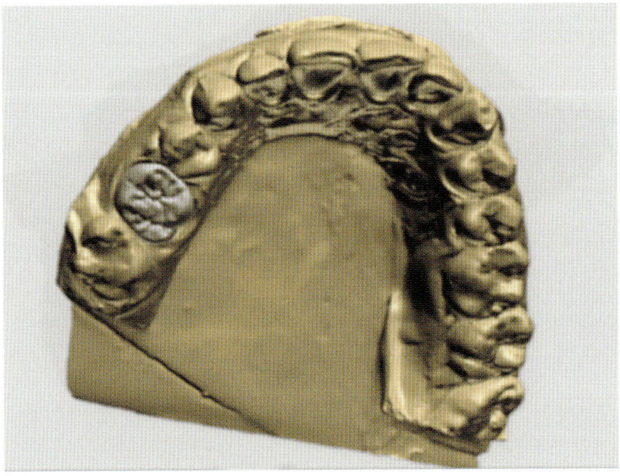

FIG 10-12 The final restoration can be virtually designed during the treatment planning phase.

Implant location and selection

To plan the treatment, the tooth or teeth in question are first virtually eliminated using the software program to allow study of the ideal implant position using the library of implant systems available in the software planning program (Fig 10-11). The aim is to plan the implant position to be in the center of the socket mesiodistally and slightly toward the lingual in the mandible and palatally in the maxilla to minimize future buccal bone loss. Unless subcrestal implant placement is planned, apicocoronally, the implant should be positioned 2.5 to 3.0 mm apical to cemento-enamel junctions of the adjacent teeth and 3.0 to 4.0 mm apical to the gingival margins of these teeth. The implant diameter should be chosen to be able to leave at least 1.8 mm of bone thickness both buccally and lingually/palatally after osteotomy preparation. To achieve the best emergence profile for the future implant prosthesis, consideration should be given to positioning it 1 to 2 mm below the bone crest buccally. The proper abutment, ideal angle of emergence, and the future crown also can be planned virtually (Fig 10-12).

Preparation of surgical guide

In order to prepare a static CAIS surgical guide, impressions and an occlusal registration must be obtained, and casts must be prepared and trimmed to allow a diagnostic wax-up of the intended final prosthesis to be prepared. This wax-up can then be used to fabricate an imaging stent to be used by the radiologist in obtaining the necessary pretreatment CBCT scan. Barium sulphate (20% concentration) is applied to the tissue side of the radiographic guide[32] to make it opaque and visible in radiographs, helping to estimate soft tissue thickness and its relation to bone (Fig 10-13).

Once the CBCT scan has been obtained, the images can be merged with either an intraoral optical scan of the patient's mouth or a laboratory scan of the wax-up

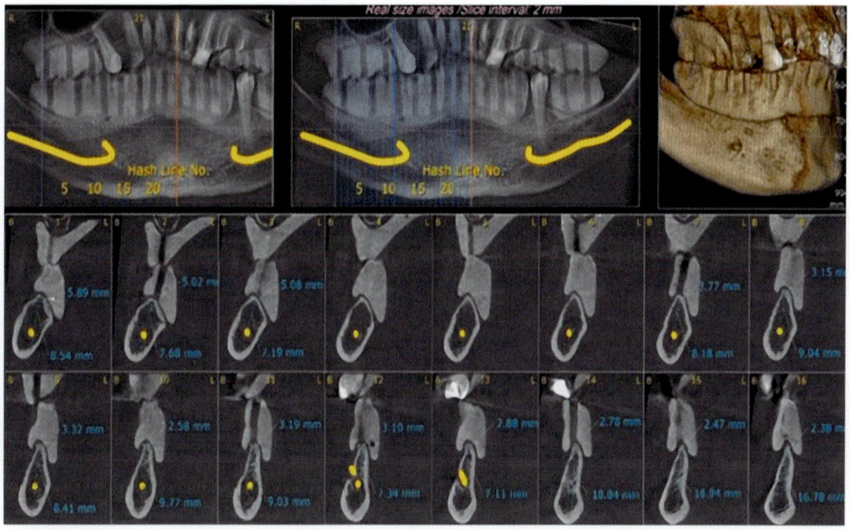

FIG 10-13 To prepare the DICOM file for the patient, a radiographic guide lined with barium sulphate is needed to obtain suitable CBCT scans.

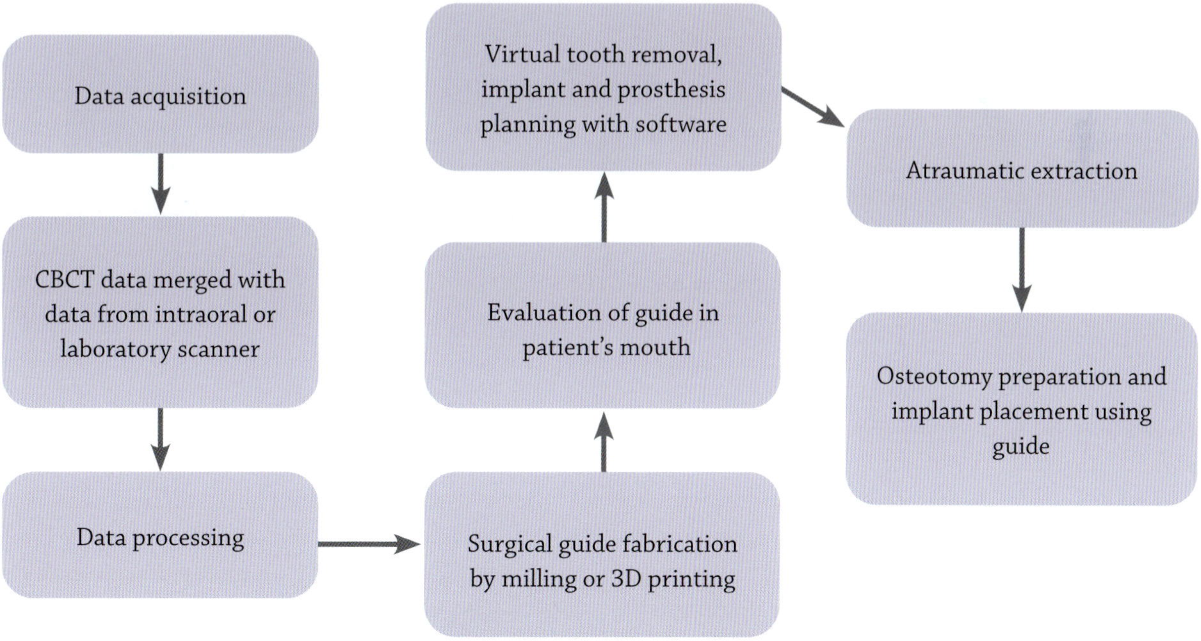

FIG 10-14 A flowchart outlining the steps involved in creating a CAIS surgical guide.

using computer software to preplan the appropriate location, diameter, length, and 3D positioning of the required implants. These data can then be used to create the CAIS surgical guide (Fig 10-14).

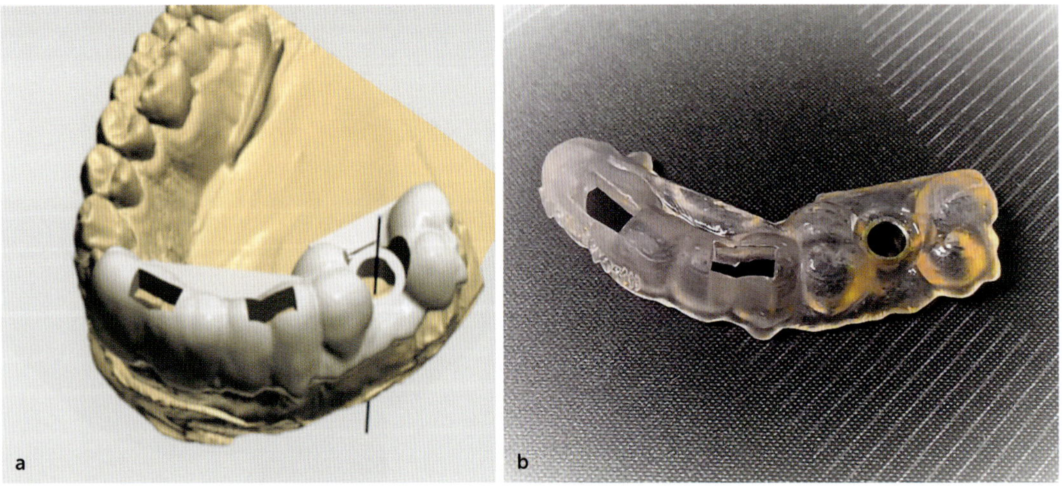

FIG 10-15 *(a)* The "wax-up" for the surgical guide is designed virtually. *(b)* A tooth-supported stent is preferred for use in IMI placement.

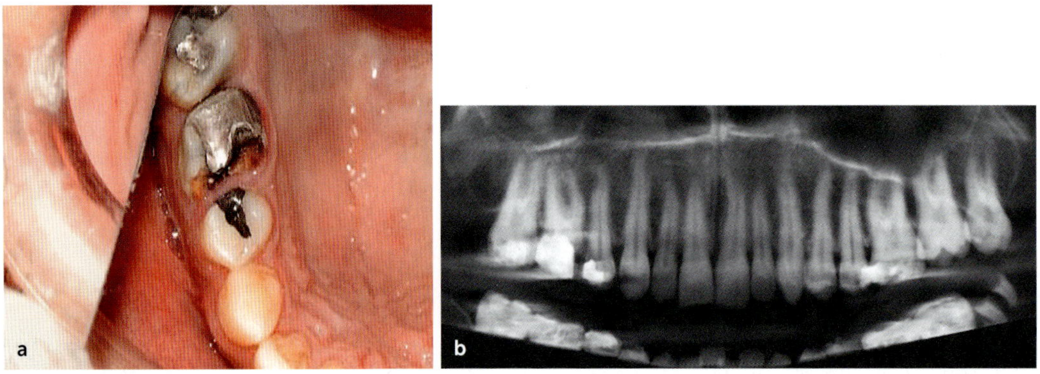

FIG 10-16 *(a)* This maxillary first molar needed to be extracted, and the plan was to replace it with an IMI. *(b)* The pretreatment panoramic radiograph showed the maxillary right first molar to have a type B IRS. →

Printing of surgical guide

After finishing the software analysis and treatment plan, the STL file is sent to either a 3D printer or laboratory with a milling apparatus to create the surgical stent/guide. With 3D printers, the guide will be made by an additive technique, whereas with a milling apparatus, it is made by a subtractive technique. An appropriate guide sleeve for the guided surgery armamentarium being used must also be added. For immediate molar implantation, ideally the neighboring teeth will still be present to permit fabrication of a fully tooth-supported stent/guide (Fig 10-15). If not, some additional mucosal or bone support for the guide may be necessary.

Surgical procedure

A sample case is presented here starting with Figs 10-16a and 10-16b. As discussed in other parts of this book, placement of IMIs should ideally employ flapless surgery. After making sharp intracrevicular incisions, the molar is first decoronated at the level of its cementoenamel junction with a high-speed handpiece and bur. This will allow access for direct visualization during separation of the molar roots and their individual removal, and it will allow the surgeon to assess the remaining IRS[13] (Fig 10-16c). The surgical guide can then be inserted into the patient's mouth, ensuring a precise fit and adequate support for stability (Fig 10-16d). This being the case, osteotomy prepa-

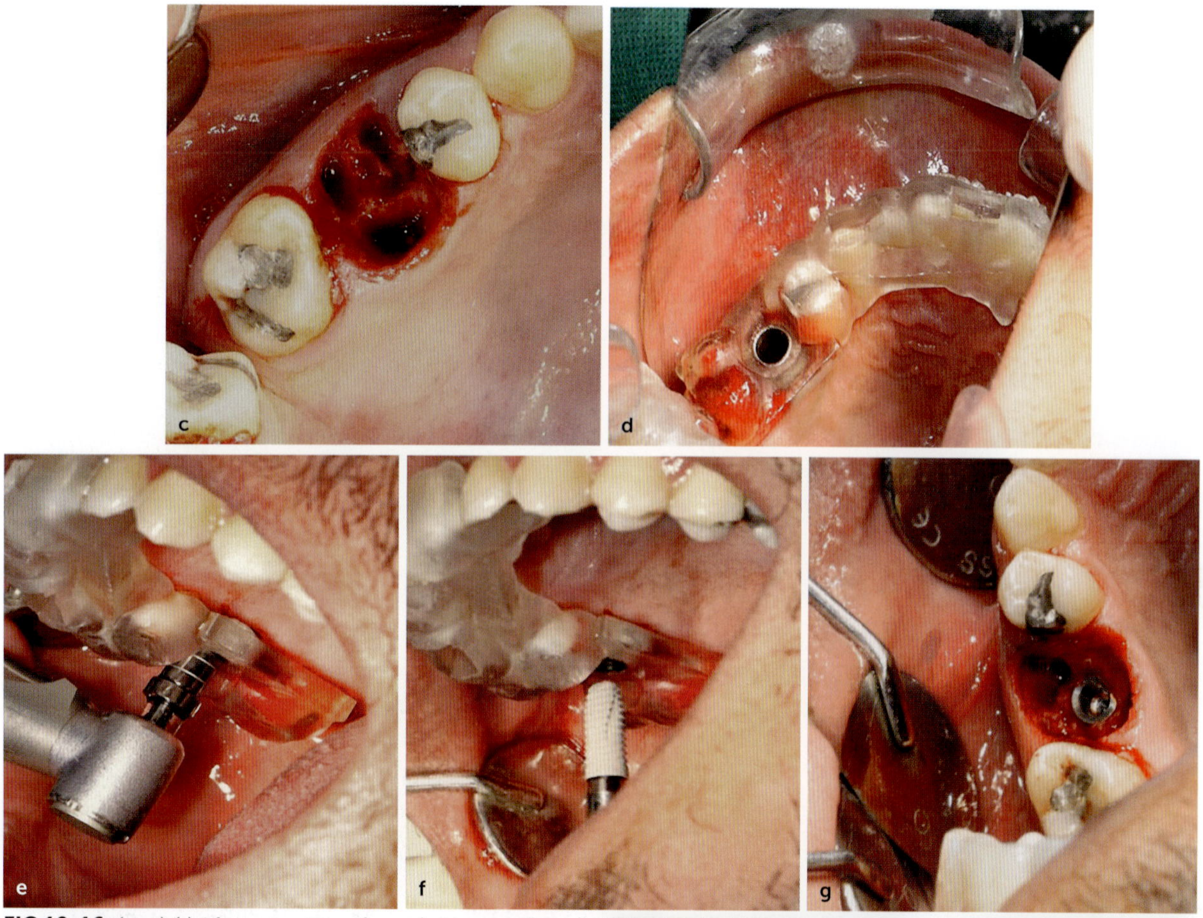

FIG 10-16 *(cont) (c)* After extraction, the socket was confirmed to be type B according to the Smith and Tarnow classification.[13] *(d)* The surgical stent was first inserted to verify that the fit was precise. *(e)* All site drilling was performed using the surgical guide. *(f)* The implant can also be inserted with the guide in place. *(g)* The implant has been fully seated in the IRS bone and is ready to receive a long healing abutment. *(h)* This immediate postoperative radiograph shows the implant in place with its added healing abutment. The tooth had had an unusually long root trunk (see part *b*), affecting the original height of IRS and final insertion depth of the implant.

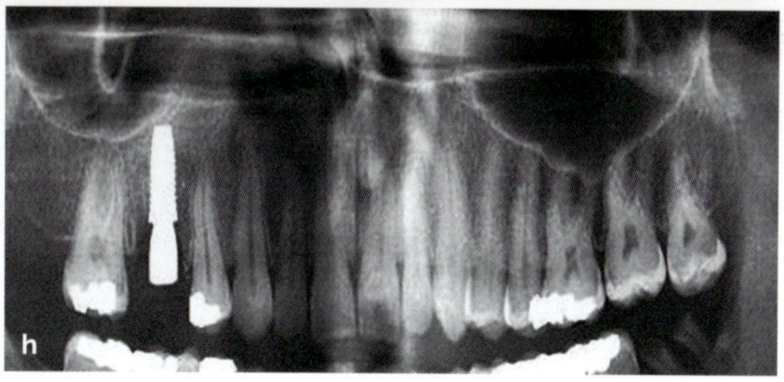

ration can then be begun with the required series of burs all being guided by the metal sleeve located over the planned implant site (Fig 10-16e). The implant can also be delivered with the assistance of the guide sleeve (Fig 10-16f). After removing the stent and ensuring that the implant has adequate stability, either a stock or a custom healing abutment or provisional restoration can be added (Figs 10-16g and 10-16h). As long as the procedure has been flapless and any gaps are sheltered by the healing abutment and thick gingival tissue, they need not necessarily be grafted according to the latest findings[33] (see also chapter 11).

The second sample case using static CAIS technique is that of a patient seeking IMI replacement of his mandibular first molar (Fig 10-17a). The IRS of the tooth was type C (Fig 10-17b), making it difficult to localize the osteotomy within bone.[13] A tooth-supported, fully guided static surgical guide was prepared (Fig 10-17c), checked for fit (Fig 10-17d),

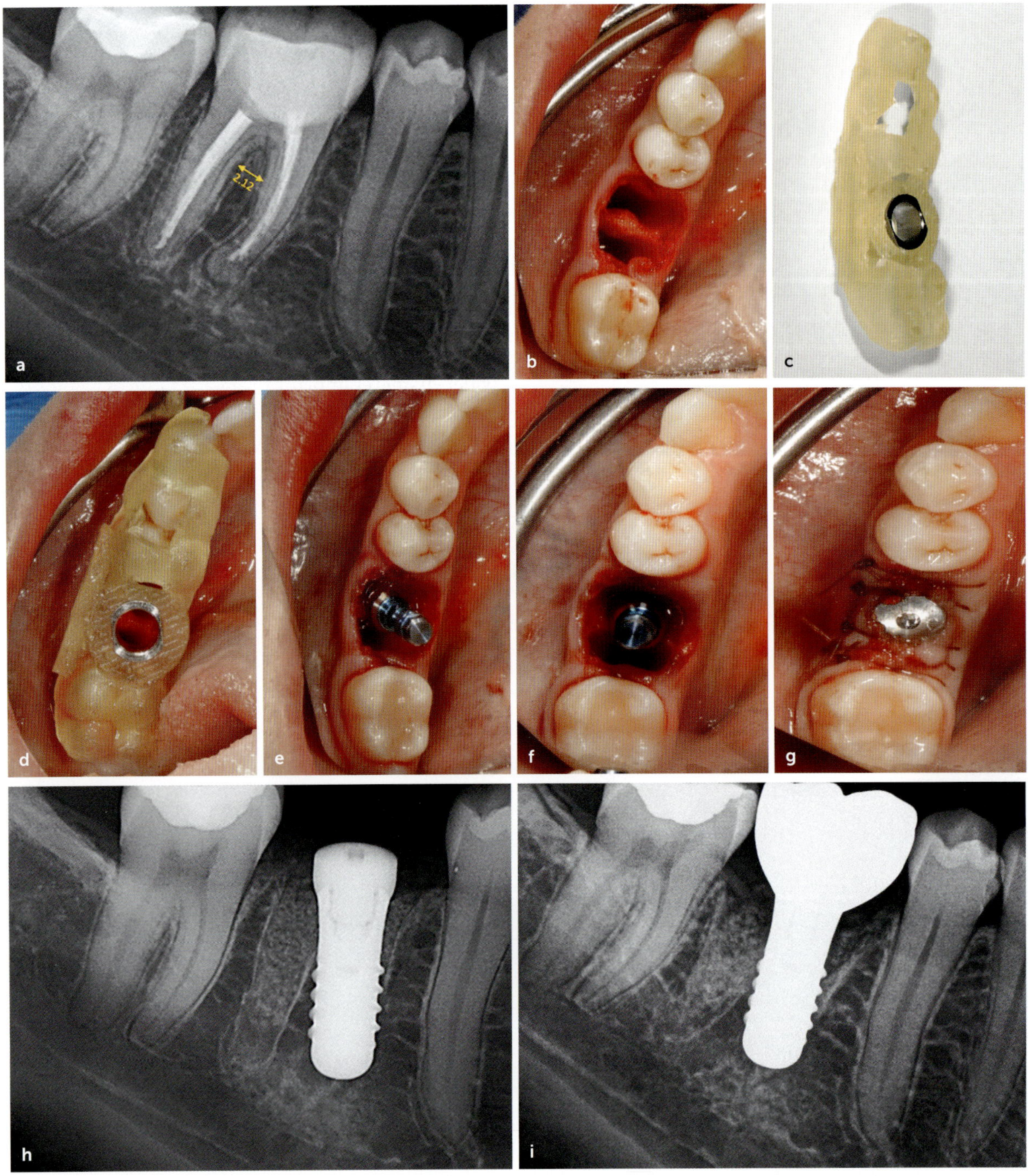

FIG 10-17 *(a)* The endodontically treated first molar was symptomatic and needed removal. *(b)* After tooth removal, the IRS can be seen to be type C. The narrowness of the IRS would have made it impossible to prepare the desired osteotomy without the assistance of a guided surgical approach. *(c)* A tooth-supported guide for fully guided surgery was prepared. *(d)* The surgical guide was first tested for appropriate fit and then used to perform the osteotomy drilling. *(e)* Osteotomy drilling and implant insertion using static fully guided CAIS resulted in optimal positioning of the IMI. *(f)* The implant can be seen to be stabilized by the remaining lingual and buccal buttresses of the instrumented IRS with large gaps mesially and distally. *(g)* After grafting the gaps with particulate allograft and adding a healing abutment, the soft tissue margins were stabilized with interproximal sutures. *(h)* The immediate postoperative radiograph shows the implant to be well-positioned and partially supported by the original narrow IRS. The gaps were grafted with particulate allograft material. *(i)* A radiograph of the restored implant.

and used to prepare the required osteotomy and implant insertion (Fig 10-17e). Because the procedure was fully guided, the final implant position was optimal and stabilized initially by contact with the buccal and lingual buttresses of bone (Fig 10-17f). The remaining peri-implant gaps were filled with allograft particulate, a healing abutment was added, and the soft tissues were stabilized with sutures (Fig 10-17g). The immediate postoperative and post-restoration radiographs show the graft material in the remaining gaps and the implant partially stabilized by what remained of the IRS (Figs 10-17h and 10-17i).

Conclusion

There are few if any reports describing outcomes with IMIs placed using CAIS methodology, but the most likely situation where it would be beneficial would be as shown in the second sample case in this chapter, ie, where a type C IRS would make optimal osteotomy preparation and implant positioning a serious challenge. The more common approaches in this situation have been either to avoid immediate implantation and perform socket preservation grafting with delayed implant placement or to remove the IRS and use a wider-diameter implant to engage more of the socket walls. Other than the added preparation and cost of a computer-generated surgical guide, CAIS offers a third viable option for this problem. However, the surgeon should beware of molars with long root trunks leading to implant overseating, as was the outcome in the case presented in Fig 10-16.

KEY POINTS

- Static CAIS is more widely used and documented than dynamic CAIS.
- Static CAIS generally is more accurate than freehand implant placement.
- Static CAIS implant placement has, until now, not been used widely for the placement of IMIs.
- Considerable extra time and costs are incurred with static CAIS, including those for software and hardware purchases, treatment planning and consultation with others (including the restorative dentist and laboratory technicians), fabricating a radiographic stent prior to ordering a CBCT scan, purchasing a reliable intraoral scanner, fabricating a precise surgical stent, and investing in implant-specific guided surgery instrumentation.
- Comparisons of static CAIS and anatomically guided IMI placement (ie, leaving the roots in situ and drilling through the molar furca and underlying bone with some or all of the necessary osteotomy drill bits) have not been done yet but may not produce significantly different outcomes.
- Static CAIS can be particularly helpful in placing IMIs in narrower-diameter type B or type C IRS bone.

References

1. Atieh MA, Payne AG, Duncan WJ, et al. Immediate placement or immediate restoration/loading of single implants for molar tooth replacement: A systematic review and meta-analysis. Int J Oral Maxillofac Implants 2010;25:401–415.
2. Ketabi M, Deporter D, Atenafu EG. A systematic review of outcomes following immediate molar implant placement based on recently published studies. Clin Implant Dent Relat Res 2016; 18:1084–1094.
3. Dawson A, Chen S (eds). The SAC Classification in Implant Dentistry. Quintessence 2009.
4. Bhola M, Neely AL, Kolhatkar S. Immediate implant placement: Clinical decisions, advantages, and disadvantages. J Prosthodont 2008;17:576–581.
5. Bover-Ramos F, Viña-Almunia J, Cervera-Ballester J, Peñarrocha-Diago M, García-Mira B. Accuracy of implant placement with computer-guided surgery: A systematic review and meta-analysis comparing cadaver, clinical, and in vitro studies. Int J Oral Maxillofac Implants 2018;33:101–115.
6. Somogyi-Ganss E, Holmes HI, Jokstad A. Accuracy of a novel prototype dynamic computer-assisted surgery system. Clin Oral Implants Res 2015;26:882–890.
7. Emery RW, Merritt SA, Lank K, Gibbs JD. Accuracy of dynamic navigation for dental implant placement-model-based evaluation. J Oral Implantol 2016;42:399–405.
8. Adell R, Lekholm U, Rockler B, Brånemark PI. A 15-year study of osseointegrated implants in the treatment of the edentulous jaw. Int J Oral Surg 1981;10:387–416.
9. Renouard F, Amalberti R, Renouard E. Are "human factors" the primary cause of complications in the field of implant dentistry? Int J Oral Maxillofac Implants 2017;32:e55–e61.
10. Tatakis DN, Chien HH, Parashis AO. Guided implant surgery risks and their prevention. Periodontol 2000 2019;81:194–208.
11. Harris D, Horner K, Gröndahl K, et al. E.A.O. guidelines for the use of diagnostic imaging in implant dentistry 2011. A consensus workshop organized by the European Association for Osseointegration at the Medical University of Warsaw. Clin Oral Implants Res 2012;23:1243–1253.
12. Tahmaseb A, Wismeijer D, Coucke W, Derksen W. Computer technology applications in surgical implant dentistry: A systematic review. Int J Oral Maxillofac Implants 2014;29 Suppl:25–42.
13. Smith RB, Tarnow DP. Classification of molar extraction sites for immediate dental implant placement: Technical note. Int J Oral Maxillofac Implants 2013;28:911–916.
14. Block MS, Emery RW. Static or dynamic navigation for implant placement-choosing the method of guidance. J Oral Maxillofac Surg 2016;74:269–277.
15. Vercruyssen M, Coucke W, Naert I, Jacobs R, Teughels W, Quirynen M. Depth and lateral deviations in guided implant surgery: An RCT comparing guided surgery with mental navigation or the use of a pilot-drill template. Clin Oral Implants Res 2015;26:1315–1320.
16. Tattan M, Chambrone L, González-Martín O, Avila-Ortiz G. Static computer-aided, partially guided, and free-handed implant placement: A systematic review and meta-analysis of randomized controlled trials. Clin Oral Implants Res 2020;31:889–916.
17. Younes F, Cosyn J, De Bruyckere T, Cleymaet R, Bouckaert E, Eghbali A. A randomized controlled study on the accuracy of free-handed, pilot-drill guided and fully guided implant surgery in partially edentulous patients. J Clin Periodontol 2018;45: 721–732.
18. Jung RE, Schneider D, Ganeles J, et al. Computer technology applications in surgical implant dentistry: A systematic review. Int J Oral Maxillofac Implants 2009;24(suppl):92–109.
19. Behneke A, Burwinkel M, Behneke N. Factors influencing transfer accuracy of cone beam CT-derived template-based implant placement. Clin Oral Implants Res 2012;23:416–423.
20. Gargallo-Albiol J, Barootchi S, Salomó-Coll O, Wang HL. Advantages and disadvantages of implant navigation surgery. A systematic review. Ann Anat 2019;225:1–10.
21. Katsoulis J, Pazera P, Mericske-Stern R. Prosthetically driven, computer-guided implant planning for the edentulous maxilla: A model study. Clin Implant Dent Relat Res 2009;11:238–245.
22. Block MS, Emery RW, Lank K, Ryan J. Implant placement accuracy using dynamic navigation. Int J Oral Maxillofac Implants 2017;32:92–99.
23. Vercruyssen M, Laleman I, Jacobs R, Quirynen M. Computer-supported implant planning and guided surgery: A narrative review. Clin Oral Implants Res 2015;26 Suppl 11:69–76.
24. Arısan V, Bölükbaşı N, Öksüz L. Computer-assisted flapless implant placement reduces the incidence of surgery-related bacteremia. Clin Oral Investig 2013;17:1985–1993.
25. D'haese J, Ackhurst J, Wismeijer D, De Bruyn H, Tahmaseb A. Current state of the art of computer-guided implant surgery. Periodontol 2000 2017;73:121–133.
26. Raico Gallardo YN, da Silva-Olivio IRT, Mukai E, Morimoto S, Sesma N, Cordaro L. Accuracy comparison of guided surgery for dental implants according to the tissue of support: A systematic review and meta-analysis. Clin Oral Implants Res 2017;28:602–612.
27. Boa K, Barrak I, Varga E Jr, Joob-Fancsaly A, Varga E, Piffko J. Intraosseous generation of heat during guided surgical drilling: An ex vivo study of the effect of the temperature of the irrigating fluid. Br J Oral Maxillofac Surg 2016;54:904–908.
28. Liu YF, Wu JL, Zhang JX, Peng W, Liao WQ. Numerical and experimental analyses on the temperature distribution in the dental implant preparation area when using a surgical guide. J Prosthodont 2018;27:42–51.
29. Kühl S, Zürcher S, Mahid T, Müller-Gerbl M, Filippi A, Cattin P. Accuracy of full guided vs. half-guided implant surgery. Clin Oral Implants Res 2013;24:763–769.
30. Arisan V, Karabuda CZ, Mumcu E, Özdemir T. Implant positioning errors in freehand and computer-aided placement methods: A single-blind clinical comparative study. Int J Oral Maxillofac Implants 2013;28:190–204.
31. Farley NE, Kennedy K, McGlumphy EA, Clelland NL. Split-mouth comparison of the accuracy of computer-generated and conventional surgical guides. Int J Oral Maxillofac Implants 2013;28:563–572.
32. Basten CH, Kois JC. The use of barium sulfate for implant templates. J Prosthet Dent 1996;76:451–454.
33. Smith RB, Tarnow DP, Sarnachiaro G. Immediate placement of dental implants in molar extraction sockets: An 11-year retrospective analysis. Compend Contin Educ Dent 2019;40:166–170.

11

MODIFICATIONS TO IMMEDIATE MOLAR IMPLANT PLACEMENT PROTOCOLS

Mohammad Ketabi
Douglas Deporter
Howard Gluckman
Charles Schwimer
Marcello Ferrer
Richard Smith
Samvel Bleyan
Ali Akbar Khoshkhounejad
Nikfam Khoshkhounejad

Some recent publications have suggested "out-of-the-box" changes to the way in which immediate molar implants (IMIs) are placed. These include management of jumping distances, ie, the gaps left around the periphery of IMIs; socket shielding to help in retaining bundle bone and alveolar ridge width; optimal choice of implant diameter in minimizing root caries risk for contiguous teeth; using osseodensification with added graft material for atraumatic indirect sinus floor elevation at maxillary IMI sites; and use of short and ultra-short implants as IMIs.

Gap Grafting and IMI Placement

During the past three decades of study and development in the field of dental implants, clinicians and researchers have constantly strived to make patient treatments easier, more natural and esthetically pleasing, faster, and—most importantly—less invasive. The introduction of IMIs with or without immediate limited loading is one of these stellar developments. Even though some of the first reports of immediate implant placement showed that grafting of peri-implant socket defects might not be necessary provided that a barrier membrane was used to cover the osteotomy site for the first few weeks of healing,[1,2] somehow these observations were overlooked for years. As dental surgeons, we felt compelled to insert particulate bone or bone substitutes into peri-implant gaps just as we had long been doing with periodontal intrabony defects, thinking that this would promote bone healing, and—having done so—to use primary wound closure with submerged implant healing.[3,4] Later, however, it was found that any added graft material (eg, allograft, xenograft, or alloplastic material) slows down the normal sequence of bone healing due to the body's need to resorb and/or adapt to the added materials, and as a result reduces the amount of new vital bone formed.[5] We also learned that we might avoid primary closure of soft tissues if the added graft material were to be covered with a nonresorbable[6] or, more recently, resorbable[7] barrier material. Who would have thought that neither of these interventions may be necessary for successful outcomes as recent reports have now shown?

Literature review

Reviewing early investigations on gap healing is appropriate here. Akimoto et al[8] studied the impact of gap size on peri-implant bone fill in dogs. Following flap elevation at healed extraction sites, gaps were created by overpreparing or enlarging osteotomies coronally but of appropriate size apically in order to obtain implant primary stability. In this way, osteotomy sites were prepared with coronal circumferential gaps of 0.5-, 1.0-, and 1.4-mm width. Primary soft tissue closure without intervening barriers was included, and after 12 weeks of submerged implant site healing, all gaps appeared clinically to have complete bone fill. However, histologic assessment revealed that fibrous connective tissue had developed between newly formed bone and the implant surface to variable depths such that the wider the initial gap, the more fibrous tissue. The likely explanation for this outcome was that the machined-surface implants used had allowed bone healing by distance osteogenesis only,[9] ie, outgrowth from the osteotomy walls. Primary soft tissue closure had also been used, but without insertion of a barrier membrane so that connective tissue repositioned over the implants without an intervening barrier membrane would have allowed fibrous tissue formation at the implant surface faster than bone cells could populate it, explaining the findings.[10]

Later, Botticelli et al[11] did similar work in dogs but with moderately rough[12] rather than machined implants and covered them with resorbable membranes before flap closure. Under these conditions, defects of 1.0 to 2.5 mm filled with bone with no fibrous tissue interface at the implant surface. The most likely explanation was that the roughened implant surface allowed for both distance and contact osteogenesis[9] and that the barriers blocked early connective tissue ingrowth into the gaps. Botticelli et al[13] also investigated spontaneous gap fill in humans. Eighteen patients requiring extraction of a total of 21 teeth (incisors, canines, or premolars) with planned immediate implant placement were included. Following flap elevation and tooth extraction, Straumann SLA (sandblasted, large-grit acid-etched) Tissue Level implants (2.8-mm-long transgingival collars) were placed such that the marginal level of the SLA portion was subcrestal relative to the buccal and lingual/palatal socket walls. Measurements of all remaining gaps had revealed 52 gaps greater than 3 mm, including 21 at buccal, 17 at lingual/palatal, and 14 at approximal surfaces. No graft materials or barriers were used with the implants being allowed to heal transgingivally, the soft tissues having been sutured about the exposed implant necks. After 4 months of healing, reentries were performed and the clinical measurements repeated. All but eight gaps originally greater than 3 mm had filled with bone.

Flapless surgery and gap grafting

A major step forward with immediate implant placement was the realization that teeth needing removal should be extracted without raising a mucogingival flap, meaning that primary soft tissue closure was not an option. The reasoning here was that if extraction sites heal naturally without soft tissue primary closure, why shouldn't sites with added dental implants do the same? Tarnow and Chu[14] tested this possibility in one patient where placement of an immediate maxillary anterior implant had left a labial gap of greater than 4-mm width. No graft or barrier materials were used, and as with normal extraction socket healing, bone filled the gap completely. In an attempt to understand this outcome, the authors noted that during normal healing at routine extraction sites, no attempt at flap closure is common so that reepithelization is delayed until the original blood clot is replaced with granulation tissue via angiogenesis from the socket bony walls, which takes 2 weeks or more. Only then can epithelium migrate over the healing wound. A peri-implant gap is merely a reduced-size extraction socket as far as the body is concerned, so why shouldn't it heal on its own with unprovoked bone fill? While the present discussion relates to IMIs, it should be noted that gap grafting may still be of value in anterior sites where esthetic outcomes are more important. Thus, in a recent review paper, Al-Kudmani et al[15] concluded that gap grafting supported superior soft tissue stability and preserved anatomical horizontal ridge dimensions when compared with no grafting.

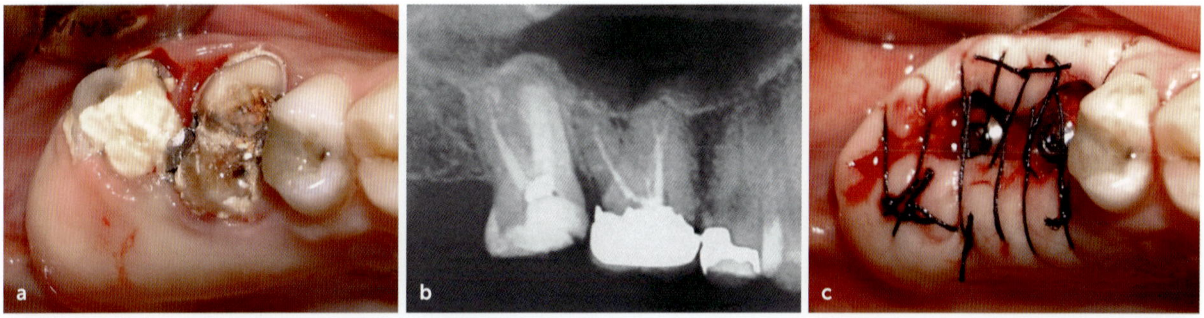

FIG 11-1 *(a)* Two heavily restored and hopeless maxillary molars required extraction. *(b)* Both teeth had received endodontic treatments in the past, and the first molar showed evidence of persistent infection. *(c)* The extraction procedure was flapless, and after socket debridement, two Dentium Superline implants with healing caps were placed. No gap grafting or barrier membranes were used, the soft tissues simply being passively secured with sutures.

More recently, Smith et al[16] reported data for 300 sites where IMIs had been installed in the same fashion, ie, flapless extraction with no gap grafting and healing by secondary intention. With time, however (the procedures were done over the period 2006 to 2014), they had learned that protection of the blood clots formed in the peri-implant gaps was a key factor, their ultimate approach being to connect a wide-diameter healing abutment or a custom temporary abutment or crown without occlusal loading at the time of implant placement. Some clinicians seek added insurance, electing to lightly pack pieces of commercially available collagen sponge over the clots that have formed in wider gaps.[17] Implants used by Smith et al[16] were all tapered, but varied per site in length, diameter, and surface texture, having been purchased from four different manufacturers. To be eligible for IMI treatment, all socket walls had to be intact, and all implants placed had to display insertion torque values (ITVs) of 15 Ncm or greater. Because mucoperiosteal flaps were not raised, no graft or barriers used, and no primary closure attempted, all gaps were simply allowed to fill with blood and heal unaided. Remarkably, as the authors had predicted, even very large gaps filled with bone, successfully integrating the IMIs. According to their own classification of socket types,[18] the majority treated had been type B (61.7%) followed by type C (31.7%), and the survival rate at the time of the report was 97% with the note that most failures had been during the early developmental stages of the procedures. A thick gingival biotype can be advantageous,[19] and it may also be beneficial to deepithelialize the soft tissue margins again to delay final wound closure.[20]

Others[21] have recently reported on a series of 210 implants placed using more or less the same approach as Smith's group while also suggesting a classification system based on location in relation to the implant periphery for predicting successful peri-implant defect fill. Seven gap types were proposed, and all but one type were reported to heal without gap grafting, provided that flapless surgery and atraumatic extraction had been used. The exception was their type II gap, which they reported happening when an implant is (in error) placed too far buccally with little to no gap remaining and possible contact with a thin buccal plate. In this case, any associated lingual/palatal gaps need not be grafted, but the buccal aspect of the implant will need hard tissue augmentation with buccal onlay grafting to avoid complications (see Fig 1-1 in chapter 1).

Further support for avoiding grafting with immediate implants comes from a recent controlled study in humans.[22] The investigators compared flapless surgery and no gap grafting with raising flaps, gap grafting with added barrier membranes, and flap closure. At least where buccal bone thickness after implant insertion was 1 mm or greater, with gaps greater than 2 mm width, no difference in outcome was found. Clearly, the flapless and no graft option would be advantageous from both time and economic aspects. Examples are shown in Figs 11-1 and 11-2.

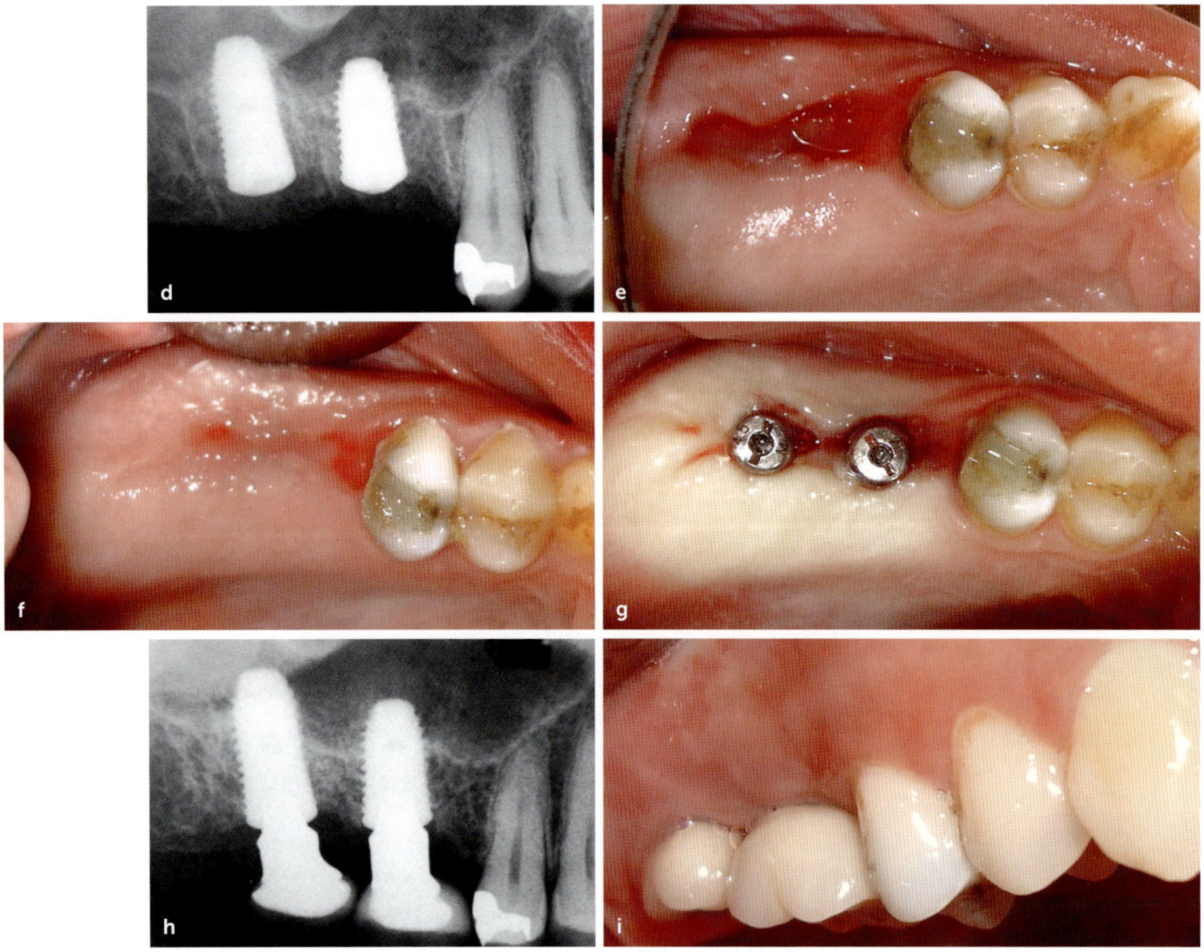

FIG 11-1 *(cont) (d)* The immediate postoperative radiograph shows two 4.8-mm-diameter implants (implant lengths of 8 mm for the mesial site and 10 mm for the distal site). No graft or barrier materials were used. *(e)* The site appearance 3 weeks later. Because of the depth of implant placement, granulation tissue had formed over the implant healing screws. Epithelial closure had begun creeping over this immature soft connective tissue and underlying osteoid. *(f)* The extent of soft tissue closure 2 months postsurgery. *(g)* A small reentry was needed at 3 months to allow connection of healing abutments. *(h)* A radiograph taken 1 year after placement of two free-standing implant crowns. Crestal bone loss is minimal due to the original subcrestal implant positioning and the incorporation of platform switching at the implant-abutment interface. *(i)* The clinical appearance of the two molar implant crowns after 1 year in function.

Case examples

In the patient shown in Fig 11-2, a hopeless maxillary right first molar was removed atraumatically without raising a flap, revealing sufficient interradicular septal (IRS) bone to receive an IMI (Fig 11-2a). There was limited subantral bone height (Fig 11-2b), and the plan was to place an 8.5-mm-long × 6-mm-diameter implant. A 2.0-mm-diameter round carbide tip connected to a piezoelectric surgery device (Surgybone, Silfradent) was used to create the initial osteotomy with the intention of breaching the sinus floor without risk of damage to the sinus membrane (Figs 11-2c and 11-2d). This allowed direct measurement of the height of bone beneath the sinus floor to be 8 mm. Site development continued with implant burs, the last being 8 mm long × 5 mm in diameter, at which time drilling was stopped (Fig 11-2e). An 8.5-mm-long × 6-mm-diameter Dentium implant was inserted and, when fully seated, registered a torque of 40 Ncm (Figs 11-2f and 11-2g). No grafting of the peri-implant gaps was done; rather, an autologous platelet-rich fibrin clot was skewered onto a healing abutment before the abutment was connected to the implant (Fig 11-2h). The fibrin clot was meant to act as a barrier,[23] and since the procedure had been flapless, no suturing was used (Fig 11-2i). The immediate postoperative radiograph showed the implant apex to

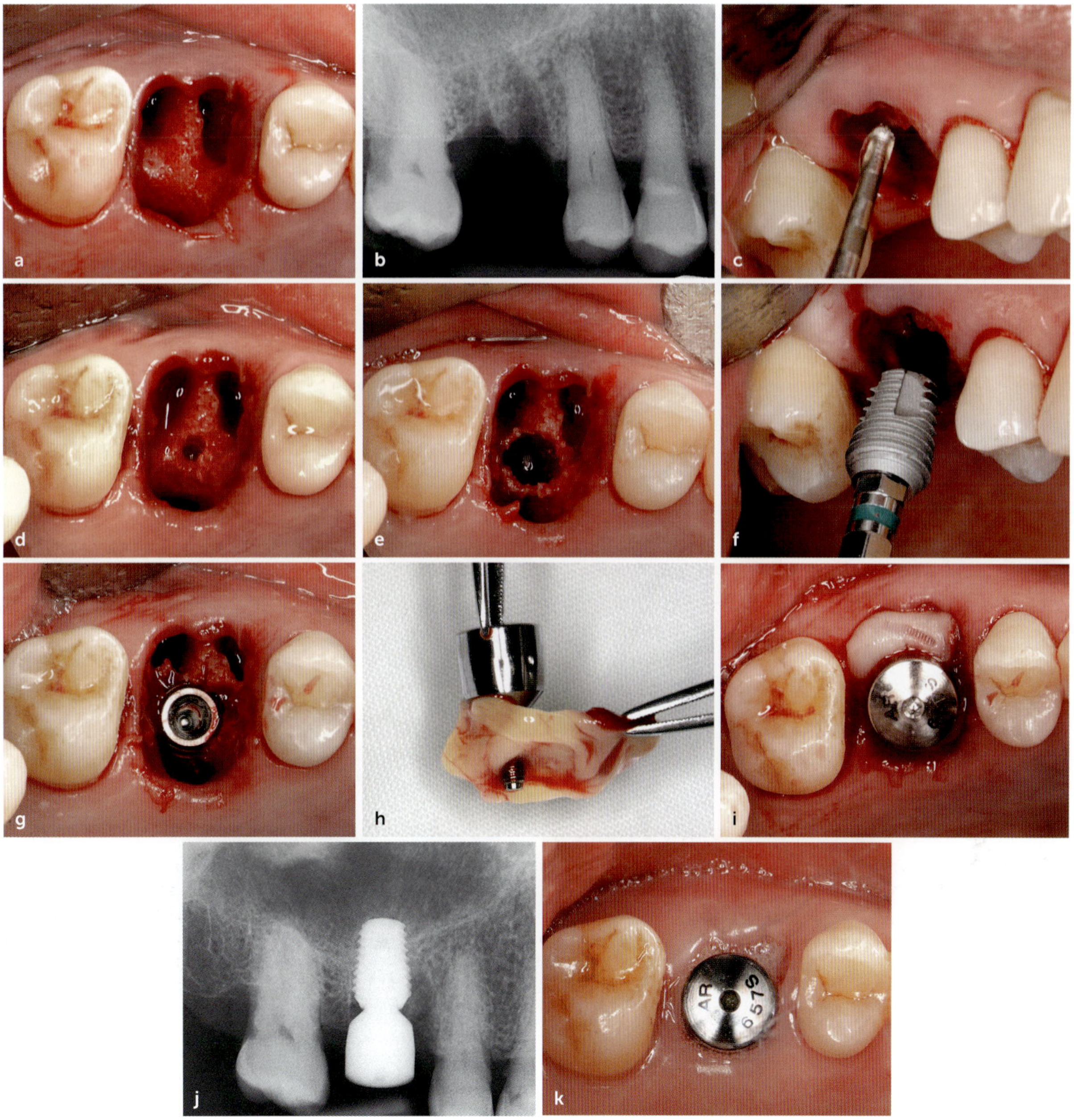

FIG 11-2 *(a)* After this hopeless maxillary first molar was removed without flap elevation, the IRS was considered adequate to stabilize an IMI. *(b)* The postextraction radiograph showed adequate bone height to receive an 8.5-mm-long implant. *(c)* A 2.0-mm-diameter round carbide tip connected to a piezoelectric surgery device (Surgybone) was used to approach the sinus floor to minimize the risk of sinus membrane perforation. *(d)* The exact IRS bone height to sinus floor was measured in this initial osteotomy site to be 8 mm. *(e)* The osteotomy was enlarged, finishing with an 8-mm-long × 5-mm-diameter bur. *(f)* The implant placed was 8.5 mm long × 6 mm wide. *(g)* Once the implant was seated and measured to have an insertion torque of 40 Ncm, no grafting of the remaining gaps was done. *(h)* An autologous platelet-rich fibrin clot[23] was skewered onto a healing abutment before the abutment was connected to the implant. *(i)* The concentrated growth factor clot acted as a barrier membrane, and no sutures were needed as the procedure had been flapless. *(j)* The immediate postoperative radiograph showing that the implant apex did extend beyond the sinus floor without consequence. *(k)* Despite no suturing, the 10-day postoperative photograph shows excellent, still nonepithelialized soft tissue closure over the site.

have penetrated beyond the sinus floor, creating a tenting effect on the sinus membrane (Fig 11-2j). By 10 days, granulation tissue had grown up to the abutment periphery (Fig 11-2k). The implant was restored after approximately 3 months of healing, and a radiograph taken at that time shows some new bone forma-

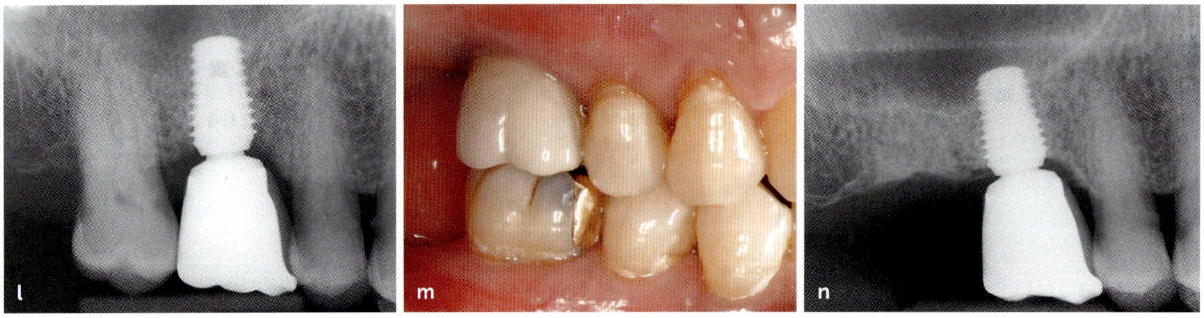

FIG 11-2 *(cont) (l)* The definitive restoration was delivered 3 months after implant insertion. Note the new bone formation at the implant apex. *(m)* The clinical status after 4 years in function. *(n)* The radiographic status after 4 years showing stable crestal bone levels.

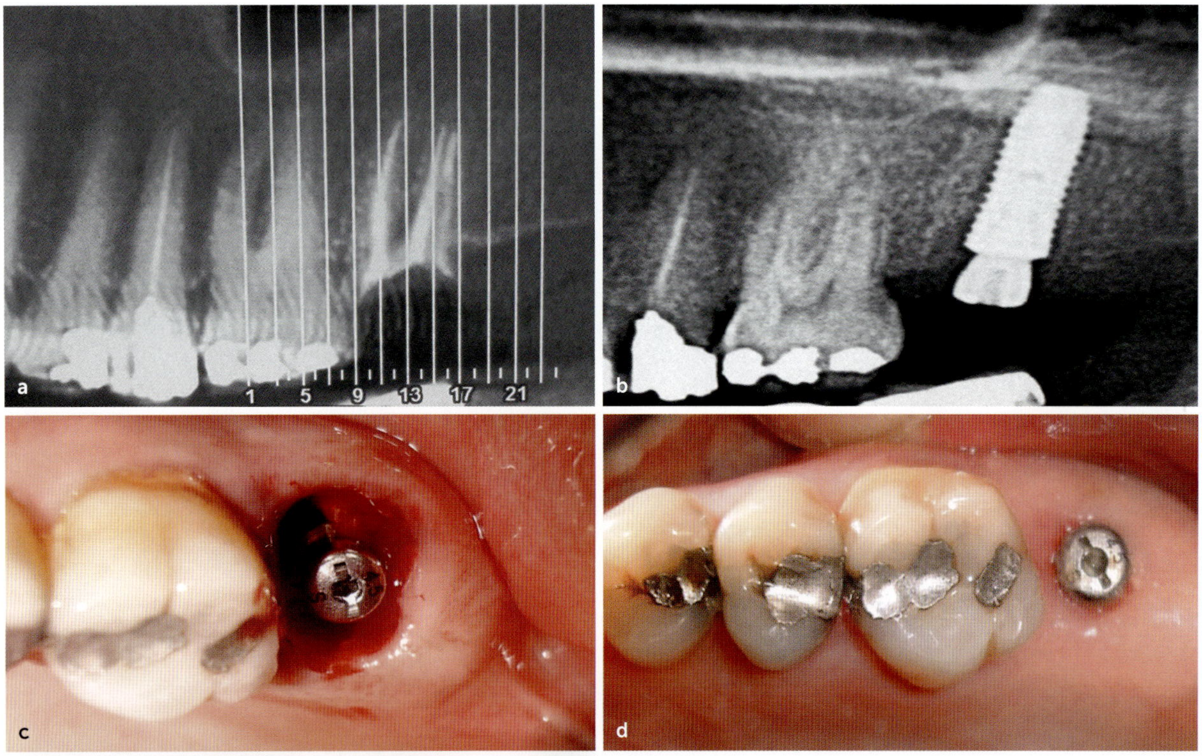

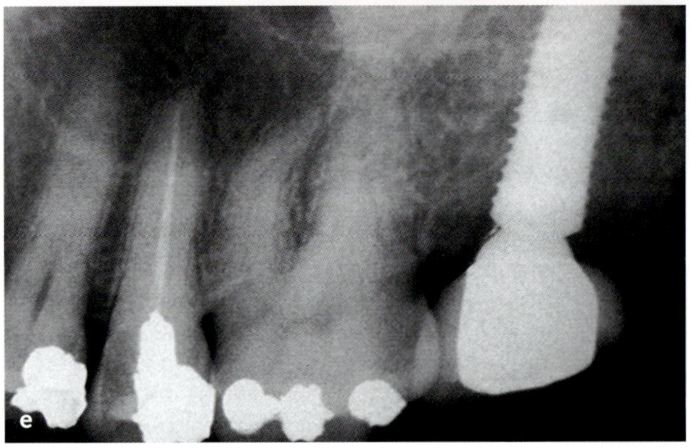

FIG 11-3 *(a)* A maxillary left second molar deemed nonrestorable was scheduled for an IMI. *(b)* The length of the chosen implant allowed engagement of native apical bone for stability, and a healing abutment was inserted at once. Note the platform-switch feature. *(c)* Since the procedure had been flapless, no grafting, barrier material, or sutures were used, the site simply being left to heal by secondary intention as an open extraction socket would do without placement of an implant. *(d)* The clinical photograph shows excellent soft tissue maturation by 3 months. *(e)* This radiograph obtained at the recall visit at 1 year in function shows excellent bone healing, including favorable crestal bone height.

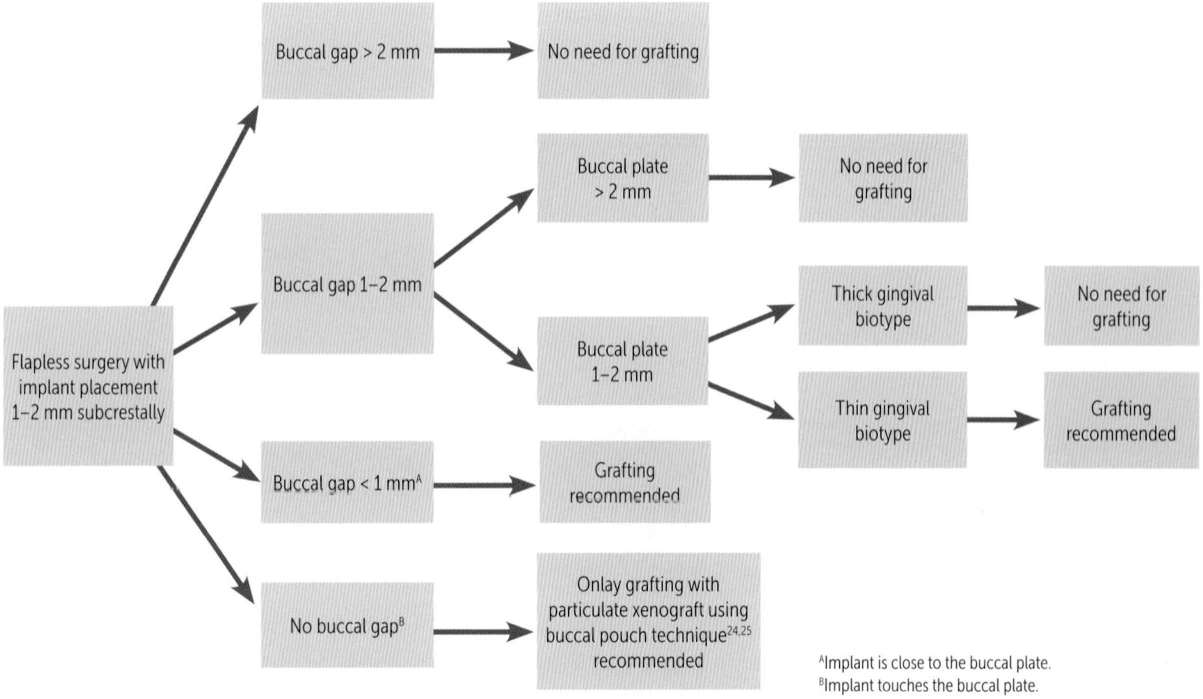

FIG 11-4 Decision flowchart regarding gap grafting with IMI placement.

tion surrounding the implant apex (Fig 11-2l). A clinical photograph and radiograph obtained at the patient's 4-year follow-up visit are shown in Figs 11-2m and 11-2n.

Remarkably, most gaps will heal spontaneously even if no sutures are used. Such a case is seen in Fig 11-3, where the maxillary left second molar required extraction. Because the IRS was type C (Fig 11-3a), it was removed and a long implant used to ensure stabilization in native bone apically (Fig 11-3b). Flapless surgery had been performed, and therefore no gap grafting, barrier material, or sutures were used, the site being allowed to heal on its own by secondary intention (Fig 11-3c). After 3 months of healing, the implant was ready for restoration (Fig 11-3d). Figure 11-3e shows a periapical radiograph of the restored implant at the patient's follow-up visit at 1 year in function.

When to graft and not to graft

In summary, provided flapless surgery is employed along with separation of roots and their atraumatic removal—if the implant is placed 1 to 2 mm subcrestally, is in the correct 3D position so as to avoid contact with the buccal socket wall, and is sufficiently stable—the majority of IMI peri-implant socket gaps, regardless of size, will fill uneventfully with bone just as if an implant had not been placed into the extraction socket. Healing will be by secondary intention, and unless the implant is intentionally overseated deep below the bone crest, soft tissue closure will not occur, leaving the top of the healing abutment readily accessible for later restoration. There may be situations, however, where gap grafting is appropriate even at IMI sites in order to optimize emergence profiles and their associated soft tissues (Fig 11-4).[24,25] If no buccal gap remains, buccal onlay/contour grafting can be of benefit. This grafting can be as straightforward as placing xenograft particles in a buccal pouch under the periosteum[24] (Fig 11-5), which should remain stable in the long term.

Finally, grafting is appropriate where, for example, there is partial loss of buccal plate with formation of a dehiscence. Traditionally, clinicians opted to raise full-thickness flaps in this situation to perform guided

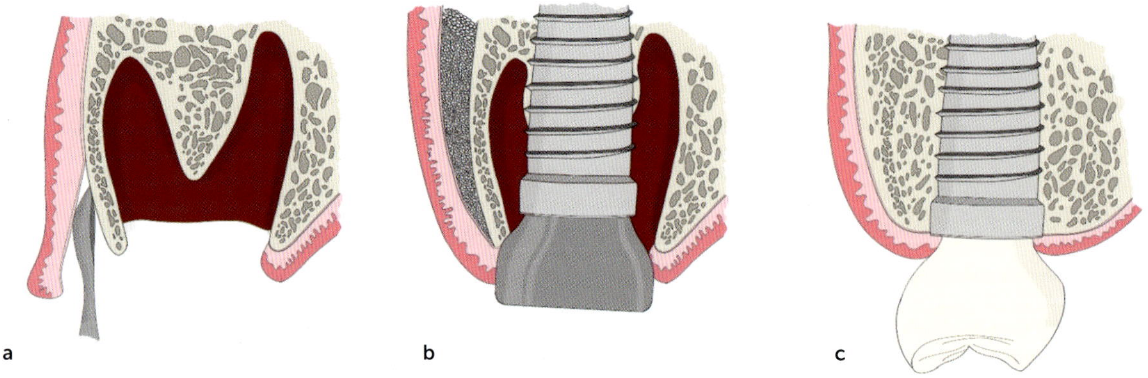

FIG 11-5 *(a to c)* To avoid buccal plate thinning and unwanted shrinkage in alveolar ridge anatomy, it can be useful to do buccal onlay grafting. This grafting can be as straightforward as placing xenograft particles in a pouch under the periosteum.

bone regeneration with graft and barriers. However, recent authors have shown that if the procedure to place the IMI was planned to be flapless, simpler options are possible. For example, Hu et al[26] managed IMI placement in sites with varying degrees of buccal dehiscence simply by densely packing xenograft particles under the buccal soft tissues and waiting 6 months for bone healing. Sicilia-Felechosa et al[27] used a similar approach for buccal dehiscences, but first placed and stabilized with sutures either an autogenous connective tissue graft or AlloDerm (AbbVie) under the buccal soft tissues.

Socket Shielding

Purpose of socket shielding

Socket shielding, intending to retain alveolar ridge anatomy, is another approach recently suggested to offer positive benefits with IMI outcomes.[28] The loss of a tooth leads to profound changes of its alveolus that may directly influence the ability to place an implant. The amount of resorption the alveolus will undergo following tooth extraction is difficult to predict, but it is generally held to be 50% or more by 1 year.[29] The main reason for this resorption is due to the "bundle bone phenomenon." *Bundle bone* is the thin (0.2- to 0.4-mm) layer of bone laid down by the developing tooth bud when a tooth's root system first develops. It forms part of the periodontal ligament (PDL) complex, and once the tooth is extracted, it quickly resorbs because of the lack of function and loss of blood supply from the PDL.

"Partial extraction therapy"[28] is an umbrella term for techniques where either the whole or part of the root is left behind to help maintain the integrity of the ridge. The technique of socket shielding, or the root membrane technique,[30] involves leaving a thin shell of buccal tooth root and periodontal attachment apparatus at the time of immediate implant placement in order to maintain buccal alveolar ridge contour, and it was first studied as a concept in one dog.[31] The investigators sectioned the dog's mandibular third and fourth premolars and decoronated the distal aspect of each crown to allow implant osteotomy preparation toward the lingual and within the remaining distal root structure. After osteotomy preparation, any remaining proximal or lingual root remnants were removed, leaving only a thin shell of intact tooth and periodontium buccally and extending approximately 1 mm coronal to the buccal bone plate. Enamel matrix derivative (Emdogain, Straumann) was applied to the internal aspect of this buccal fragment, presumably to encourage new cementum formation,[32] followed by placement of an immediate implant. Four implants were placed, with two intentionally in direct contact with the buccal root fragment and two not. Placement of 4-mm-long healing abutments then allowed nonsubmerged site healing. After 4 months, specimens were retrieved and examined by backscatter scanning electron and light microscopy. With the two implants intentionally installed in contact with the retained shell of tooth, new cementum did in fact form at the implant-to–tooth fragment interface. The removal of the palatal or lingual portion of the root, including its root canal contents, apex, and any pathology,

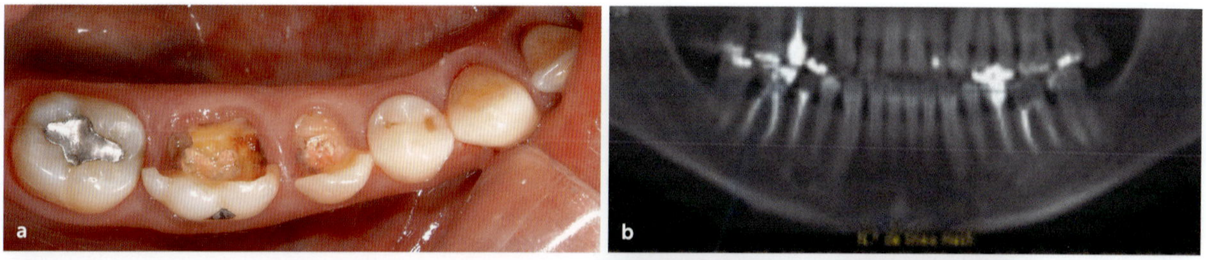

FIG 11-6 *(a to c)* Both the mandibular second premolar and first molar in this patient were condemned with the plan to place immediate implants.

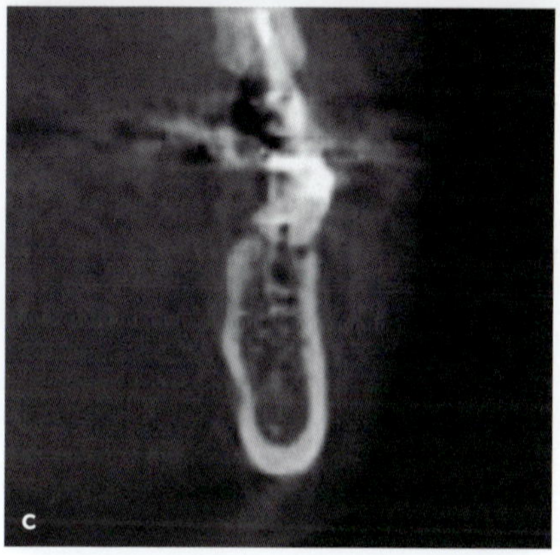

combined with the maintenance of the thin section of buccal root and periodontium, was seen to maintain and nourish the thin buccal plate and bundle bone. Following this proof-of-principle study, investigators[33] undertook clinical studies confirming at 5 years that there were minimal changes in local ridge dimensions. A large cohort retrospective study by Gluckman et al[34] confirmed the viability of the technique despite limitations.[35]

The original socket shield was intended to contribute to esthetically pleasing immediate implants placed in the anterior maxilla, and this has proved to be the case. However, the technique is highly technical and likely not appropriate for use by the average clinician without training. Nevertheless, with adequate experience, it has now been shown to be applicable with IMI placement. The concept of the molar shield was first published by Schwimer[36] and coworkers, showing excellent maintenance and emergence of alveolar bone and soft tissue morphology both clinically and radiologically. The thinness and curvatures of molar roots, however, can make it difficult to resect the lingual or palatal portions and to eliminate apical pathology. If successful, the rewards are stunning. Contraindications include molars with marked curvatures in the root, lack of buccal plate, periodontal attachment loss, mobile roots, and inaccessible apical infection.

Socket shielding procedure

A molar should be prepared for socket shielding as shown in Fig 11-6. The authors recommend raising a conservative flap to enable visualization of the buccal bone crest (Figs 11-6a to 11-6c). Following decoronation, the root trunk is sectioned mesiodistally at the level of the furcation using a long-shank, straight diamond bur at high speed and with copious irrigation (Figs 11-6d and 11-6e). The length and depth of cut needed are determined from the pretreatment radiographs. This sectioning will allow separation of the buccal from the lingual/palatal root portions. Thereafter, a similar mesiodistal cut is made in the buccal half of the first cut (Fig 11-6f). The unwanted root fragments are removed, leaving only the two future socket shields, which then can be thinned and shaped with the same long shank diamond bur[18] (Figs 11-6g and 11-6h). Next, a round 2-mm-diameter diamond bur is used at high speed to reduce the crestal portion of the two socket shields to bone level and create a 2-mm internal chamfer bevel to provide prosthetic space for the crown margin (Figs 11-6i and 11-6j).

At this point, the root sockets should be meticulously curetted apically and rinsed vigorously using sterile saline. One or more periapical radiographs should be taken to verify that all endodontic root

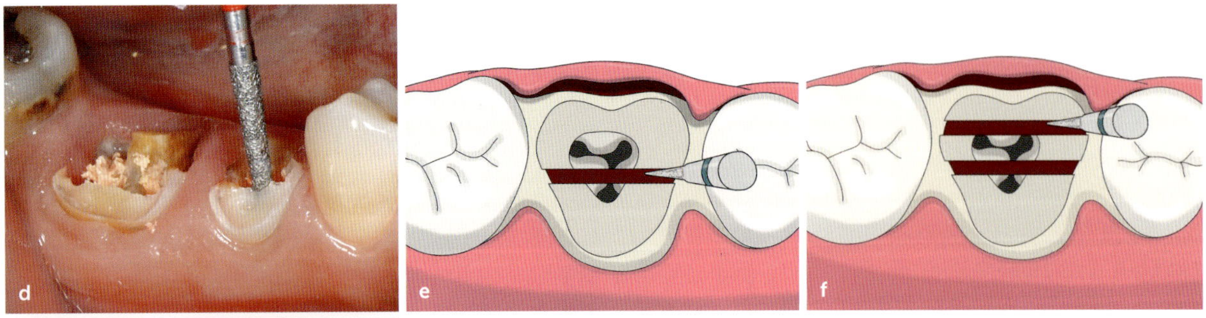

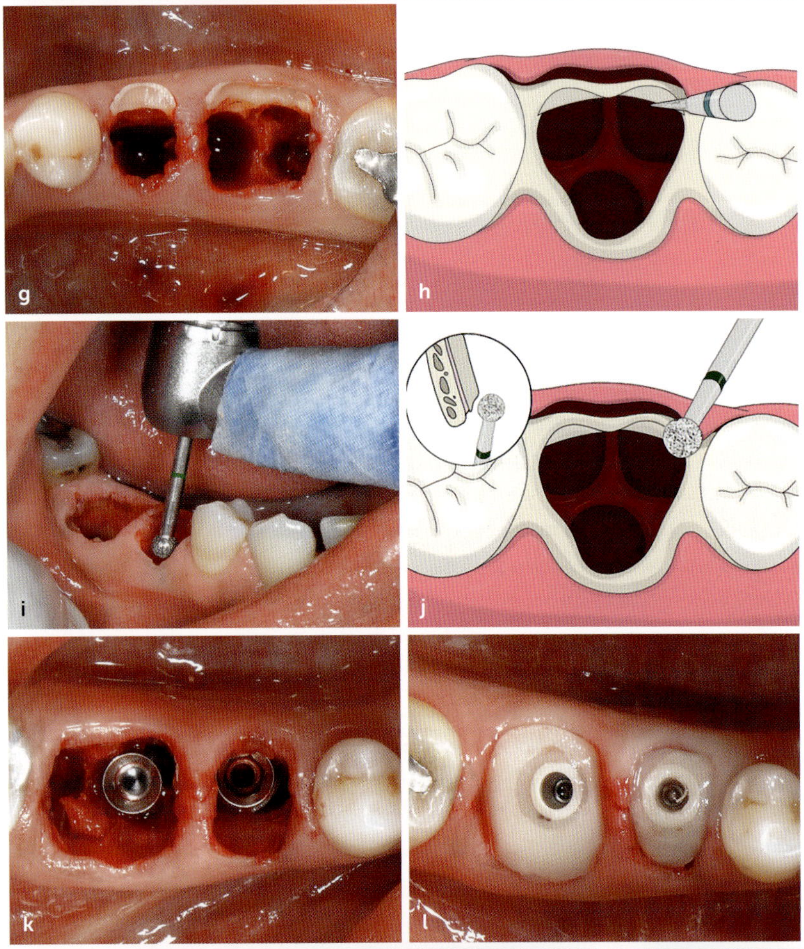

FIG 11-6 *(cont) (d)* After decoronation, the teeth are sectioned into buccal and lingual halves. *(e)* Illustration of the first cut. *(f)* The second cut is made to separate the buccal half into two pieces. *(g)* After removal of the unwanted root fragments, the two "shields" can be thinned further using a long-shanked diamond pencil bur. The remaining IRS can be seen to be type C.[18] *(h)* The pencil bur is used to thin and shape the buccal root shields. *(i)* A high-speed, large-diameter round diamond bur is then used to reduce the crestal portion of the two socket shields to bone level and create a 2-mm internal chamfer bevel to provide prosthetic space for the crown margin. *(j)* The round bur is used to reduce the height and create a chamfer in the two buccal shields. *(k)* The two implants were successfully placed and stabilized. *(l)* Custom healing abutments were fabricated chairside to isolate the peri-implant gaps and shape the surrounding soft tissues during site healing. No suturing of the tissues was needed. *(m)* When the implants were ready for restoration, the soft tissue contours were seen to have been maintained by the custom healing abutments. *(n)* A clinical photograph at the time of insertion of the implant restorations. (Illustrations courtesy of Dr Ryan Noh, University of Toronto.)

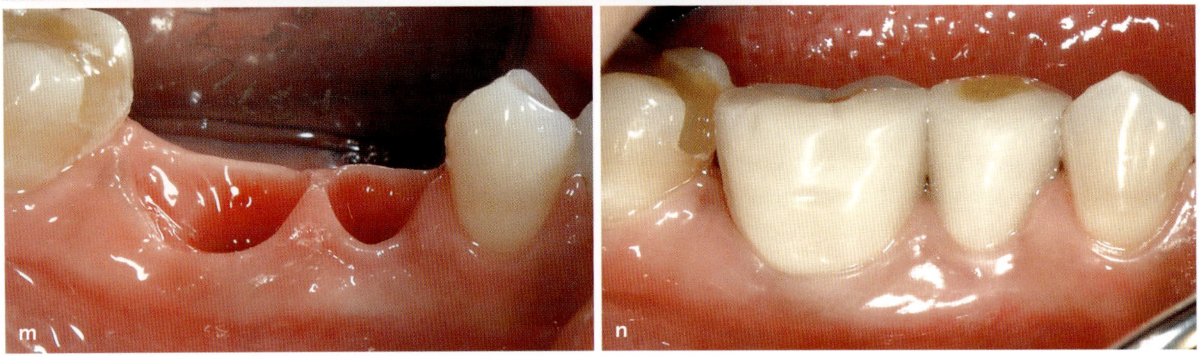

canals and obturation material and granulation tissue have been eradicated. Knowing this and that there is absolutely no mobility of the buccal root shields after checking their internal surfaces with a sharp probe, the implant osteotomy preparation can proceed. Wherever possible, the authors prefer to use the osseodensification protocol described by Huwais and Meyer[37] (see chapter 7).

After inserting the implants and verifying them to have adequate stability (Fig 11-6k), the buccal gaps between implant and shields were grafted with a particulate bone allograft. Finally, custom transgingival healing abutments were prepared onto PAEK (polyaryletherketone) temporary prosthetic abutments, taking care to capture and support the soft tissues with a flaring emergence profile that conformed to the socket circumference (Fig 11-6l; see also chapter 12).

Explicit postoperative instructions are necessary. Typically, patients are prescribed a regimen of a 0.2% chlorhexidine oral rinse twice daily for 2 weeks. Generally, systemic antibiotics are unnecessary and not prescribed. A short checkup appointment is made for the patient 48 hours postsurgery, and again at 2 weeks for removal of any sutures used. Assuming that no adverse healing events are reported by the patient, the implant should be ready for restoration (resonance frequency value > 70) after approximately 3 months, preferably with a screw-retained crown (Figs 11-6m and 11-6n).

IMI Placement and Risk of Interproximal Caries

Matching implant diameter to the mesiodistal space of a molar extraction site, ie, the distance from the implant's coronal margin (implant-to-abutment interface) from the proximal surfaces of contiguous teeth is a crucial consideration. Thus, Smith et al[38] observed that when the implant-abutment interface is placed too far from an adjacent tooth root surface, an unusually high incidence of caries on this tooth is a risk, likely due to frequent food impaction/collection. The cited critical implant-tooth distance (ITD) was found by the author to be 4 mm (Fig 11-7). Cases in which the ITD was 4 mm or more showed a clinically and statistically significant jump in decay rates, with rates continuing to rise as distance increased.

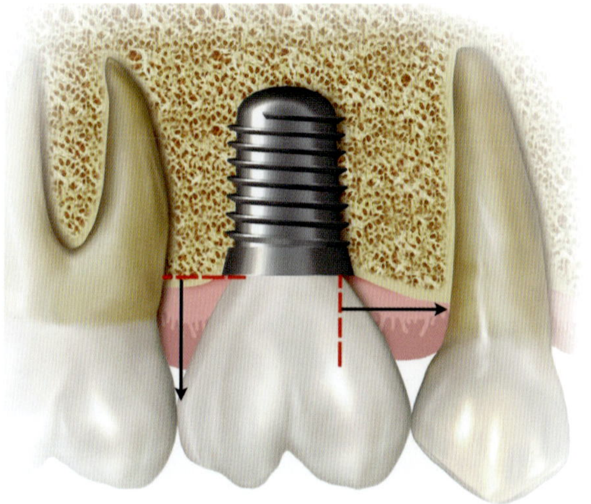

FIG 11-7 ITD is measured horizontally at the level of the crest of bone from the implant-abutment interface to the adjacent root surface.

The distance from tooth to tooth as measured at the alveolar crest across an edentulous molar site will vary between arches and with the sex of the patient. For example, mean mesiodistal widths of mandibular first molars have been recorded as 11.5 mm in men and 10.9 mm in women, while the same measurements for mandibular second molars are 10.9 mm in men and 10.1 mm in women.[39] Therefore, with typical mandibular molar sites (mesiodistal width up to 11 mm) having type A or B septa, appropriate implant diameters would be 4.5 to 6.0 mm. With a 6-mm-diameter implant, the ITD would be approximately 2.5 mm from each adjacent tooth. On the other hand, with type C septa or when mesiodistal width of the site is significantly greater than 11 mm, an implant of wider diameter may be needed to reduce risk of root caries. With some of these situations, an ultra-wide-diameter implant (> 6 mm) can be helpful (Fig 11-8; see also chapter 8).

Rarely, the distance between the teeth on either side of an IMI may be too great even for an ultra-wide implant to allow the ITD to be less than 4 mm on either side. In these cases, two narrower-diameter implants placed in the root sockets and within the acceptable ITD range may be preferable (Fig 11-9). The

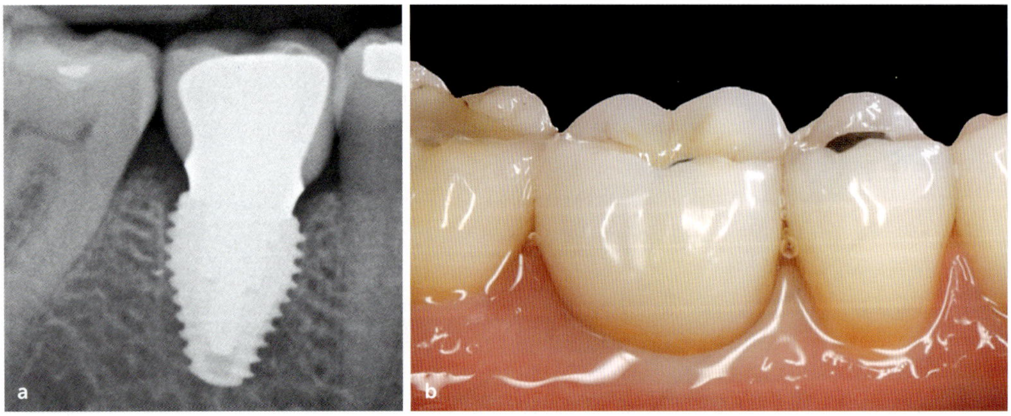

FIG 11-8 *(a)* An ultra-wide implant was used in this site to ensure appropriate ITD. *(b)* Use of an ultra-wide-diameter implant will allow for an anatomically accurate molar restoration.

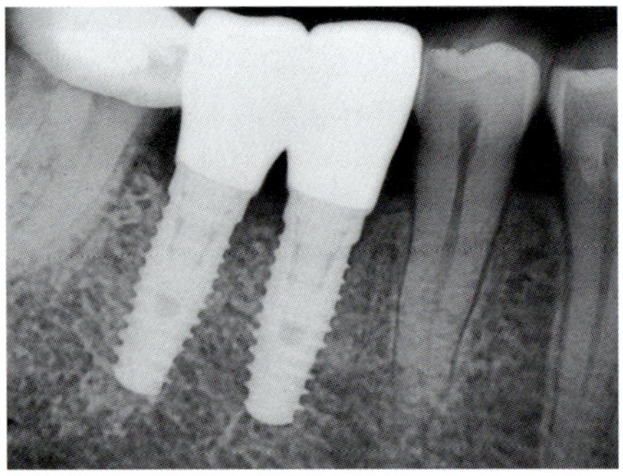

FIG 11-9 Two 4.1-mm-diameter implants were placed at this mandibular molar site in order not to exceed favorable ITD distances.

restoration then can be designed as either two premolars or as a "fluted" molar with a cleansable gingival embrasure between the two implants. If the implant is to replace the terminal molar in the arch, it is more important to place the implant within an acceptable ITD to the tooth mesial to it than it is to place it in the center of the socket.

Osseodensification for Indirect Sinus Floor Elevation

As discussed elsewhere in this book (see chapter 7), unlike traditional implant burs that remove bone in order to create an osteotomy, osseodensification burs run at high speed in reverse (ie, noncutting) mode, creating osteotomies by compacting bone laterally and apically. The autograft collected and pushed apically by these burs can create a minor (2 to 3 mm), localized, indirect sinus floor elevation not unlike that achievable with hand osteotomes,[40,41] but in a much less traumatic way for the patient and less stressful manner for the clinician. However, the approach can be further modified for sites requiring more than 3 mm of sinus elevation using a well-tested protocol provided by the manufacturer. Sites selected should have 4 to 5 mm of residual subantral bone height measured from CBCT scans. The surgery should be flapless, as is usual with IMI procedures. Following decoronation of the molar crown at the level of the tooth's furcation, the three roots should be sectioned and removed individually.

The case shown is one with a maxillary first molar needing replacement (Figs 11-10a to 11-10c). After extraction, a type A IRS suitable to receive an IMI remained (Fig 11-10d). The plan was to place a 10-mm-long × 6-mm-diameter implant, meaning that around 6 mm of sinus membrane elevation was needed. Rather than initiating the osteotomy with a pilot bur, the smallest diameter (2.0-mm) Densah bur (Versah) was used in cutting mode (clockwise) to the approximate depth of the sinus floor. The same bur then was used in reverse (counterclockwise [CCW]

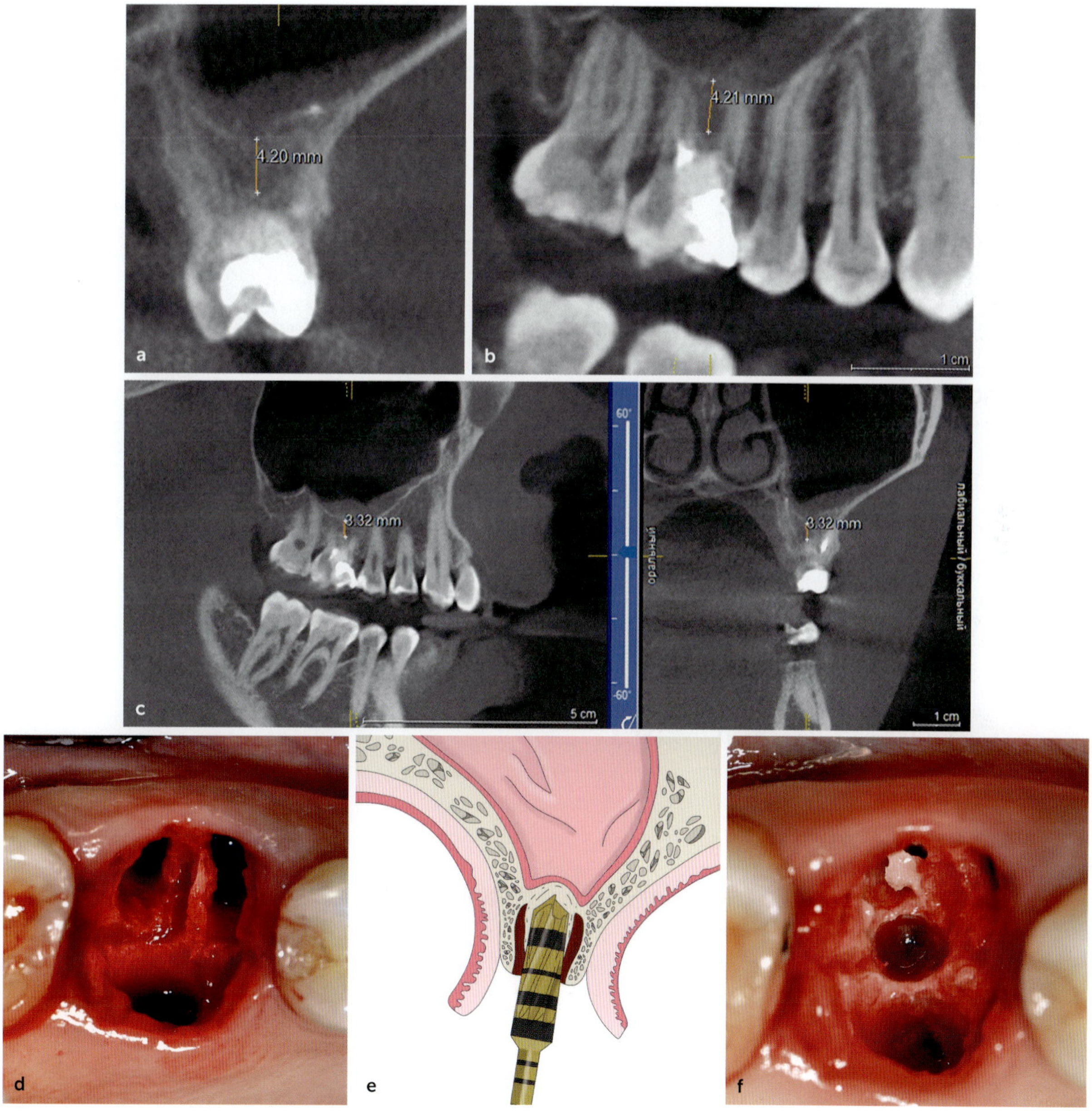

FIG 11-10 *(a)* Residual bone height of the IRS ranged from 3.2 to 4.21 mm. *(b)* Type A IRS of 4.21-mm height was seen. *(c)* The lowest measurement of residual IRS was measured as 3.32 mm. *(d)* The tooth roots were removed without raising a mucoperiosteal flap to reveal a type A socket. *(e)* Osseodensification burs were used in reverse mode to propel autogenous bone shavings from the osteotomy walls apically, ultimately upfracturing the sinus floor. *(f)* The initial osteotomy included intentional upfracture of the sinus floor, reaching 3 mm into the sinus domain without damaging the sinus membrane by driving autogenous bone shavings upward. →

mode) at 800 to 1,500 rpm to locate the sinus floor with haptic feedback and then upfracture it, leaving an intact sinus membrane (Figs 11-10e and 11-10f). Osteotomy development is then continued in sequence with Densah burs of 3-, 4-, and 5-mm diameter in CCW mode, each entering the sinus domain 1 mm at a time to a final depth of 3 mm, all the while employing a modulating pressure and pumping motion with the handpiece.

Sticky bone was prepared as the graft material by combining the patient's platelet-rich plasma with particulate allograft material[23] (Fig 11-10g). This

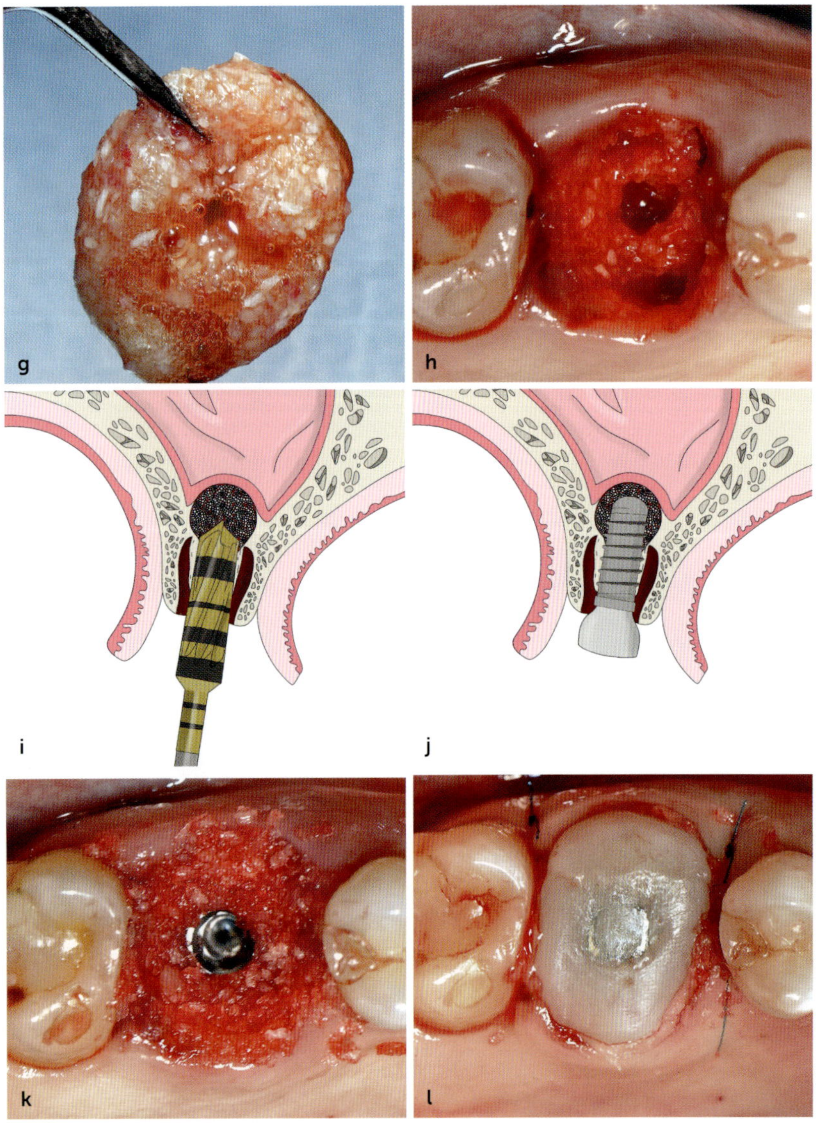

FIG 11-10 *(cont) (g)* Sticky bone was created by mixing the patient's venous platelet-rich plasma with particulate allograft.[23] *(h)* Small bits of sticky bone were added to the site and propelled apically with the bur used in CCW mode at 100 rpm without irrigation to elevate the sinus floor to the desired level. *(i)* Small bits of sticky bone were added in a stepwise fashion and propelled apically using the bur in reverse mode without saline at 100 rpm. Never did the actual bur tip penetrate more than 1 to 2 mm beyond the sinus floor. *(j)* Once the sinus membrane had been elevated approximately 6 mm, a 10-mm-long implant was inserted. *(k)* Following implant placement, all gaps were filled with sticky bone as a means of supporting the soft tissue profile during site healing. *(l)* A chairside customized abutment was used to shelter the grafted gaps and support the healing soft tissues.

biomaterial has the advantages of immediately sealing any undetected minor membrane tears, having anti-inflammatory/antibacterial properties, and containing growth factors that promote vascular ingrowth and osteogenesis. The sticky gelatinous preparation was cut into small pieces, which were then packed into the osteotomy one at a time and propelled apically into the sinus domain using the 5.0-mm Densah bur in CCW mode at 100 rpm and without irrigation (Fig 11-10h). While the bur propelled the graft material apically, the actual bur tip was not allowed to penetrate more than 1 to 2 mm into the graft material, after which the procedure was repeated with more sticky bone. This sequence was repeated sufficient times to achieve the desired elevation of the sinus membrane, which in this case was approximately 6 mm beyond the original sinus floor in order to receive a 10-mm-long × 6-mm-diameter implant (Figs 11-10i to 11-10r). Once inserted, the implant stability was measured with resonance frequency analysis to be 75, as measured with an Osstell resonance frequency device.

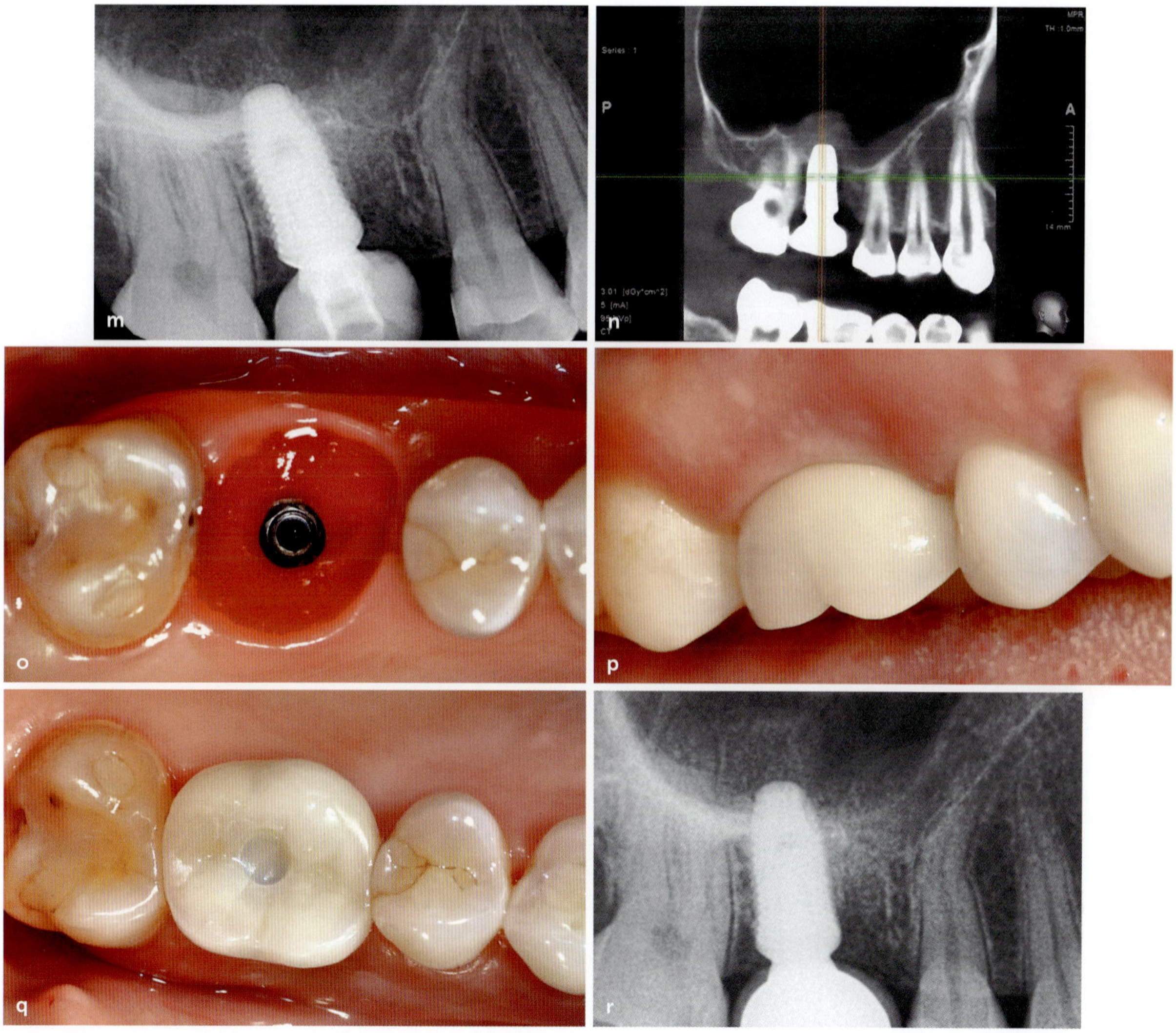

FIG 11-10 *(cont) (m)* The immediate postoperative radiograph of the implant and abutment. *(n)* A CBCT image of the implant immediately after placement. A well-circumscribed dome of sticky bone can be seen holding up the sinus membrane. *(o)* The soft tissue profile after 3 months of site healing. *(p)* A photograph of the definitive restoration. *(q)* An occlusal image of the screw-retained implant crown. *(r)* The radiograph of the restored implant.

Short Implants as IMIs

While short threaded implants (≤ 7 mm) had a checkered history in the past,[42] considerable evidence has now accumulated to verify that with proper technique and implant design, implant length is rarely a primary consideration[43] since functional loading primarily affects only the most coronal three to five threads regardless of implant length.[44] Accordingly, many implant manufacturers now offer short (6 to 8 mm) and even ultra-short (< 6 mm) implants for use in replacing molars, particularly in the mandible, where proximity to the neurovascular canal is a hazard.[45] Many of these were originally offered as "rescue" implants and were made with diameters of 5 mm or greater, generally for use at healed extraction sockets.[45,46] The present authors have used both short and ultra-short threaded implants frequently, initially in healed extraction sites, but more recently as IMIs. Several sample IMI cases will be shown.

Case 1

A first example involved a patient needing replacement of his left maxillary right second premolar and first and second molars (Fig 11-11a). The three teeth

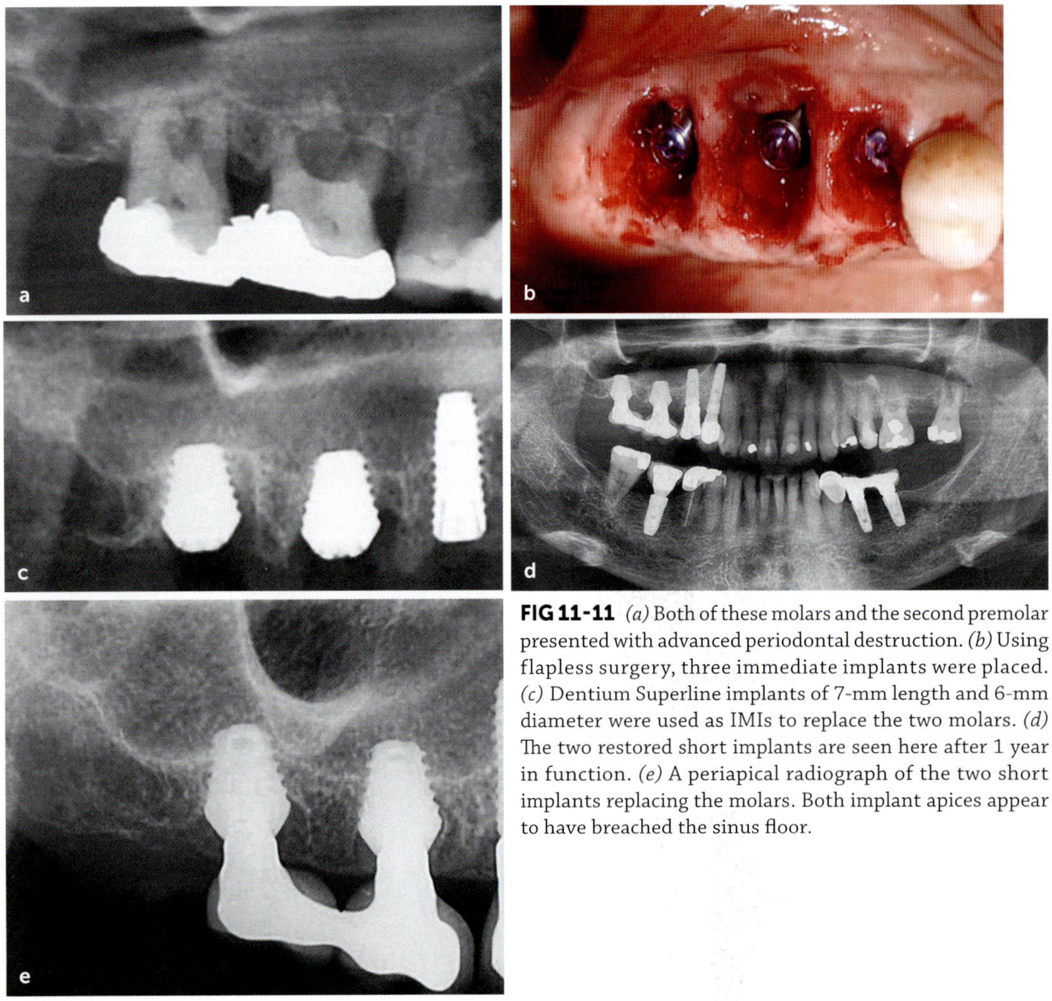

FIG 11-11 *(a)* Both of these molars and the second premolar presented with advanced periodontal destruction. *(b)* Using flapless surgery, three immediate implants were placed. *(c)* Dentium Superline implants of 7-mm length and 6-mm diameter were used as IMIs to replace the two molars. *(d)* The two restored short implants are seen here after 1 year in function. *(e)* A periapical radiograph of the two short implants replacing the molars. Both implant apices appear to have breached the sinus floor.

were removed using flapless surgery, and three immediate implants were placed (Figs 11-11b and 11-11c), the two molar implants being short Dentium Superline implants (7 mm long × 6 mm diameter). No gap grafting was done, and the implants were left with healing caps rather than healing abutments. Healing was uneventful, and after 3 months, the molar implants were used to support a two-unit fixed partial denture, while the premolar implant received a single crown (Figs 11-11d and 11-11e).

Case 2

The second example is of a single hopeless maxillary first molar (Fig 11-12a). While minimal subantral bone height remained, the socket walls were all intact, and the septum was type B (Fig 11-12b). Therefore it was decided to place an IMI with dimensions 5 × 5 mm (Fig 11-12c). The immediate postoperative radiograph of this implant can be seen in Fig 11-12d. No transcrestal sinus grafting was used, and while large peri-implant gaps remained, these were left ungrafted. A healing cap rather than a healing abutment was used, and healing by secondary intention was uneventful (Fig 11-12e). The implant was successfully restored, but the patient has not yet been available for a current image of the restored implant.

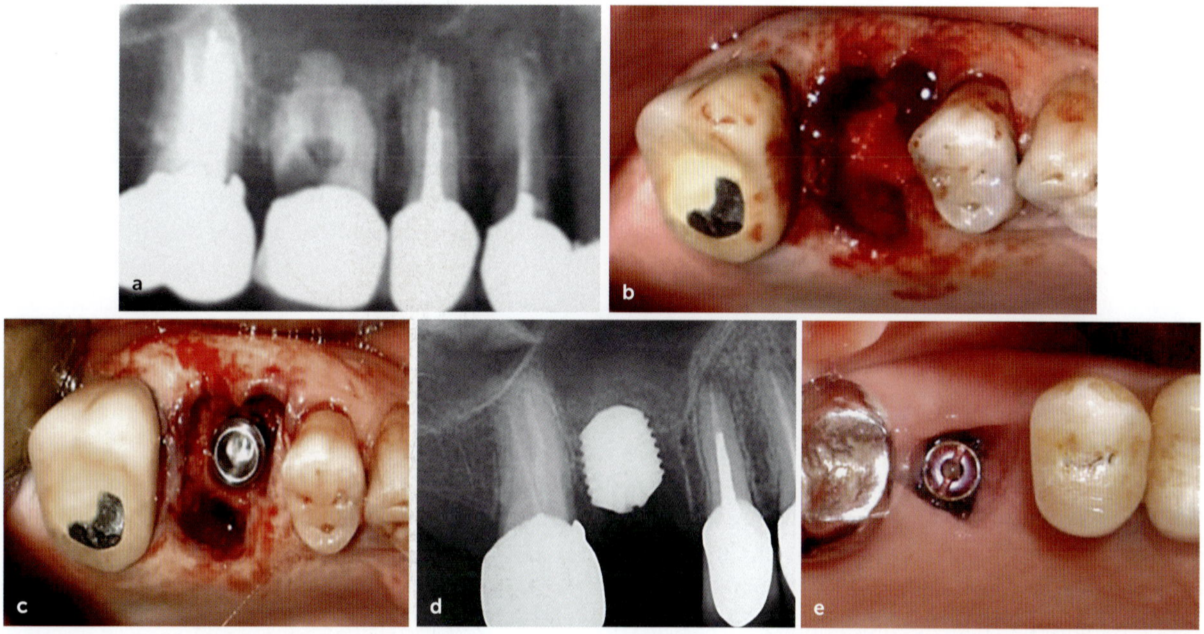

FIG 11-12 *(a)* The maxillary right first molar was deemed hopeless. *(b)* After removing the tooth remnants, a type B IRS was seen. *(c)* The implant was stabilized by the IRS, and no gap grafting was needed. *(d)* An immediate postoperative radiograph of the implant. *(e)* By 3 weeks, the peri-implant gaps showed advanced healing by secondary intention.

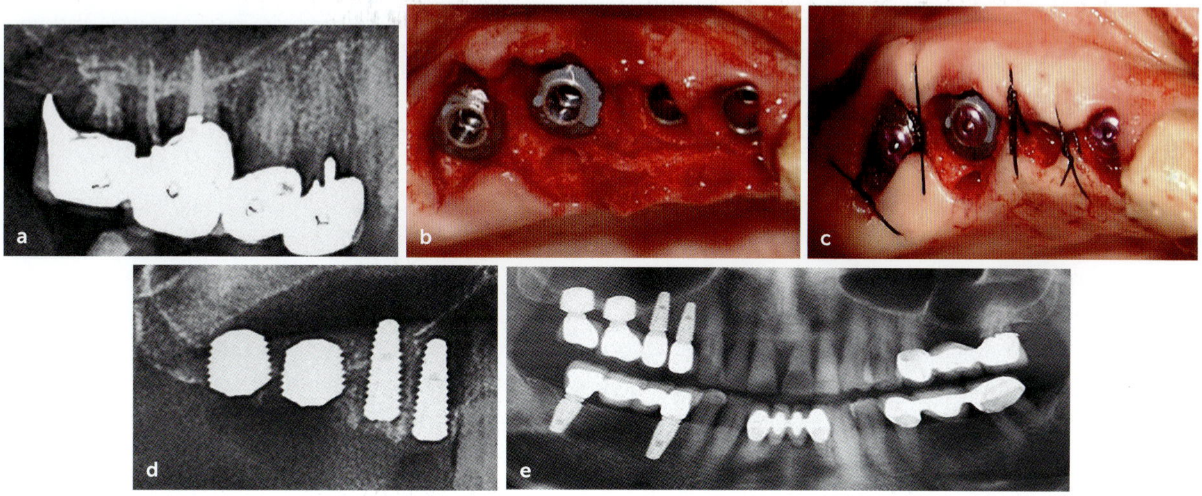

FIG 11-13 *(a)* All four posterior teeth in this quadrant were hopeless. *(b)* All four sites received immediate implants. *(c)* No gap grafting was performed. *(d)* An immediate postoperative radiograph shows that the two molar sites received ultra-short, ultra-wide threaded implants. *(e)* A panoramic radiograph of the completed case after 1 year in function.

Case 3

A third case involved a patient requiring the replacement of his maxillary right first and second premolars and first and second molars (Fig 11-13a). Immediate implants were planned for all four sites. MegaGen Rescue implants (5 × 5 mm) were selected for the two molar sites, as there was very limited subantral bone height (Figs 11-13b and 11-13c). Healing caps only were used. No gap grafting was done, and the soft tissue margins were secured with sutures. As can be seen in the postoperative radiograph (Fig 11-13d), both implant apices penetrated through the sinus floor, but the implants were stable (Fig 11-13e).

Short implant research

Wide ultra-short threaded implants have been shown to perform well as delayed molar implants placed in healed edentulous sites,[45,47] although the longest follow-up interval reported thus far is only 5 years, and time in function is a known risk factor for failure of threaded implants that are 6 mm or shorter.[48] However, limited documentation is available on the use of ultra-short implants as IMIs. One study that we identified was that of Checchi et al.[49] These investigators treated 50 patients, each requiring replacement of one or two hopeless molars. Patients received 5-mm-long × 6- to 8-mm-diameter implants as IMIs. The teeth were extracted atraumatically to preserve the buccal alveolar bone and the interdental septa, without flap elevation when possible. One or two 6- to 8-mm diameter Rescue implants (MegaGen) of various lengths (5, 6, 7, 8.5, 10, and 11.5 mm), all with external connections, were placed in each patient.

Seventeen (31.5%) of the IMIs placed were of 5 mm length, and an example of one of these cases is shown in Fig 11-14. The first molar site showed approximately 5 mm of subantral bone height, an intact buccal socket wall, and a sufficiently wide ridge to ensure that following implant placement and gap grafting a buccal bone thickness of approximately 3 mm could be predicted (Figs 11-14a and 11-14b). A 5-mm-diameter (internal diameter of 4 mm) trephine bur with a vertical stop was used to initialize the osteotomy at the first molar site. Subsequent drilling with twist burs left the osteotomy site one bur size smaller in diameter than the implant, which in this case was 7 mm in diameter (Fig 11-14c). Acceptable torque was considered to be 20 Ncm. All implants were placed 1.0 to 2.0 mm subcrestal to the palatal bone level. Cover screws only were connected to the implants, and residual gaps between bony walls and implants grafted with autogenous bone chips retrieved elsewhere with a trephine (Figs 11-14d and 11-14e). A surgical hemostatic collagen dressing of equine origin (Gingistat, Acteon) was used to cover the grafted gaps. Finally, the soft tissue margins were secured using sutures but with no attempt at primary wound closure.

Healing by secondary intention was uneventful, as shown at the 1-week postoperative visit (Figs 11-14f and 11-14g). Provisional restorations were placed after 4 months of healing (Fig 11-14h), and another 4 months later were replaced with definitive ones. The final radiographic and clinical images are shown in Fig 11-14i and 11-14j.

Reliability of short implants as IMIs

While the authors of this chapter have treated many patients using ultra-short implants as IMIs, the approach must be considered experimental and will require verification of its reproducibility and predictability in further large-scale prospective clinical trials. Their use as IMIs could be a next milestone in the step toward normalizing IMIs treatments, as it would avoid the need for sophisticated, higher risk, costly, and invasive grafting procedures and could at the very least in the future be offered to patients as one treatment option with the understanding that, if failure occurred after 5 or more years in function, more invasive treatments could be contemplated.[50]

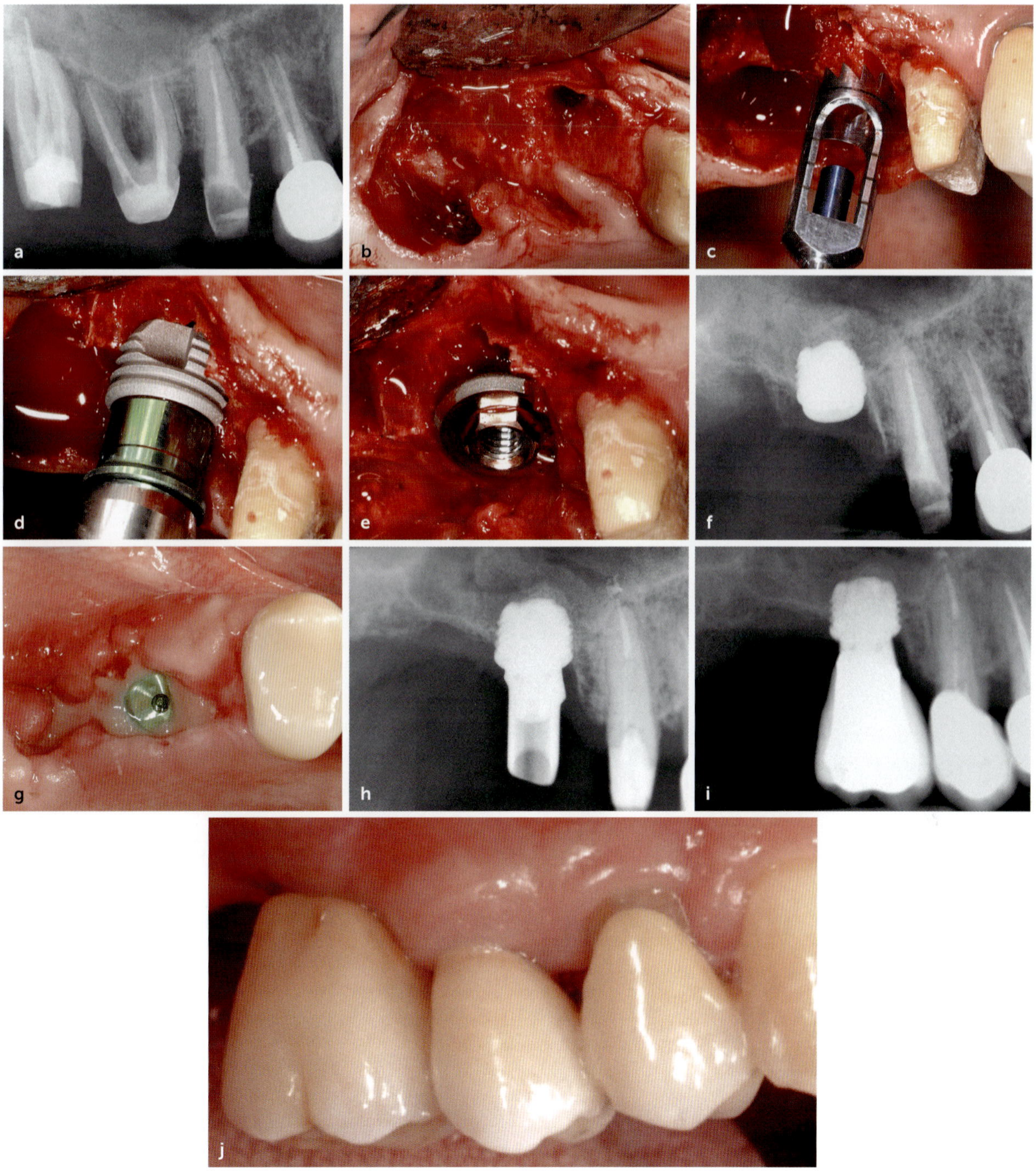

FIG 11-14 *(a)* The patient's maxillary right first and second molars required extraction. The requisite 5 mm of subantral bone height was present. *(b)* The two teeth were removed using flapless surgery, which confirmed the ridge to be sufficiently wide buccopalatally to receive an ultra-wide implant at the first molar site. *(c)* Preparation began by using a 5-mm-diameter (internal diameter of 4 mm) trephine to establish the osteotomy partially in the IRS. *(d)* During implant seating, a minimum torque of 20 Ncm was required for satisfactory initial stability. *(e)* A 5-mm-long × 7-mm-diameter implant was inserted with the platform 1 mm apical to the palatal bone height. The remaining large buccal gap was subsequently grafted with autogenous bone chips covered by a collagen sponge. *(f)* The radiographic status after 1 week of site healing. *(g)* The clinical status of the soft tissues at 1 week postsurgery. *(h)* After 4 months of site healing, the implant was ready to receive a transitional prosthesis. *(i)* A periapical radiograph taken 1 year after the implant was loaded with its definitive prosthesis. *(j)* The clinical condition of the implant restoration after 1 year in function.

Conclusion

With time and experience, clinicians have continued to refine the protocols for successful usage of IMIs. Several examples have been shared here, including the options of gap grafting or not, proper proximal spacing, socket shielding, using Densah burs for indirect sinus floor elevation, and the use of short and ultra-short implants as IMIs.

KEY POINTS

- Provided that optimal 3D implant positioning is achieved at sites with thick buccal bone plates and large buccal gaps, grafting of these gaps may not be necessary.
- Optimal proximal spacing from teeth adjacent to IMIs seems to be 4 mm or less to reduce the risk of interproximal caries.
- Osseodensification burs can be used for IMI placement with concomitant sinus floor elevation.
- While further investigations are needed, it seems possible that short and ultra-short implants may be used as IMIs.

References

1. Dahlin C, Sennerby L, Lekholm U, Linde A, Nyman S. Generation of new bone around titanium implants using a membrane technique: An experimental study in rabbits. Int J Oral Maxillofac Implants 1989;4:19–25.
2. Lazzara RJ. Immediate implant placement into extraction sites: Surgical and restorative advantages. Int J Periodontics Restorative Dent 1989;9:332–343.
3. Fugazzotto PA. Implant placement at the time of maxillary molar extraction: Technique and report of preliminary results of 83 sites. J Periodontol 2006;77:302–309.
4. Fugazzotto PA, Hains FO. Immediate implant placement in posterior areas: The mandibular arch. Compend Contin Educ Dent 2012;33:494–510.
5. Santos FA, Pochapski MT, Martins MC, Zenóbio EG, Spolidoro LC, Marcantonio E Jr. Comparison of biomaterial implants in the dental socket: Histological analysis in dogs. Clin Implant Dent Relat Res 2010;12:18–25.
6. Bartee BK. The use of high-density polytetrafluoroethylene membrane to treat osseous defects: Clinical reports. Implant Dent 1995;4:21–26.
7. Holtzclaw D, Tofe R. An updated primer on the utilization of amnion-chorion allografts in dental procedures. J Implant Adv Clin Dent 2017;9(2):16–37.
8. Akimoto K, Becker W, Persson R, Baker DA, Rohrer MD, O'Neal RB. Evaluation of titanium implants placed into simulated extraction sockets: A study in dogs. Int J Oral Maxillofac Implants 1999;14:351–360.
9. Davies JE. Understanding peri-implant endosseous healing. J Dent Educ 2003;67:932–949.
10. El Helow K, El Askary Ael S. Regenerative barriers in immediate implant placement: A literature review. Implant Dent 2008;17:360–371.
11. Botticelli D, Berglundh T, Lindhe J. Resolution of bone defects of varying dimension and configuration in the marginal portion of the peri-implant bone. An experimental study in the dog. J Clin Periodontol 2004;31:309–317.
12. Albrektsson T, Wennerberg A. Oral implant surfaces: Part 1—Review focusing on topographic and chemical properties of different surfaces and in vivo responses to them. Int J Prosthodont 2004;17:536–543.
13. Botticelli D, Berglundh T, Lindhe J. Hard-tissue alterations following immediate implant placement in extraction sites. J Clin Periodontol 2004;31:820–828.
14. Tarnow DP, Chu SJ. Human histologic verification of osseointegration of an immediate implant placed into a fresh extraction socket with excessive gap distance without primary flap closure, graft, or membrane: A case report. Int J Periodontics Restorative Dent 2011;31:515–521.
15. Al-Kudmani H, Al Jasser R, Andreana S. Is bone graft or guided bone regeneration needed when placing immediate dental implants? A systematic review. Implant Dent 2017;26:936–944.
16. Smith RB, Tarnow DP, Sarnachiaro G. Immediate placement of dental implants in molar extraction sockets: An 11-year retrospective analysis. Compend Contin Educ Dent 2019;40:166–170.
17. Amato F, Polara G. Immediate implant placement in single-tooth molar extraction sockets: A 1- to 6-year retrospective clinical study. Int J Periodontics Restorative Dent 2018;38:495–501.
18. Smith RB, Tarnow DP. Classification of molar extraction sites for immediate dental implant placement: Technical note. Int J Oral Maxillofac Implants 2013;28:911–916.

19. Grassi FR, Grassi R, Rapone B, Alemanno G, Balena A, Kalemaj Z. Dimensional changes of buccal bone plate in immediate implants inserted through open flap, open flap and bone grafting and flapless techniques: A cone-beam computed tomography randomized controlled clinical trial. Clin Oral Implants Res 2019;30:1155–1164.
20. Clementini M, Agostinelli A, Castelluzzo W, Cugnata F, Vignoletti F, De Sanctis M. The effect of immediate implant placement on alveolar ridge preservation compared to spontaneous healing after tooth extraction: Radiographic results of a randomized controlled clinical trial. J Clin Periodontol 2019;46:776–786.
21. Deporter D, Khoshkhounejad AA, Khoshkhounejad N, Ketabi M. A new classification of peri implant gaps based on gap location (a case series of 210 immediate implants). Dent Res J (Isfahan) 2021;18:29.
22. Naji BM, Abdelsameaa SS, Alqutaibi AY, Said Ahmed WM. Immediate dental implant placement with a horizontal gap more than two millimetres: A randomized clinical trial. Int J Oral Maxillofac Surg 2021;50:683–690.
23. Sohn DS, Huang B, Kim J, Park EW, Park CC. Utilization of autologous concentrated growth factors (CGF) enriched bone graft matrix (sticky bone) and CGF-enriched fibrin membrane in implant dentistry. J Implant Adv Clin Dent 2015;7(10):11–29.
24. Caiazzo A, Brugnami F, Galletti F, Mehra P. Buccal plate preservation with immediate implant placement and provisionalization: 5-year follow-up outcomes. J Maxillofac Oral Surg 2018; 17:356–361.
25. Brugnami F, Caiazzo A. Efficacy evaluation of a new buccal bone plate preservation technique: A pilot study. Int J Periodontics Restorative Dent 2011;31:67–73.
26. Hu C, Gong T, Lin W, Yuan Q, Man Y. Immediate implant placement into posterior sockets with or without buccal bone dehiscence defects: A retrospective cohort study. J Dent 2017;65:95–100.
27. Sicilia-Felechosa A, Pereira-Fernández A, García-Lareu J, Bernardo-González J, Sicilia-Blanco P, Cuesta-Fernández I. Flapless immediate implant placement and provisionalization in periodontal patients: A retrospective consecutive case-series study of single-tooth sites with dehiscence-type osseous defects. Clin Oral Implants Res 2020;31:229–238.
28. Gluckman H, Salama M, Du Toit J. Partial extraction therapies (PET) Part I: Maintaining alveolar ridge contour at pontic and immediate implant sites. Int J Periodontics Restorative Dent 2016;36:681–687.
29. Schropp L, Wenzel A, Kostopoulos L, Karring T. Bone healing and soft tissue contour changes following single tooth extraction: A clinical and radiographic 12-month prospective study. Int J Periodontics Restorative Dent 2003;23:313–323.
30. Siormpas K, Mitsias M, Kontsiotou-Siormpa E, Garber D, Kotsakis G. Immediate implant placement in the esthetic zone utilizing the "root-membrane" technique: Clinical results up to 5 years postloading. Int J Oral Maxillofac Implants 2014;29:1397–1405.
31. Hürzeler MB, Zuhr O, Schupbach P, Rebele SF, Emmanouilidis N, Fickl S. The socket-shield technique: A proof-of-principle report. J Clin Periodontol 2010;37:855–862.
32. Al-Hezaimi K, Al-Askar M, Al-Rasheed A. Characteristics of newly formed cementum following Emdogain application. Int J Oral Sci 2011;3:21–26.
33. Baumer D, Zuhr O, Rebele S, Hurzeler M. Socket shield technique for immediate implant placement: Clinical, radiographic and volumetric data after 5 years. Clin Oral Implants Res 2017: 28:1450–1458.
34. Gluckman H, Salama M, Du Toit J. A retrospective evaluation of 128 socket-shield Cases in the esthetic zone and posterior sites: Partial extraction therapy with up to 4 years follow-up. Clin Implant Dent Rel Res 2018;20:122–129.
35. Gluckman H, Salama M, Du Toit J. Partial extraction therapies (PET) Part 2: Procedures and technical aspects. Int J Periodontics Restorative Dent 2017;37:377–385.
36. Schwimer CW, Gluckman H, Salama M, Nagy K, Du Toit J. The socket-shield technique at molar sites: A proof-of-principle technique report. J Prosthet Dent 2019;121:229–233.
37. Huwais S, Meyer E. A novel osseous densification approach in implant osteotomy preparation to increase biomechanical primary stability, bone mineral density, and bone to implant contact. Int J Oral Maxillofac Implants 2017;32:27–36.
38. Smith RB, Rawdin SB, Kagan V. Influence of implant-tooth proximity on incidence of caries in teeth adjacent to implants in molar sites: A retrospective radiographic analysis of 300 consecutive implants. Compend Contin Educ Dent 2020;41:e1–e5.
39. Malkoç S, Basçiftçi FA, Nur M, Catalbas B. Maxillary and mandibular mesiodistal tooth sizes among different malocclusions in a sample of the Turkish population. Eur J Orthod 2011;33: 592–596.
40. Si MS, Shou YW, Shi YT, Yang GL, Wang HM, He FM. Long-term outcomes of osteotome sinus floor elevation without bone grafts: A clinical retrospective study of 4-9 years. Clin Oral Implants Res 2016;27:1392–1400.
41. Summers RB. The osteotome technique: Part 3—Less invasive methods of elevating the sinus floor. Compendium 1994;15: 698–710.
42. Hagi D, Deporter DA, Pilliar RM, Arenovich T. A targeted review of study outcomes with short (< or = 7 mm) endosseous dental implants placed in partially edentulous patients. J Periodontol 2004;75:798–804.
43. Deporter D (ed). Short and Ultra-Short Implants. Chicago: Quintessence, 2018.
44. Pierrisnard L, Renouard F, Renault P, Barquins M. Influence of implant length and bicortical anchorage on implant stress distribution. Clin Implant Dent Relat Res 2003;5:254–262.
45. Esposito M, Barausse C, Pistilli R, et al. Posterior atrophic jaws rehabilitated with prostheses supported by 5 × 5 mm implants with a nanostructured calcium-incorporated titanium surface or by longer implants in augmented bone. Five-year results from a randomised controlled trial. Int J Oral Implantol (Berl) 2019;12:39–54.
46. Esposito M, Pellegrino G, Pistilli R, Felice P. Rehabilitation of postrior atrophic edentulous jaws: Prostheses supported by 5 mm short implants or by longer implants in augmented bone? One-year results from a pilot randomised clinical trial. Eur J Oral Implantol 2011;4:21–30.
47. Felice P, Barausse C, Pistilli R, Ippolito DR, Esposito M. Five-year results from a randomised controlled trial comparing prostheses supported by 5-mm long implants or by longer implants in augmented bone in posterior atrophic edentulous jaws. Int J Oral Implantol (Berl) 2019;12:25–37.
48. Vazouras K, de Souza AB, Gholami H, Papaspyridakos P, Pagni S, Weber HP. Effect of time in function on the predictability of short dental implants (≤6 mm): A meta-analysis. J Oral Rehabil 2020;47:403–415.
49. Checchi V, Felice P, Zucchelli G, et al. Wide diameter immediate post-extractive implants vs delayed placement of normal-diameter implants in preserved sockets in the molar region: 1-year post-loading outcome of a randomised controlled trial. Eur J Oral Implantol 2017;10:263–278.
50. Nisand D, Renouard F. Short implant in limited bone volume. Periodontol 2000 2014;66:72–96.

12

PROSTHETIC CONSIDERATIONS AND LOADING PROTOCOLS FOR IMMEDIATE MOLAR IMPLANTS

Adriano Piattelli
Margherita Tumedei
Samvel Bleyan
Richard Smith

Literature Review

Early research on immediate loading

Starting in the early 1990s with almost a decade of experience using titanium threaded endosseous implants, investigators began to challenge established protocols. The original Brånemark protocols[1] for successful osseointegration dictated the need for submerged initial site healing and delayed loading after at least 4 months of healing. However, these protocols had been conceived after testing machine-turned, threaded screw implants used under demanding conditions in fully edentulous mandibles by fairly inexperienced clinicians, a nonoptimized implant design, nonoptimized surgical protocols, and biomechanically nonoptimized prosthesis designs.[2] Therefore, these original tenets slowly began to unravel with a growing knowledge and understanding of the interactions of bone and implant during the osseointegration process. Soon, clinicians were reporting that—provided sufficient bone had been available at implant placement to achieve good initial stability (generally torque ≥ 35 Ncm)—implants placed in healed edentulous sites did not require submerged healing and could be subjected to some loading earlier than had been originally recommended. Indeed, even immediate loading was sometimes attempted.[2–15] Researchers then began publishing findings from animal and human studies showing positive outcomes both clinically and histologically.[16–22]

In humans, immediate loading protocols for implants placed in healed extraction sites were first described for the completely edentulous mandible, where bone is typically dense. However, using rigid, cross-arch-stabilized fixed immediate prostheses gave excellent outcomes in both fully edentulous

BOX 12-1 Contraindications for immediate loading[36]

Local factors
- Absence of adequate primary stability
- Need for extensive bone grafting
- Severe maxillomandibular skeletal discrepancy
- Heavy smoking
- Uncontrolled bruxism
- History of severe periodontitis
- Existing acute infection
- Lack of adequate posterior occlusal support

Systemic factors
- Drug and/or alcohol abuse
- History of radiotherapy of the head or neck within the previous 2 years
- Recent chemotherapy
- Severe chronic liver or renal disease
- Uncontrolled diabetes
- Recent myocardial infarction
- Immune-compromised status
- Pregnancy
- Bleeding disorders

mandibles and maxillae.[6,7,23,24] Prosthetic considerations for immediate loading were proposed by Morton et al[25] and included the following:

- Limiting and distributing occlusal contact in centric occlusion, ie, maximum intercuspation
- Removing all excursive contacts from the provisional restorations
- Limiting the effects of cantilevers and off-axis loading
- Splinting implants together where possible
- Leaving provisional restorations in place and undisturbed throughout the process of healing

Dietary modifications also were considered appropriate in order to minimize the risk of the restorations loosening during initial site healing.[26] Immediate loading of single implant restorations, including those placed at healed mandibular molar extraction sites,[27–32] also showed some success, despite the fact that biting forces experienced by molars (especially first molars) are the highest in the mouth.[33] A meta-analysis of results from 13 prospective clinical trials with various prosthetic modalities published in 2005 revealed failure rates for immediately loaded implants placed at healed extraction sites to be similar to those with conventionally loaded ones.[34] As a result, experienced clinicians started opting to load implants much earlier in order to decrease treatment time, increase patient acceptance, and maintain optimal soft tissue esthetics.[35] Both local and systemic contraindications for immediate loading have been suggested by Peñarrocha-Oltra et al[36] (Box 12-1).

Terminology

Different definitions exist in the literature as to what constitutes *immediate* loading of implants, but generally it is defined as loading within 48 hours post-implantation, although loading up to 1 week post-implantation is considered "immediate" by some clinicians.[27,37–39] Both immediate *occlusal* loading and immediate *nonocclusal* loading have been investigated. Immediate nonocclusal loading applies to those situations where standard or custom healing abutments[40,41] or transitional restorations, freed from both centric and eccentric occlusal contacts (eg, using 200-µm-thick articulating paper[42]) are placed immediately. With immediate molar implants (IMIs), since esthetics is not usually an issue, it may be safer to take the custom abutment approach.[43,44] *Early* occlusal loading, on the other hand, is specified as prosthesis insertion in centric contact at more than 48 hours but less than 3 months after implant placement, while *delayed* occlusal loading refers to situations where the implants are loaded only after 3 or more months of initial osseointegration.

Importance of primary stability

In a very recent literature review and meta-analysis comparing levels of crestal bone loss after 1 year of implant function in humans, Sommer et al[45] reported that the least crestal bone loss at 1 year was found for immediate nonocclusal loading with immediate occlusal loading a close second, while the greatest bone loss at 1 year was seen with conventional delayed loading. Others have shown that immediate nonocclusal loading increases implant stability earlier than delayed loading.[46] This might seem counterintuitive, except that some level of controlled implant loading during healing can be beneficial by actually stimulating bone formation.[37,47] Thus, histologic findings from both monkey and human studies have documented a higher percentage of bone-to-implant contact with immediately loaded implants than implants allowed submerged healing and delayed loading.[19,48] High initial stability of single-tooth implants or rigid splinting of multiple implants, including cross-arch stabilization in bone of low density, will limit nonaxial loading. Provided that micromotion at the bone-implant interface under axial loading is within the critical threshold of 50 to 150 μm, bone formation will actually be stimulated.[49–51] Splinting might not always be essential, as recent histologic investigations in monkey mandibles showed similar findings (average bone-to-implant contact and average bone density up to 1 mm from the implant-bone interface) with immediate or delayed loading of nonsplinted implants.[52] Again, however, adequate primary stability is key and will vary according to local bone quality.

Primary implant stability is generally assessed by measuring implant insertion torque with a torque wrench and/or with resonance frequency assessment (ie, ISQ or implant stability quotient) using commercially available instruments (eg, Osstell). Most clinicians rely on insertion torque of 35 Ncm or greater and ISQ values of 68 or greater[53] as appropriate for immediate implant loading. Excessively high insertion torque, however, should be avoided as it may result in complications due to delayed bone remodeling. For example, Rea et al[54] performed a study in dogs to evaluate the influence of different insertion torques on outcomes with implants placed in healed sites and either loaded immediately or left unloaded. All mandibular premolars and molars were extracted, and implants (two per side of mandible) were placed 4 months later. Osteotomies were prepared either following the manufacturer's protocol or undersized by 0.3 mm. This resulted in insertion torques of ~ 30 Ncm for the control implants compared to more than 70 Ncm at the undersized sites. Healing abutments (nonocclusal loading) were applied to implants on the left side of the mandible, but transmucosal abutments were placed on the right side. Then, within 20 hours, crowns were cemented to the implant abutments on the right side (occlusal loading). After 4 months in function, the experiment was terminated and histomorphometric assessment of retrieved samples performed. Results showed greater buccal crestal bone loss with occlusal loading along with greater bone-to–implant surface contact (BIC) and quantity of peri-implant mineralized tissue. Further, higher BIC was found with implants prepared using a standard protocol compared with those where osteotomies had been underprepared with much higher insertion torque.

The specific mechanical signals detected by bone cells following acceptable levels of micromotion with immediate loading protocols and the way in which the signals are converted into cellular activity are still unknown but most likely involve strain-mediated fluid flow through the canalicular channels and responses by osteocytes.[55,56] Support for this is added by the finding of statistically significant greater numbers of osteocytes in peri-implant bone around immediately loaded implants compared with nonloaded ones.[57] The same investigators found a correlation between percentage of BIC and osteocyte density for immediately loaded but not for submerged implants. This all could help to explain Sommer's findings linking type of load and peri-implant bone loss. Work in a minipig model by others[58] has shown differences in bone collagen orientation and mineralization between immediately loaded and nonloaded implants, with the former showing greater transverse bone collagen orientation and higher mineralization.

Immediate loading of molar implants

There are several advantages of immediate or early loading of molar implants, as follows:

- Some occlusal function is established faster.
- Optimal soft tissue esthetics may be developed with custom healing abutments or temporary crowns.[59,60]
- There is no need for temporary removable dentures with their risk of unfavorably affecting integration.
- Patient comfort and satisfaction is improved.
- Speech is improved.
- As already stated, there is reduced marginal bone loss with nonocclusal loading.

However, a strong initial contact of the implant with peri-implant bone and careful management of the prosthesis are essential to avoid inhibition of bone and formation of a fibrous tissue interface with failed integration. Other contributing factors include the anatomical characteristics of the molar socket after tooth removal; implant size, shape, and surface properties; methodology of implant placement (eg, with traditional burs, hand osteotomes, or osseodensification[61]), 3D implant positioning in a prosthetically favorable location, and of course, adequate implant stability. Certainly, higher masticatory forces will be experienced in the posterior jaw sites, making the combination of immediate function with IMI placement particularly challenging.

As already stated, results with immediate occlusally loaded and nonocclusally loaded molar implants placed in previously healed extraction sites have been reported to give comparable clinical short-term outcomes to similar implants loaded using conventional delayed protocols.[27,38] Vogl et al[62] reported 3-year results following the use of immediate nonocclusal (control) and immediate occlusal (test) loading of implants placed into healed extraction sockets in posterior sites of partially edentulous patients. Minimum initial stability of 20 Ncm was required for all implants in the study, and all restorations (an unspecified number of which were splinted) were installed within 72 hours of implant placement but torqued only to 14 Ncm. Twenty patients were randomly assigned each to receive one or other of the two loading conditions. Of the 59 implants planned, 1 implant could not be inserted due to a bone deficiency, while 3 were left unrestored due to inadequate primary stability. One implant was lost 24 months after surgery, and with that, the investigators reported 3-year survival rates as 97.1% in the control and 100% in the test group, or 98.2% overall based on both groups.

Favorable outcomes also have been reported for single mandibular molar implants placed in healed extraction sites and then loaded immediately with or without occlusal contact or with delayed loading.[63,64] These latter two reports were from the same randomized controlled split-mouth trial, but reported after different time intervals in function. Implants were inserted into healed healthy bone with an insertion torque between 35 and 45 Ncm. One first molar in each patient was restored within 24 hours using either an occluding or a nonoccluding temporary crown, while the contralateral first molar in each patient was restored only with a definitive crown placed 4 to 5 months after implant insertion. A total of 20 patients (8 men and 12 women) agreed to participate in the study, and after 5 years in function, all implants had survived with similar and minimal mean crestal bone loss among the loading protocols.

Longer-term outcomes (≥ 10 years) from trials where investigators have focused on immediate versus delayed loading of molar implants placed in healed extraction sites are currently not available. Results from the first planned 10-year prospective study comparing immediate versus delayed loading of Brånemark-type implants placed in healed extraction sites of edentulous mandibles appeared in 1990. It was undertaken more or less as a proof-of-principle study, was generally shocking to experts at the time, but offered surprisingly favorable early outcomes. However, this was pioneering work, and after the study patients had reached 10 years in function, the immediately loaded implants had performed significantly less well than originally submerged implants loaded in the traditional delayed fashion (84.7% vs 100% survival).[65] It must be pointed out, however, that the study was with the original machine-turned Brånemark implant, which is no longer in use.

More recently, Degidi et al[66] reported the 10-year outcome of a group of patients treated with fixed two- to four-unit partial provisional restorations supported by immediately loaded, moderately rough implants placed in healed sites in various regions of the mouth. The provisionals were replaced with gold alloy/ceramic restorations approximately 28 weeks after implant insertion. Of the 284 implants placed in 114 patients, 78 (27.5%) implants placed in 30 (26.3%) patients were lost over the 10-year follow-up period. Eight implant failures were reported, seven of which were due to peri-implantitis. Moreover, using a 2008 consensus conference reference guide,[67] 121 (61.4%) of the remaining implants were considered healthy (no pain, mobility, or tenderness with < 2 mm of radiographic bone loss from baseline). But then, 21 (10.9%) implants were considered as "satisfactory survivals" (no pain or tenderness, but 2 to 4 mm crestal bone loss), while 49 (25.49%) were classified as having "compromised survival" status. The implants in this last group showed slight to moderate peri-implantitis along with greater than 4 mm of crestal bone loss and increasing probing depths with periods of suppuration. This outcome could hardly be considered favorable, but it may have been related to factors other than the use of immediate loading, although this could not be concluded because there had been no controls (ie, implants loaded in a delayed fashion in the same patient pool).

Chen et al[68] performed a meta-analysis on mostly short-term results from only randomized controlled clinical trials (RCTs) comparing immediate to conventional loading of dental implants placed in healed extraction sites. Study quality assessment included estimation of investigator bias using dichotomous and continuous variables that were pooled and analyzed for risk ratios and weighted mean differences with 95% confidence intervals. Thirty-nine RCTs were identified, although the majority showed medium to high risk of investigator bias. In 9 of the 39 trials, survival rates for both groups were 100%, while in the remaining 29 trials significant differences were found, with immediate loading showing poorer performance (risk ratio of 0.974; 95% confidence interval [CI], 0.954, 0.994; $P = .012$), stressing once more the challenges of immediate loading. When results from the whole group of 39 trials were assessed using implant as the statistical unit, immediate loading showed 96.8% survival compared to 98.6% survival for delayed loading.

Results from another systematic review[69] were more encouraging. The authors compared outcomes after at least 5 years of immediate (occlusal or nonocclusal) versus conventional loading of implants placed in healed extraction sites. Thirty-four prospective studies published between 2007 and 2017 were identified and had reported on 5,349 implants placed in 1,738 patients. A total of 135 implant failures were reported, most of which occurred early after loading or during the first year. This would suggest that inadequate primary stability may have been the issue. Cumulative implant survival rates with immediate loading at up to 5 and 10 years were 97.7% and 96.9%, respectively, although results were significantly better for immediate loading in the mandible vs maxilla. Interestingly, implant length may not be an issue with immediate loading. For example, Weerapong et al[70] recently reported results from a study in which 6-mm-long or conventional-length implants were placed in healed extraction sites of mandibular molars and loaded immediately. High survival rates for both groups were reported, likely because both groups showed high stability at placement (short: mean ISQ value 73.86 ± 2.38; conventional length: mean ISQ value 75.05 ± 3.26, $P = .088$).

Wider implant diameter as factor for success

Clearly, to be considered for immediate nonocclusal or occlusal loading, an IMI must have adequate initial (ie, mechanical) stability, and in this vein, some investigators have favored the use of wider-diameter implants. *Wide implants* have been identified as those with diameters 4.5 mm or greater,[71] while *ultra-wide implants* have been proposed to be those greater than 6 mm.[72] Wider-diameter implants can achieve greater initial stability given that they will allow greater initial contact of the implant with the socket walls in addition to the interradicular septum (IRS) bone.[73] Other advantages with wider-diameter implants relevant to IMI placement include the possibility of more prosthetically friendly implant positioning, reduction of critical tooth-implant distance to minimize the risk of decay on adjacent tooth surfaces,[74] increased implant surface area helping to overcome limited bone height where shorter implants are planned, more favorable emergence profiles for molar crowns given the wider prosthetic platforms, better distribution of occlusal forces, and lower stress on crestal bone.[75] While stress on crestal bone has not been shown to cause marginal bone loss, excessive stress can cause catastrophic sudden and complete microfracture of the bone-to-implant interface with implant loss.

Immediate loading in combination with immediate placement

Combining IMI placement with immediate loading obviously will further increase the challenges for success, as it adds an extra level of difficulty. It is important to realize that researchers reporting positive outcomes with this approach are generally highly talented and specialized clinicians working in teams under strict protocols. In addition to adequate primary stability, achieving optimal prosthetically favorable molar implant positioning will also be important to ensure that only axial forces are in play if immediate occlusal loading is the goal.[76] This is particularly the case for men, where higher occlusal forces will be a factor. Indeed, a case might be made for using computer-guided implant placement surgery to optimize IMIs intended for immediate function (see chapter 10). Certainly, risk of mechanical overload might be expected if an IMI is placed into one of the root sockets rather than into the molar IRS.

The combination of immediate implantation followed by immediate loading has been particularly well documented in the anterior maxilla.[77] However, higher occlusal loads are present in posterior regions of the jaws with increased risk of eccentric biomechanical stress.[63] Degidi et al[78] undertook a retrospective study on a large series of immediately loaded implants that had been placed immediately in a variety of extraction sites, including some molars and premolars. In total, 416 implants had been inserted immediately after extraction, and 658 implants had been placed at healed edentulous sites. Implants from a variety of manufacturers were used. Provisional restorations were cemented on or screwed to each implant to allow loading within 1 to 2 hours postsurgery. Occlusal contact, when possible, was avoided in centric and lateral excursions (ie, nonocclusal loading). After 24 weeks, the provisional restorations were replaced with their permanent counterparts, and all patients were enrolled in a strict hygiene recall. The mean follow-up was reported to be 3 years. Only 8 of the 1,074 implants were lost (survival rate of 99.3%), and no statistically significant differences were detected among the study variables, suggesting that immediate loading of immediate implants is feasible.

More supportive evidence was recently provided by Bettach et al.[79] In their study, 133 patients received 261 implants inserted into fresh postextraction sockets, including some molar sites of either jaw. There were 165 implants in the immediately loaded (IL) group, while 96 underwent delayed loading (DL). Fifty-six (34%) implants were immediately loaded as single crowns. By 3 years in function, two IL and one DL implant had failed in three patients, and the survival rates were given as 98.8% and 99% for the IL and DL groups, respectively.

Measuring implant stability

Returning for the moment to primary implant stability and its usefulness in deciding whether or not to load an implant immediately, clinicians do vary on their preferences to rely on ITVs (insertion torque values) or on ISQ values. Unfortunately, the two methods are completely independent and not comparable in measuring primary implant stability: A high torque does not mean a high ISQ, and vice versa. ISQ is a measure of three distinct variables: stiffness of the implant itself, rigidity of the implant-tissue interface, and stiffness of the surrounding bone.[80] The common instrument used to determine ISQ is the Osstell device, consisting of a wireless receptor fastened into the implant and a handheld probe placed in close proximity to the wireless transducer. Bavetta et al[81] compared the suitability of ISQ versus ITVs in decision making regarding adoption of immediate loading in fresh extraction sockets. Implants placed either immediately or after 3 months postextraction were all assessed initially for ITV and ISQ values. Results showed significantly lower ISQ values at immediately placed implants compared to implants placed after 3 months of socket healing. This was explained as being due to the peri-implant gaps present at immediate implant sites. It was proposed that ITV measurements are likely more appropriate in deciding whether or not to undertake immediate loading. However, ISQ monitoring can be a useful method to choose the best time to move from the provisional to the definitive restoration with an immediate implant that has been loaded immediately based on an adequate ITV value, and this would agree with earlier findings of others.[82] However, as long as the ISQ of an immediately placed implant is greater than a threshold of 65, it is generally considered a candidate for immediate loading.

Clinical Protocols for Immediate Loading of IMIs

To be successful with immediate loading of immediately placed molar implants, strict surgical and prosthodontic protocols must be followed. Site selection is crucial. Thus, pretreatment CBCT scans need to

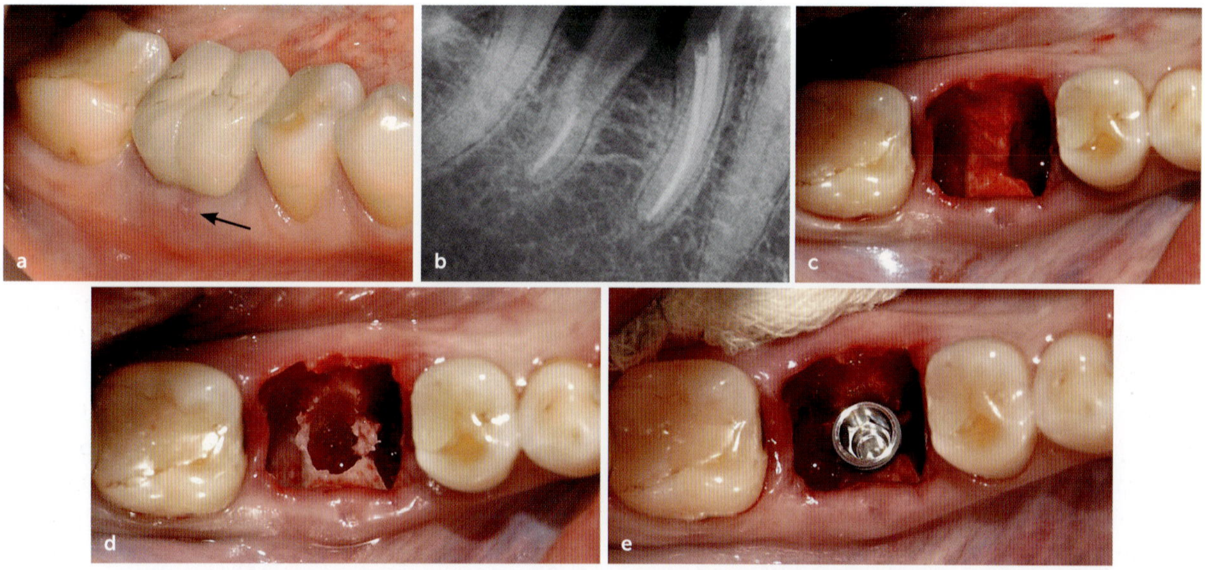

FIG 12-1 *(a)* The initial clinical photograph did not reveal that advanced recurrent decay had made the mandibular right first molar hopeless, but the patient complained of a recurrent fistula at the bifurcation zone *(arrow)*. *(b)* A pretreatment periapical radiograph was taken after removal of the restoration and separation of the two roots for atraumatic removal. The site can be seen to have adequate IRS bone to stabilize an IMI. *(c)* After the crown was removed, the tooth roots were removed using flapless surgery without damage to the IRS bone or socket walls. *(d)* An osteotomy was created in the IRS bone following the principles of osseodensification (see chapter 7), ie, compacting and retaining rather than removing bone. *(e)* A 12 × 4–mm Dentium Superline implant was inserted into the osteotomy with good initial stability. Note that the seated implant was largely housed within the IRS bone and that thick buccal and lingual buttresses of bone remained. Indeed, the site could have accommodated a 5-mm-diameter implant, helping to reduce the distances between the implant and adjacent teeth.

confirm that there is adequate IRS bone to allow good initial implant stability (ie, ITV ≥ 35 Ncm and ISQ ≥ 65). Flapless, atraumatic tooth extraction is essential to minimize damage to the socket walls, which should all be intact. Osteotomy development should follow the protocols described in previous chapters of this book. Ideally, an implant with a diameter of 4.5 mm or greater will be used to allow the development of a suitable molar emergence profile, and the prosthetic platform should be submerged subcrestally to a level where at least 1.5 mm of buccal bone thickness is present. The distance at the crest measured between the teeth adjacent to the planned molar implant is crucial.[74] Ideally, an implant-to–adjacent tooth distance of 4 mm or less should be planned, and if this cannot be achieved with a single wide-diameter implant, two smaller-diameter implants should be considered.

Case 1

This patient was a 52-year-old woman (no smoking or other bad habits, good hygiene) who presented with a hopeless mandibular right first molar due to recurrent caries and recurrent fistula and bone resorption of the furcation zone under an existing prosthetic crown (Fig 12-1a). The crown was removed, and the two roots were separated with a high-speed handpiece. A radiograph taken at that time revealed substantial IRS bone that widened apically and was thought to be suitable for placement of an IMI (Figs 12-1b and 12-1c).

The IRS bone was classified as type B and felt to be suitable for osteotomy preparation using osseodensification burs (Fig 12-1d; see also chapter 7). A 12 × 4–mm Dentium Superline implant was subsequently inserted with insertion torque of 30 Ncm and ISQ of 69, making it sufficiently stable to receive immediate nonocclusal loading (Fig 12-1e).

Significant peri-implant gaps remained and were grafted with particulate allograft material, the socket being overfilled in order to provide support for the surrounding soft connective tissue walls (Figs 12-1f and 12-1g). After connecting a temporary titanium abutment to the implant, a chairside custom large-diameter healing abutment was created. To do this, a spiderweb-like outline of the required abutment

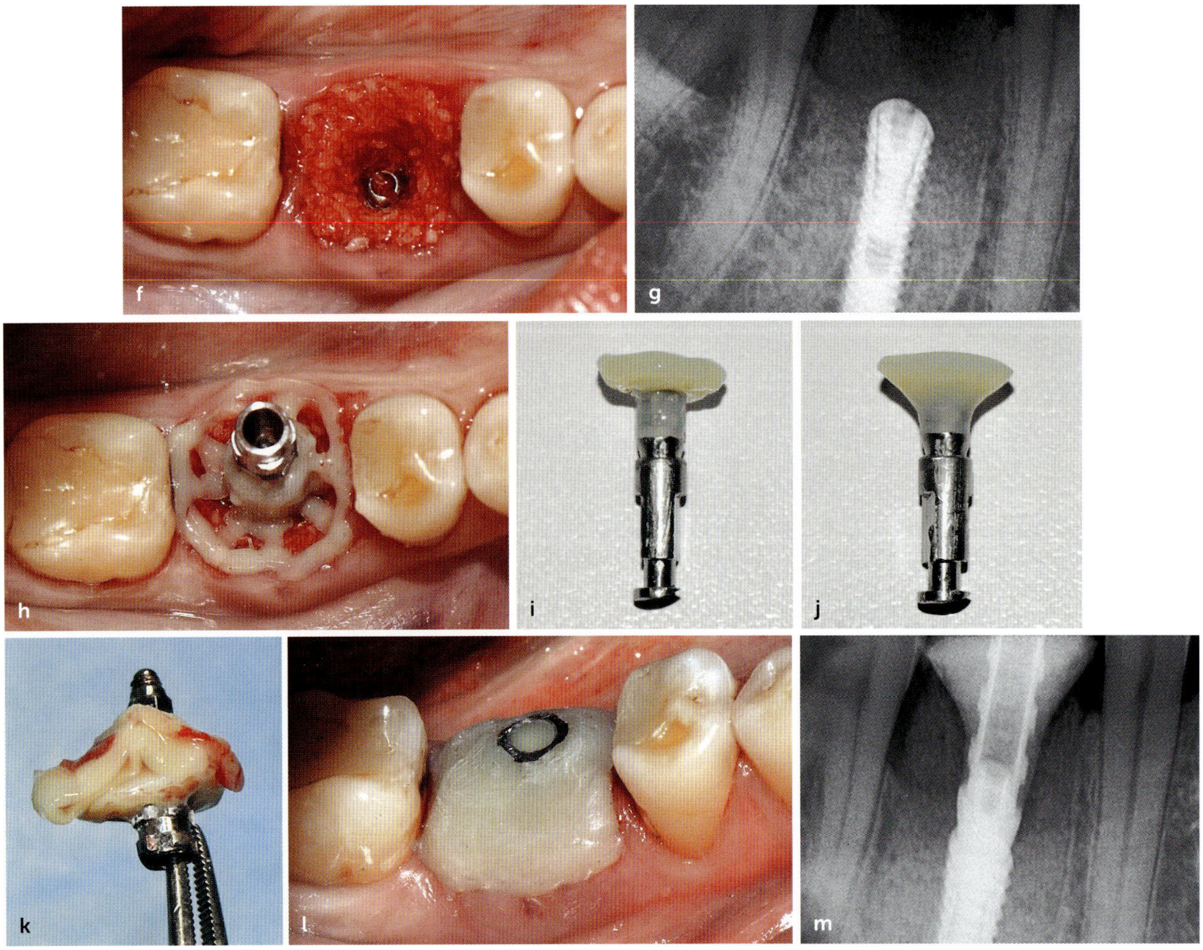

FIG 12-1 *(cont) (f)* Particulate allograft was used to fill all peri-implant gaps with overfill to help to support the peri-implant soft tissues. Many clinicians prefer to use xenograft for this gap grafting, as it is felt to provide more long-term stability of local ridge anatomy. *(g)* This postgrafting radiograph shows the gaps and intended crestal overfill with particulate allograft. *(h)* After connecting a stock prosthetic abutment to the implant, a flowable composite (Estelite Flow Quick) is used to create a spiderweb-like framework in situ. *(i)* After the web outline had set, it was removed with the prosthetic abutment and attached to a stock implant analog. *(j)* The custom healing abutment was shaped by the addition of more composite to form a mushroom-shaped prosthesis meant to seal the tooth socket, protecting and compressing the allograft material. *(k)* Before connecting the custom healing abutment to the implant, a platelet-rich fibrin clot was skewered over the retaining screw to provide a biologic seal, separating the abutment material from the underlying particulate graft and delivering platelet-derived growth factors known to promote revascularization. *(l)* The custom healing abutment was connected to the implant and had three functions: to provide some immediate nonocclusal loading of the implant, to protect and compress the allograft material beneath, and to promote guided soft tissue healing by dynamic compression. *(m)* The immediate post-treatment radiograph shows the custom healing abutment compressing the overfill of allograft material.

shape was begun using flowable composite material (Estelite Flow Quick, Tokuyama; Fig 12-1h). Once this material had set in situ (Fig 12-1i), it was removed along with the prosthetic abutment and further developed by adding more of the same composite (Fig 12-1j). Next, an autologous platelet-rich fibrin clot prepared from the patient's own venous blood was skewered over the retention screw of the custom healing abutment (Fig 12-1k) to provide a biologic seal for the implant site, separating the abutment underface from the underlying particulate graft material. This was then connected to the implant with further addition of composite material in the mouth if necessary (Fig 12-1l). A radiograph taken at the time of connection of the custom healing abutment confirmed that it was wide enough to protect the underlying allograft material (Fig 12-1m).

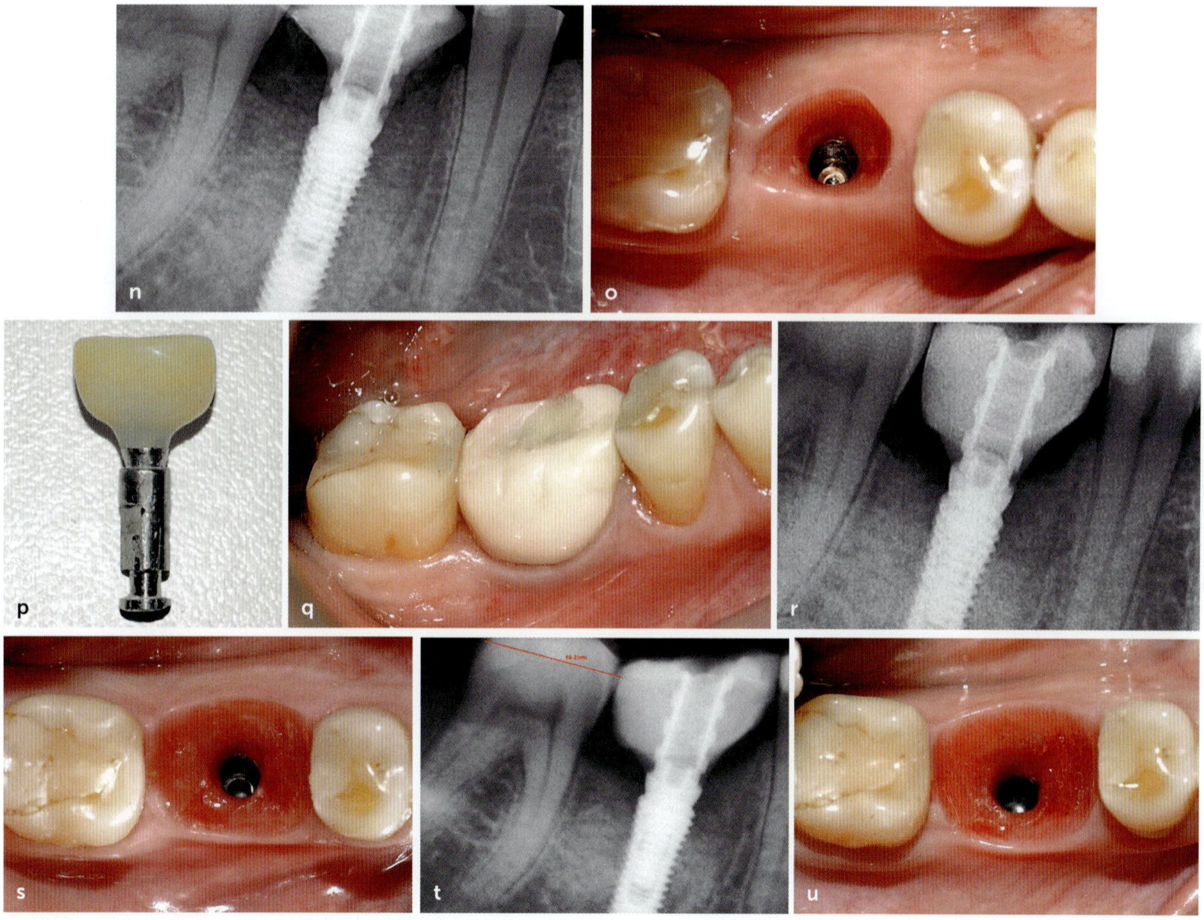

FIG 12-1 *(cont)* *(n)* A periapical radiograph taken after 2 months of site healing shows some allograft particulate material resorption. *(o)* The healing abutment was removed at 2 months, revealing thick healthy peri-implant keratinized tissues. Note that some allograft particles can be seen in the soft tissue. This commonly happens and is self-resolving. However, if the situation persists as healing progresses, any remaining isolated particles should be removed to reduce the risk of soft tissue abscess formation. *(p)* After 2 months' site healing, the healing abutment was enlarged with the addition of more composite to form a molar-shaped provisional crown intended to further refine the peri-implant soft tissues to ensure a favorable emergence profile for the definitive crown. *(q)* The molar-shaped provisional composite crown was prepared and inserted at the 2-month recall visit. *(r)* A radiograph taken of the new transitional restoration, which can be modified as need be during further site healing to finish sculpting the soft tissues by dynamic compression. *(s)* The clinical status of the soft tissue profile 10 days after inserting the transitional crown. Allograft particles can no longer be seen in the soft tissue. *(t)* Additional composite material was added subgingivally to further refine the soft tissue profile prior to taking impressions for the final crown. *(u)* The final soft tissue profile at the time of impression taking. Note the absence of any exfoliating graft particles and the thick soft tissue profile.

The radiographic appearance of the site can be seen in Fig 12-1n after 2 months' healing, at which time the abutment was removed to show the soft tissue healing that had already occurred (Fig 12-1o). With the addition of more composite, the healing abutment was enlarged into a molar-sized provisional crown meant to continue shaping the peri-implant soft tissues prior to impression taking for the definitive prosthesis (Figs 12-1p to 12-1r). Figure 12-1s shows the condition and shape of the soft tissues at the site 10 days later. More composite was again added, and after a further 3 weeks of healing (Figs 12-1t and 12-1u), the site was ready for impressions to be taken and for fabrication and delivery of the definitive crown (Figs 12-1v and 12-1w). Figure 12-1x shows the implant site after 2 months in function.

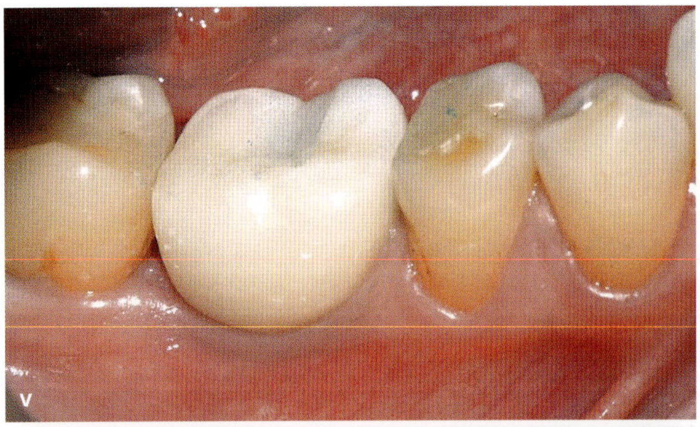

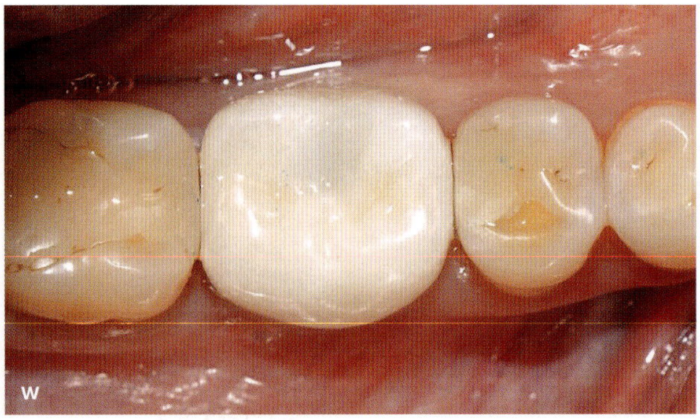

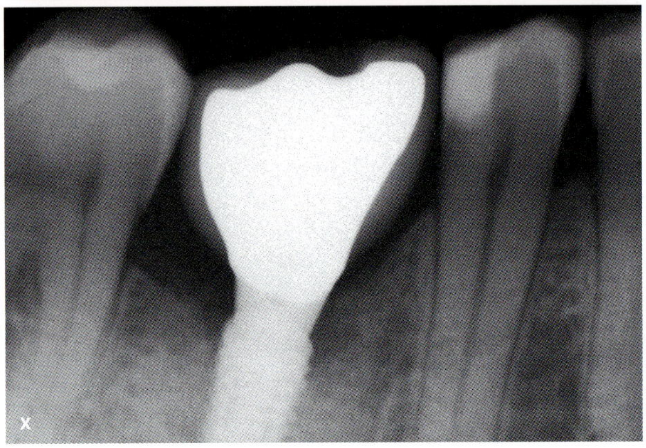

FIG 12-1 *(cont) (v)* The definitive zirconia crown at the time of insertion. Note the favorable emergence crown profile, the reformation of interdental papillae, and the healthy band of keratinized tissue. *(w)* An occlusal view of the definitive restoration. *(x)* A periapical radiograph of the definitive prosthesis 5 months after the original implant surgery. Note the continued remodeling of the allograft material. (Treatment by Dr Samvel Bleyan, Moscow, Russia.)

Case 2

This 70-year-old woman presented with a periodontally hopeless maxillary right first molar (Figs 12-2a and 12-2b). As can be seen in the pretreatment radiograph, the IRS was type B, ie, with adequate bone to stabilize an immediate implant suitable for replacement of a molar. A 10 × 6–mm Zimmer Biomet implant was inserted into the IRS (Fig 12-2c) with large gaps all around the perimeter that were left nongrafted.[83] A custom healing abutment was used to maintain soft tissue architecture.

To prepare this abutment, a polyaryletherketone (PAEK) cylinder was connected to the implant (Fig 12-2d) and acrylic added incrementally with a brush to outline the existing soft tissue profile (Fig 12-2e). Further acrylic was added outside the mouth to finalize the abutment shape and contours (Figs 12-12f and 12-2g) before returning the polished and steam-cleaned abutment to the implant (Figs 12-2h and 12-2i). No suturing was required as the procedure had been flapless and minimally traumatic. An immediate posttreatment radiograph (Fig 12-2j) shows the implant to be well positioned and unaffecting the maxillary sinus. The implant was ready for fabrication of the definitive prosthesis after 3 months of site healing (Figs 12-2k and 12-2l). After removing the healing abutment, a pickup-type impression coping was placed (Fig 12-2m) and the soft tissue contours captured by the addition of acrylic in the mouth (Figs 12-2n and 12-2o). The master cast was then fabricated with accurate soft tissue representation. Figure 12-2p shows the soft tissue profile on the day of crown insertion (Fig 12-2q). The final radiograph after crown insertion is depicted in Fig 12-2r.

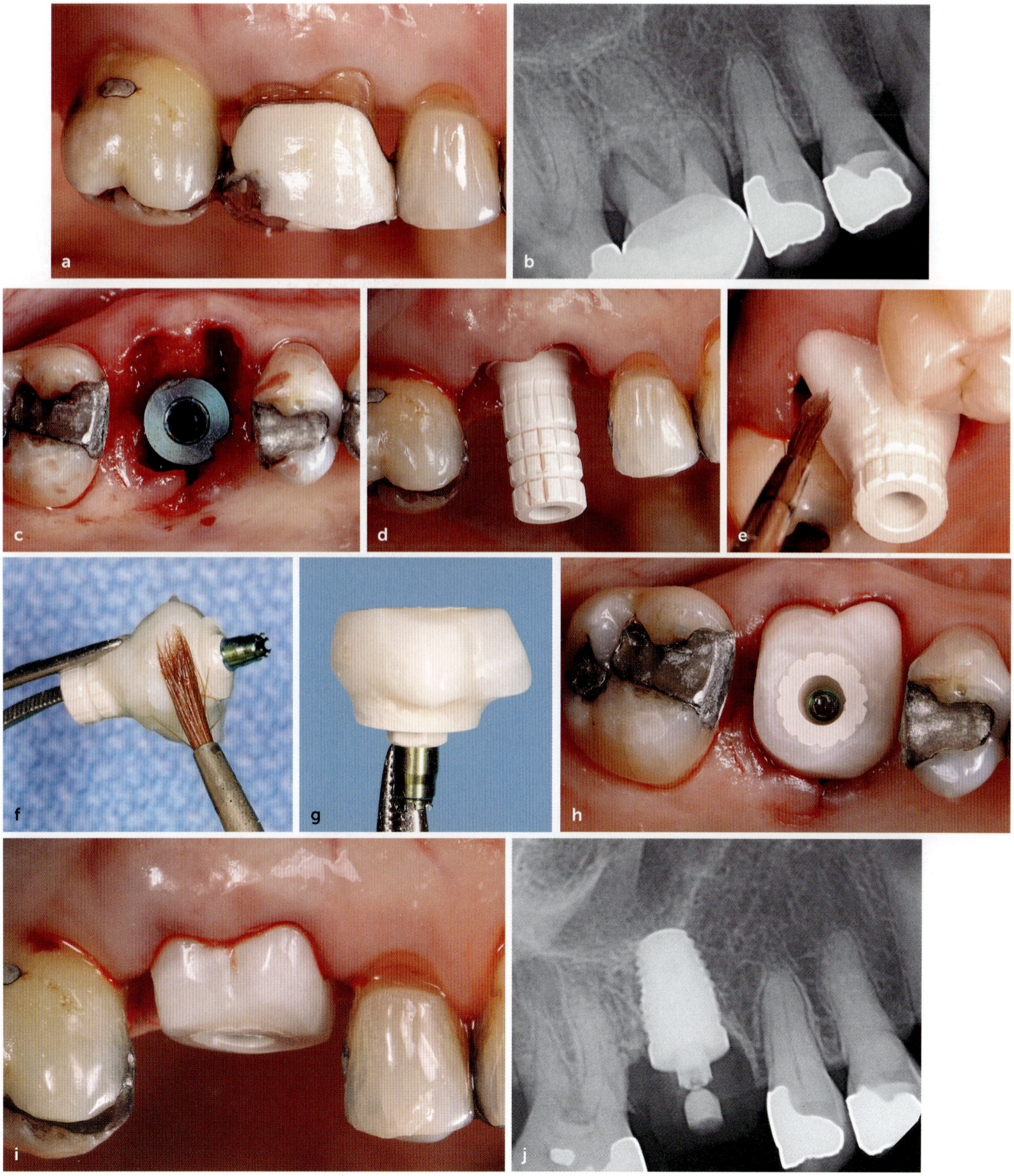

FIG 12-2 *(a)* The patient's maxillary right first molar was periodontally condemned. *(b)* The maxillary first molar required extraction due to an advanced periodontal attachment loss affecting both buccal roots and the furcation. *(c)* Following flapless atraumatic tooth extraction, a 6-mm-diameter implant was inserted into the type B socket.[83] All outer walls were intact, and no gap grafting was performed. Because the buccal wall was thick and the surgery flapless, there was little concern about potential buccal architecture collapse. *(d)* An engaging stock temporary PAEK cylinder served as the foundation for a custom healing abutment. *(e)* Acrylic was added intraorally to allow pickup of the soft tissue marginal profile. *(f)* The PAEK cylinder was removed to permit the subgingival root-form contours of the custom abutment to be developed outside the mouth. *(g)* The root-form and cervical region contours as completed and the buccal surface marked for easy orientation at insertion. *(h)* Once inserted, the custom healing abutment provided protection for the blood clots that had formed in the gaps beneath and served to maintain soft tissue architecture during site healing for future esthetic and functional purposes. *(i)* The custom healing abutment matched the shape and contours of the natural tooth at its cervical region and was left shy of occlusal contacts. *(j)* The immediate postoperative radiograph shows the implant just beneath the sinus floor and the custom healing abutment in place.

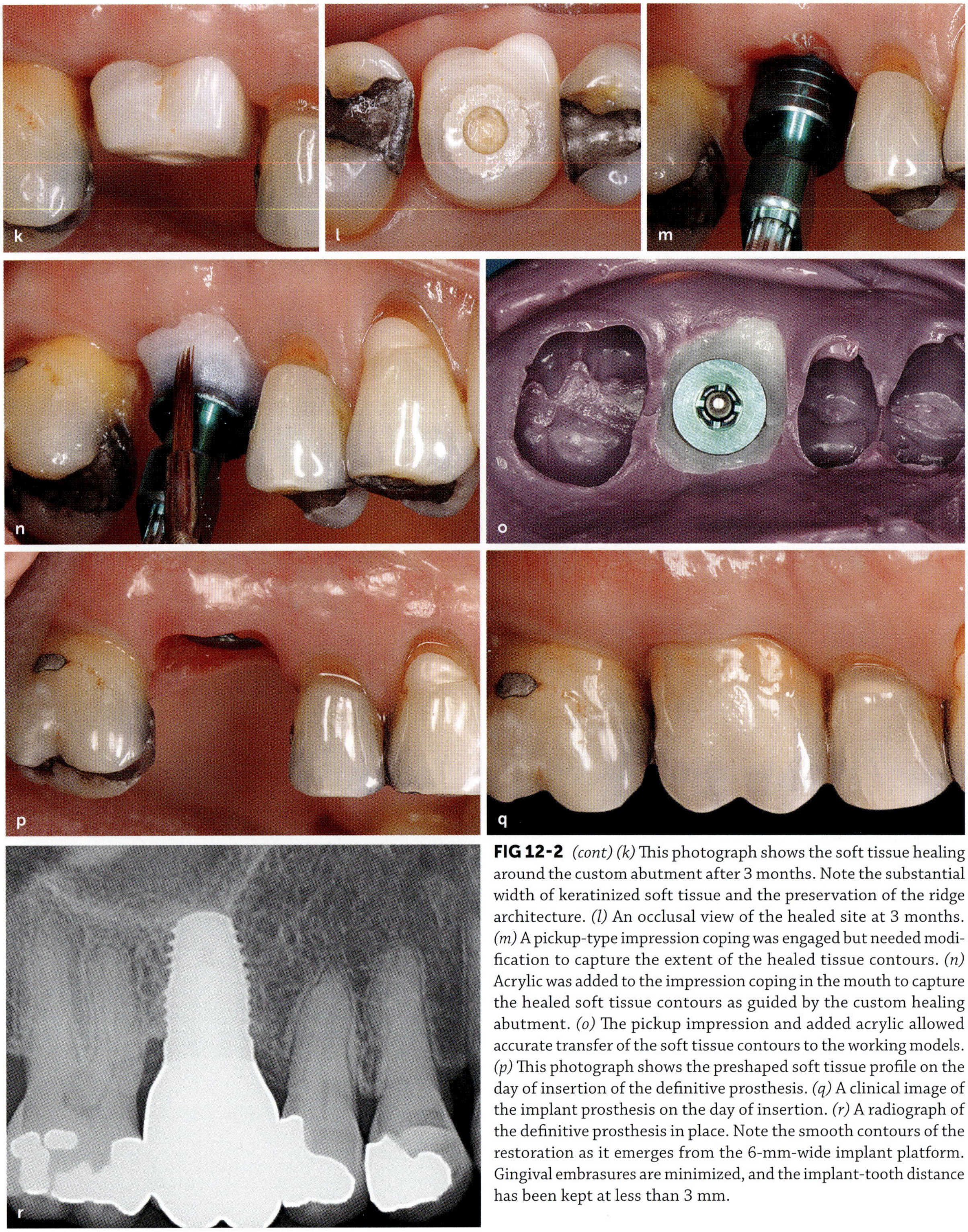

FIG 12-2 *(cont) (k)* This photograph shows the soft tissue healing around the custom abutment after 3 months. Note the substantial width of keratinized soft tissue and the preservation of the ridge architecture. *(l)* An occlusal view of the healed site at 3 months. *(m)* A pickup-type impression coping was engaged but needed modification to capture the extent of the healed tissue contours. *(n)* Acrylic was added to the impression coping in the mouth to capture the healed soft tissue contours as guided by the custom healing abutment. *(o)* The pickup impression and added acrylic allowed accurate transfer of the soft tissue contours to the working models. *(p)* This photograph shows the preshaped soft tissue profile on the day of insertion of the definitive prosthesis. *(q)* A clinical image of the implant prosthesis on the day of insertion. *(r)* A radiograph of the definitive prosthesis in place. Note the smooth contours of the restoration as it emerges from the 6-mm-wide implant platform. Gingival embrasures are minimized, and the implant-tooth distance has been kept at less than 3 mm.

Conclusion

Immediate loading of immediately placed molar implants, while once considered an impossibility, has now become a reality for many patients and their treating clinicians. The preferred approach for single molar replacements is to use nonocclusal loading by adding a standard, wide-diameter, or custom healing abutment or a transitional custom crown relieved of all centric and eccentric contacts.

KEY POINTS

- Adequate initial implant stability is advisable with ITV ≥ 35 Ncm and/or ISQ ≥ 65.
- The most favorable approach in terms of minimizing early crestal bone loss is to use nonocclusal loading.
- Nonocclusal loading ideally will be with the use of custom healing abutments that will shelter any peri-implant gaps and provide some stimulation of osteogenesis.
- A carefully made custom healing abutment also will maintain soft tissue architecture for the eventual definitive prosthesis.

References

1. Adell R, Lekholm U, Rockler B, Brånemark PI. A 15-year study of osseointegrated implants in the treatment of the edentulous jaw. Int J Oral Surg 1981;10:387–416.
2. Szmukler-Moncler S, Piattelli A, Favero GA, Dubruille JH. Considerations preliminary to the application of early and immediate loading protocols in dental implantology. Clin Oral Implants Res 2000;11:12–25.
3. Schnitman PA, Wohrle PS, Rubenstein JE. Immediate fixed interim prostheses supported by two-stage threaded implants: Methodology and results. J Oral Implantol 1990;16:96–105.
4. Sagara M, Akagawa Y, Nikai H, Tsuru H. The effects of early occlusal loading on one-stage titanium alloy implants in beagle dogs: A pilot study. J Prosthet Dent 1993;69:281–288.
5. Chiapasco M, Gatti C, Rossi E, Haefliger W, Markwalder TH. Implant-retained mandibular overdentures with immediate loading. A retrospective multicenter study on 226 consecutive cases. Clin Oral Implants Res 1997;8:48–57.
6. Tarnow DP, Emtiaz S, Classi A. Immediate loading of threaded implants at stage 1 surgery in edentulous arches: Ten consecutive case reports with 1- to 5-year data. Int J Oral Maxillofac Implants 1997;12:319–324.
7. Balshi TJ, Wolfinger GJ. Immediate loading of Brånemark implants in edentulous mandibles: A preliminary report. Implant Dent 1997;6:83–88.
8. Ledermann PD, Schenk RK, Buser D. Long-lasting osseointegration of immediately loaded, bar-connected TPS screws after 12 years of function: A histologic case report of a 95-year-old patient. Int J Periodontics Restorative Dent 1998;18:552–563.
9. Jaffin RA, Kumar A, Berman CL. Immediate loading of implants in partially and fully edentulous jaws: A series of 27 case reports. J Periodontol 2000;71:833–838.
10. Romanos GE, Toh CG, Siar CH, Wicht H, Yacoob H, Nentwig GH. Bone-implant interface around titanium implants under different loading conditions: A histomorphometrical analysis in the *Macaca fascicularis* monkey. J Periodontol 2003;74:1483–1490.
11. Rocci A, Martignoni M, Burgos PM, Gottlow J, Sennerby L. Histology of retrieved immediately and early loaded oxidized implants: Light microscopic observations after 5 to 9 months of loading in the posterior mandible. Clin Implant Dent Relat Res 2003;5 Suppl 1:88–98.
12. Dilek O, Tezulas E, Dincel M. Required minimum primary stability and torque values for immediate loading of mini dental implants: An experimental study in nonviable bovine femoral bone. Oral Surg Oral Med Oral Pathol Oral Radiol Endod 2008;105:e20–e27.
13. Kim SH, Choi BH, Li J, et al. Peri-implant bone reactions at delayed and immediately loaded implants: An experimental study. Oral Surg Oral Med Oral Pathol Oral Radiol Endod 2008;105:144–148.
14. Glauser R, Ruhstaller P, Windisch S, et al. Immediate occlusal loading of Brånemark System TiUnite implants placed predominantly in soft bone: 4-year results of a prospective clinical study. Clin Implant Dent Relat Res 2005;7 Suppl 1:S52–S59.
15. Cannizzaro G, Leone M. Restoration of partially edentulous patients using dental implants with a microtextured surface: A prospective comparison of delayed and immediate full occlusal loading. Int J Oral Maxillofac Implants 2003;18:512–522.

16. Piattelli A, Trisi P, Romasco N, Emanuelli M. Histologic analysis of a screw implant retrieved from man: Influence of early loading and primary stability. J Oral Implantol 1993;19:303–306.
17. Piattelli A, Corigliano M, Scarano A. Microscopical observations of the osseous responses in early loaded human titanium implants: A report of two cases. Biomaterials 1996;17:1333–1337.
18. Piattelli A, Paolantonio M, Corigliano M, Scarano A. Immediate loading of titanium plasma-sprayed screw-shaped implants in man: A clinical and histological report of two cases. J Periodontol 1997;68:591–597.
19. Piattelli A, Corigliano M, Scarano A, Costigliola G, Paolantonio M. Immediate loading of titanium plasma-sprayed implants: An histologic analysis in monkeys. J Periodontol 1998;69:321–327.
20. Degidi M, Petrone G, Iezzi G, Piattelli A. Histologic evaluation of a human immediately loaded titanium implant with a porous anodized surface. Clin Implant Dent Relat Res 2002;4:110–114.
21. Degidi M, Petrone G, Lezzi G, Piattelli A. Histologic evaluation of 2 human immediately loaded and 1 titanium implants inserted in the posterior mandible and submerged retrieved after 6 months. J Oral Implantol 2003;29:223–229.
22. Degidi M, Scarano A, Petrone G, Piattelli A. Histologic analysis of clinically retrieved immediately loaded titanium implants: A report of 11 cases. Clin Implant Dent Relat Res 2003;5:89–93.
23. Salama H, Rose LF, Salama M, Betts NJ. Immediate loading of bilaterally splinted titanium root-form implants in fixed prosthodontics: A technique reexamined: two case reports. Int J Periodontics Restorative Dent 1995;15:344–361.
24. Grunder U. Immediate functional loading of immediate implants in edentulous arches: Two-year results. Int J Periodontics Restorative Dent 2001;21:545–551.
25. Morton D, Jaffin R, Weber HP. Immediate restoration and loading of dental implants: Clinical considerations and protocols. Int J Oral Maxillofac Implants 2004;19(suppl):103–108.
26. Misch CE, Wang HL, Misch CM, Sharawy M, Lemons J, Judy KW. Rationale for the application of immediate load in implant dentistry: Part II. Implant Dent 2004;13:310–321.
27. Moraschini V, Porto Barboza E. Immediate versus conventional loaded single implants in the posterior mandible: A meta-analysis of randomized controlled trials. Int J Oral Maxillofac Surg 2016;45:85–92.
28. Calandriello R, Tomatis M. Immediate occlusal loading of single lower molars using Brånemark System Wide Platform TiUnite implants: A 5-year follow-up report of a prospective clinical multicenter study. Clin Implant Dent Relat Res 2011;13:311–318.
29. Abboud M, Koeck B, Stark H, Wahl G, Paillon R. Immediate loading of single-tooth implants in the posterior region. Int J Oral Maxillofac Implants 2005;20:61–68.
30. Rao W, Benzi R. Single mandibular first molar implants with flapless guided surgery and immediate function: Preliminary clinical and radiographic results of a prospective study [published correction appears in J Prosthet Dent 2008;99:167]. J Prosthet Dent 2007;97(6 suppl):S3–S14.
31. Güncü MB, Aslan Y, Tümer C, Güncü GN, Uysal S. In-patient comparison of immediate and conventional loaded implants in mandibular molar sites within 12 months. Clin Oral Implants Res 2008;19:335–341.
32. Schincaglia GP, Marzola R, Giovanni GF, Chiara CS, Scotti R. Replacement of mandibular molars with single-unit restorations supported by wide-body implants: Immediate versus delayed loading. A randomized controlled study. Int J Oral Maxillofac Implants 2008;23:474–480.
33. Ferrario VF, Sforza C, Serrao G, Dellavia C, Tartaglia GM. Single tooth bite forces in healthy young adults. J Oral Rehabil 2004; 31:18–22.
34. Ioannidou E, Doufexi A. Does loading time affect implant survival? A meta-analysis of 1,266 implants. J Periodontol 2005; 76:1252–1258.
35. Werbitt MJ, Goldberg PV. The immediate implant: Bone preservation and bone regeneration. Int J Periodontics Restorative Dent 1992;12:206–217.
36. Peñarrocha-Oltra D, Soto-Peñaloza D, Peñarrocha-Diago M. Immediate loading in implantology. Clin Dent Rev 2020;4:15.
37. Barndt P, Zhang H, Liu F. Immediate loading: From biology to biomechanics. Report of the Committee on Research in Fixed Prosthodontics of the American Academy of Fixed Prosthodontics. J Prosthet Dent 2015;113:96–107.
38. Gallardo YNR, da Silva-Olivio IR, Gonzaga L, Sesma N, Martin W. A systematic review of clinical outcomes on patients rehabilitated with complete-arch fixed implant-supported prostheses according to the time of loading. J Prosthodont 2019;28:958–968.
39. Gallucci GO, Hamilton A, Zhou W, Buser D, Chen S. Implant placement and loading protocols in partially edentulous patients: A systematic review. Clin Oral Implants Res 2018;29 (suppl 16):106–134.
40. Akin R. A new concept in maintaining the emergence profile in immediate posterior implant placement: The anatomic harmony abutment. J Oral Maxillofac Surg 2016;74:2385–2392.
41. Hu C, Lin W, Gong T, Zuo Y, Qu Y, Man Y. Early healing of immediate implants connected with two types of healing abutments: A prospective cohort study. Implant Dent 2018;27:646–652.
42. Grandi T, Guazzi P, Samarani R, Garuti G. Immediate positioning of definitive abutments versus repeated abutment replacements in immediately loaded implants: Effects on bone healing at the 1-year follow-up of a multicentre randomised controlled trial. Eur J Oral Implantol 2012;5:9–16.
43. Mihali SG, Freiman PC, Bratu EA. Maintaining tissue architecture in immediate implant placement following extraction of natural teeth using custom healing screw. Biomed J Sci Tech Res 2018;7:6096–6101.
44. Ruales-Carrera E, Pauletto P, Apaza-Bedoya K, Volpato CAM, Özcan M, Benfatti CAM. Peri-implant tissue management after immediate implant placement using a customized healing abutment. J Esthet Restor Dent 2019;31:533–541.
45. Sommer M, Zimmermann J, Grize L, Stübinger S. Marginal bone loss one year after implantation: A systematic review of different loading protocols. Int J Oral Maxillofac Surg 2020; 49:121–134.
46. Brizuela-Velasco A, Chávarri-Prado D. The functional loading of implants increases their stability: A retrospective clinical study. Clin Implant Dent Relat Res 2019;21:122–129.
47. Chavarri-Prado D, Brizuela-Velasco A, Álvarez-Arenal Á, et al. The bone buttress theory: The effect of the mechanical loading of bone on the osseointegration of dental implants. Biology (Basel) 2020;10:12.
48. Degidi M, Piattelli A, Shibli JA, Perrotti V, Iezzi G. Bone formation around immediately loaded and submerged dental implants with a modified sandblasted and acid-etched surface after 4 and 8 weeks: A human histologic and histomorphometric analysis. Int J Oral Maxillofac Implants 2009;24:896–901.
49. Szmukler-Moncler S, Salama H, Reingewirtz Y, Dubruille JH. Timing of loading and effect of micromotion on bone-dental implant interface: Review of experimental literature. J Biomed Mater Res 1998;43:192–203.
50. Vandamme K, Naert I, Geris L, Sloten JV, Puers R, Duyck J. Histodynamics of bone tissue formation around immediately loaded cylindrical implants in the rabbit. Clin Oral Implants Res 2007;18:471–480.

51. Vandamme K, Naert I, Geris L, Vander Sloten J, Puers R, Duyck J. The effect of micro-motion on the tissue response around immediately loaded roughened titanium implants in the rabbit [published correction appears in Eur J Oral Sci 2007;115:167]. Eur J Oral Sci 2007;115:21–29.
52. Stokholm R, Isidor F, Nyengaard JR. Histologic and histomorphometric evaluation of peri-implant bone of immediate or delayed occlusal-loaded non-splinted implants in the posterior mandible: An experimental study in monkeys. Clin Oral Implants Res 2014;25:1311–1318.
53. Meredith N, Alleyne D, Cawley P. Quantitative determination of the stability of the implant-tissue interface using resonance frequency analysis. Clin Oral Implants Res 1996;7:261–267.
54. Rea M, Botticelli D, Ricci S, Soldini C, González GG, Lang NP. Influence of immediate loading on healing of implants installed with different insertion torques: An experimental study in dogs. Clin Oral Implants Res 2015;26:90–95.
55. Burr DB, Robling AG, Turner CH. Effects of biomechanical stress on bones in animals. Bone 2002;30:781–786.
56. Skerry TM, Bitensky L, Chayen J, Lanyon LE. Early strain-related changes in enzyme activity in osteocytes following bone loading in vivo. J Bone Miner Res 1989;4:783–788.
57. Barros RR, Degidi M, Novaes AB, Piattelli A, Shibli JA, Iezzi G. Osteocyte density in the peri-implant bone of immediately loaded and submerged dental implants. J Periodontol 2009;80: 499–504.
58. Traini T, Neugebauer J, Thams U, Zöller JE, Caputi S, Piattelli A. Peri-implant bone organization under immediate loading conditions: Collagen fiber orientation and mineral density analyses in the minipig model. Clin Implant Dent Relat Res 2009;11:41–51.
59. Wang J, Lerman G, Bittner N, Fan W, Lalla E, Papapanou PN. Immediate versus delayed temporization at posterior single implant sites: A randomized controlled trial. J Clin Periodontol 2020;47:1281–1291.
60. González-Martín O, Lee E, Weisgold A, Veltri M, Su H. Contour management of implant restorations for optimal emergence profiles: Guidelines for immediate and delayed provisional restorations. Int J Periodontics Restorative Dent 2020;40:61–70.
61. Huwais S, Meyer EG. A novel osseous densification approach in implant osteotomy preparation to increase biomechanical primary stability, bone mineral density, and bone-to-implant contact. Int J Oral Maxillofac Implants 2017;32:27–36.
62. Vogl S, Stopper M, Hof M, Theisen K, Wegscheider WA, Lorenzoni M. Immediate occlusal vs nonocclusal loading of implants: A randomized prospective clinical pilot study and patient centered outcome after 36 months. Clin Implant Dent Relat Res 2019;21:766–774.
63. Meloni SM, De Riu G, Pisano M, De Riu N, Tullio A. Immediate versus delayed loading of single mandibular molars. One-year results from a randomised controlled trial. Eur J Oral Implantol 2012;5:345–353.
64. Meloni SM, Baldoni E, Duvina M, Pisano M, De Riu G, Tallarico M. Immediate non-occlusal versus delayed loading of mandibular first molars. Five-year results from a randomised controlled trial. Eur J Oral Implantol 2018;11:409–418.
65. Schnitman PA, Wöhrle PS, Rubenstein JE, DaSilva JD, Wang NH. Ten-year results for Brånemark implants immediately loaded with fixed prostheses at implant placement. Int J Oral Maxillofac Implants 1997;12:495–503.
66. Degidi M, Nardi D, Piattelli A. 10-year prospective cohort follow-up of immediately restored XiVE implants. Clin Oral Implants Res 2016;27:694–700.
67. Misch CE, Perel ML, Wang HL, et al. Implant success, survival, and failure: The International Congress of Oral Implantologists (ICOI) Pisa Consensus Conference. Implant Dent 2008;17:5–15.
68. Chen J, Cai M, Yang J, Aldhohrah T, Wang Y. Immediate versus early or conventional loading dental implants with fixed prostheses: A systematic review and meta-analysis of randomized controlled clinical trials. J Prosthet Dent 2019;122:516–536.
69. Del Fabbro M, Testori T, Kekovic V, Goker F, Tumedei M, Wang HL. A systematic review of survival rates of osseointegrated implants in fully and partially edentulous patients following immediate loading. J Clin Med 2019;8:2142.
70. Weerapong K, Sirimongkolwattana S, Sastraruji T, Khongkhunthian P. Comparative study of immediate loading on short dental implants and conventional dental implants in the posterior mandible: A randomized clinical trial. Int J Oral Maxillofac Implants 2019;34:141–149.
71. Renouard F, Nisand D. Impact of implant length and diameter on survival rates. Clin Oral Implants Res 2006;17(suppl 2):35–51.
72. Ketabi M, Deporter D, Atenafu EG. A systematic review of outcomes following immediate molar implant placement based on recently published studies. Clin Implant Dent Relat Res 2016; 18:1084–1094.
73. Hattingh AC, De Bruyn H, Ackermann A, Vandeweghe S. Immediate placement of ultrawide-diameter implants in molar sockets: Description of a recommended technique. Int J Periodontics Restorative Dent 2018;38:17–23.
74. Smith RB, Rawdin SB, Kagan V. Influence of implant-tooth proximity on incidence of caries in teeth adjacent to implants in molar sites: A retrospective radiographic analysis of 300 consecutive implants. Compend Contin Educ Dent 2020;41:e1–e5.
75. Lee CT, Chen YW, Starr JR, Chuang SK. Survival analysis of wide dental implant: Systematic review and meta-analysis. Clin Oral Implants Res 2016;27:1251–1264.
76. Anitua E, Flores C, Flores J, Alkhraisat MH. Clinical effectiveness of 6.5-mm-long implants to support two-implant fixed prostheses in premolar-molar region: The influence of immediate loading and the length of splinting implant. J Prosthodont 2019;28:e688–e693.
77. Kan JYK, Rungcharassaeng K, Deflorian M, Weinstein T, Wang H-L, Testori T. Immediate implant placement and provisionalization of maxillary anterior single implants. Periodontol 2000 2018;77:197–212.
78. Degidi M, Piattelli A, Carinci F. Immediate loaded dental implants: Comparison between fixtures inserted in postextractive and healed bone sites. J Craniofac Surg 2007;18:965–971.
79. Bettach R, Taschieri S, Mortellaro C, Del Fabbro M. Immediate implant placement into fresh extraction sites using single-drilling bur and two loading procedures: Follow-up results. J Craniofac Surg 2018;29:2135–2142.
80. Sennerby L, Meredith N. Implant stability measurements using resonance frequency analysis: Biological and biomechanical aspects and clinical implications. Periodontol 2000 2008;47: 51–66.
81. Bavetta G, Bavetta G, Randazzo V, et al. A retrospective study on insertion torque and implant stability quotient (ISQ) as stability parameters for immediate loading of implants in fresh extraction sockets. Biomed Res Int 2019;2019:9720419.
82. Atieh MA, Alsabeeha NH, Payne AG, de Silva RK, Schwass DS, Duncan WJ. The prognostic accuracy of resonance frequency analysis in predicting failure risk of immediately restored implants. Clin Oral Implants Res 2014;25:29–35.
83. Smith RB, Tarnow DP. Classification of molar extraction sites for immediate dental implant placement: Technical note. Int J Oral Maxillofac Implants 2013;28:911–916.

13

COMMON COMPLICATIONS WITH IMMEDIATE MOLAR IMPLANT PLACEMENT

Stuart J. Froum
Mohammad Ketabi
Tanatorn Asvaplungprohm
Hyongsup Kimm
Yung Cheng Paul Yu
Sang-Choon Cho

Postextraction implant placement can be classified according to the timing of the placement as follows: immediate, early, and delayed placement.[1] A delayed implant placement protocol was utilized in the early 1960s when endosseous root-form threaded implant designs were first introduced by the Brånemark group.[2] This original protocol mandated that implants be placed at least 6 to 12 months postextraction in order to ensure that full socket healing had occurred.[3] Eight-year follow-up using this approach was reported to give cumulative success rates of 99.1% in the mandible and 84.9% in the maxilla. However, waiting this long resulted in extensive biologic bone remodeling and alveolar ridge shrinkage[4] that often necessitated subsequent guided bone regeneration (GBR) before or along with implant placement.[5] As a result, earlier placement protocols were later introduced by the International Team for Implantology (ITI) Consensus Group[1] and classified into two time frames depending on the extent of biologic healing: at 4 to 8 weeks after soft tissue healing or at 12 to 16 weeks with healed soft tissue and significant new bone formation.

In 1989, *immediate implant placement*—referred to as placement on the day of extraction—was first described by Lazzara[6] and later reported by others to result in success rates comparable with those of early and delayed placement.[7] One study using an immediate implant protocol for molar sites reported a 96% survival rate with a sample size of 1,925 implants delivered over the course of a 16-year follow-up period.[8] With its shortened overall treatment time, reduced number of office visits, and comparatively high success rates, immediate implant placement is certain to become more widespread. However, it may be associated with complications, some of which are discussed in this chapter.

Placement of immediate molar implants (IMIs) requires a good working knowledge of anatomy and careful treatment planning, including the use of CBCT radiographs and appropriate computer software (see chapter 2). A

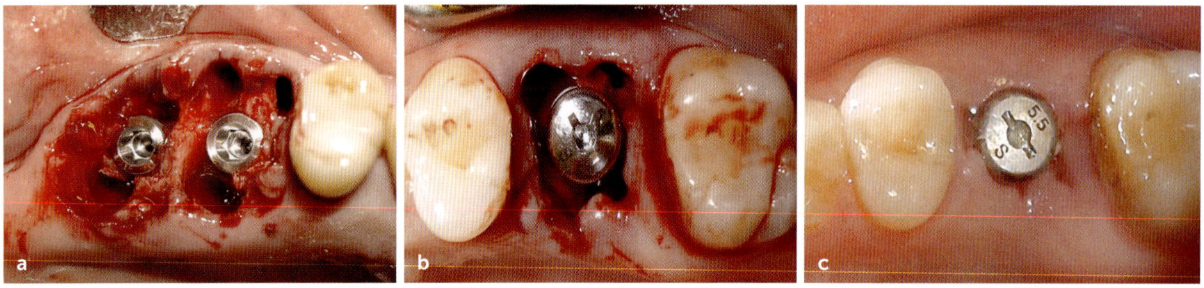

FIG 13-1 *(a)* Both of these IMIs were well positioned within the IRS and stabilized by the remaining bone buttresses. Thick buccal bone and large gaps will lead to optimal site healing without gap grafting. *(b)* This IMI is well positioned centrally, secured by remaining buttresses of the IRS with large buccal gaps that will fill in with new bone without issue. *(c)* Site healing several weeks postimplantation. Note the maintenance of buccal ridge anatomy at this early stage.

favorable outcome is best achieved by adhering to the following principles:

- Determining the amount of interradicular septum (IRS) bone remaining following extraction and whether it will be sufficient to house or at least stabilize an IMI
- Flapless surgery and atraumatic tooth extraction
- Developing the osteotomy in a prosthetically friendly location in all of the mesiodistal, buccolingual/palatal, and coronoapical vectors
- Choosing the appropriate implant diameter
- Achieving good initial implant stability without compromising vital structures, in particular the inferior alveolar nerve bundle and maxillary sinus

Complications may include the following:

- Placing the implant too close to the buccal plate of bone
- Failing to place the implant centrally in the socket
- Overseating the implant
- Leaving inappropriate spaces between the IMI and adjacent teeth or implants
- Having inadequate width and thickness of keratinized tissue to minimize long-term buccal hard and soft tissue recession
- Damaging the sinus or inferior alveolar nerve
- Perforating the lingual plate of bone in mandible
- Failure of regenerative procedures meant to deal with the loss of one or more socket walls

These complications are preventable with proper implant planning and surgical technique.

Complications with Implant Positioning

Malpositioning an IMI too close to the buccal plate

Immediate implant placement requires proper positioning so that the implant is not too close to the buccal plate. For anterior teeth, the implant should be placed at the cingulum for screw-retained restorations or in the incisal area for cemented restorations. For posterior teeth, the implant should be placed in the location of the central fossa for both screw-retained and cemented restorations. Engagement of the implant should be made at the palatal incline of a maxillary anterior tooth socket, at the socket apex for premolars, and in the IRS for molars. Placing molar implants in the IRS will not only result in the most favorable position for the ultimate prosthetic crown, but will also aid in avoiding violation of the mandibular canal.[9] Currently, this is most commonly done by leaving the molar roots in situ until part or all of the osteotomy drilling has been completed.[10,11] To do this, the tooth is first decoronated to expose its furcation. For mandibular molar sites, drilling should then begin centrally but slightly toward the lingual to minimize buccal bur drift; in the maxilla, drilling should start slightly mesiopalatal to the midpoint to avoid distal bur drift. In all cases, the greatest concern should be to avoid any direct contact between implant and buccal bone. Ideally, the implant will be stabilized by contact with what remains of the buccal and linguopalatal buttresses of the prepared IRS, leaving large buccal gaps (≥ 2 mm) in what remains of the root sockets

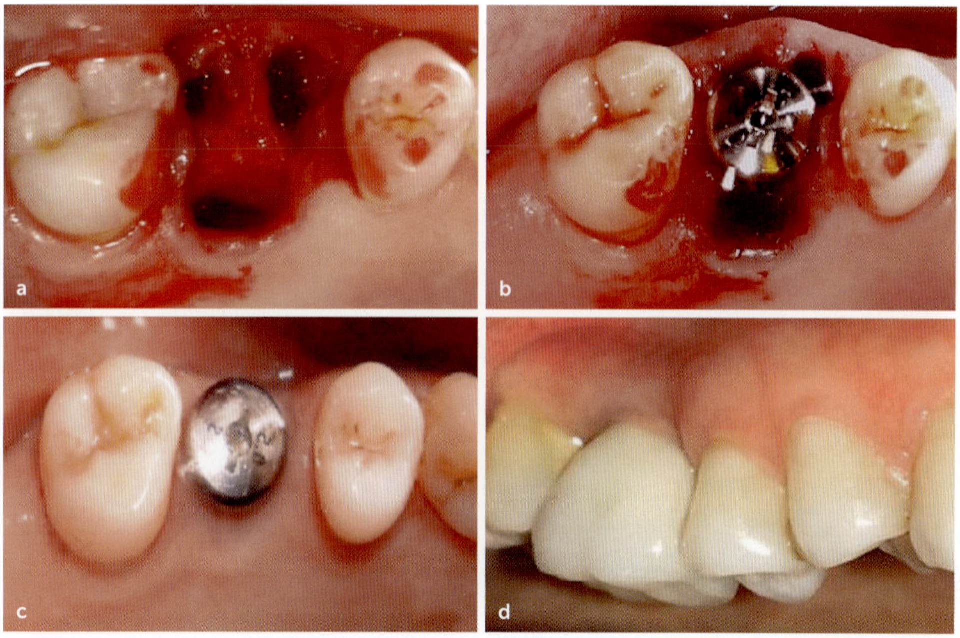

FIG 13-2 *(a)* After extraction of this maxillary first molar, the IRS was seen to be adequate to receive a 6-mm-diameter implant, but the operator developed the osteotomy too far buccally. *(b)* Once inserted, a large gap existed palatally rather than buccally. *(c)* After 3 months of healing, significant buccal bone loss with anatomical collapse can be seen. *(d)* Once restored, a noticeable buccal depression was the outcome, a situation likely to cause further buccal bone loss and soft tissue recession.

(Fig 13-1). These gaps will fill naturally with bone, and provided that the buccal wall itself is reasonably thick (≥ 2 mm), drastic reductions in local anatomy are unlikely to occur.[12–16] If, on the other hand, the buccal plate is thin, the remaining buccal gaps should definitely be grafted with a stable bone substitute such as a xenograft—again to reduce the risk of unfavorable buccal bone remodeling with loss in buccolingual/palatal dimension and subsequent soft tissue recession (Fig 13-2). Hu et al,[17] for example, successfully managed buccal plate dehiscences at IMI sites using flapless surgery and condensing a xenograft (Bio-Oss, Geistlich) into the buccal peri-implant gaps. Alexopoulou et al[18] likewise minimized alveolar ridge shrinkage with IMIs by packing the peri-implant gaps and the overlying intact buccal bone with Bio-Oss and then sheltering the grafted gaps with custom healing abutments.

While an implant with a wider diameter will provide a better prosthetic platform for a molar crown, clinicians should avoid the trap of choosing a diameter so wide that it will obliterate any buccal gaps. As well, should the IMI (regardless of the diameter) inadvertently end up too far buccally, either the procedure should be aborted, or as recommended by Alexopoulou, the buccal plate should be augmented with a xenograft. Provided that the overlying soft tissues are thick and well-keratinized, this augmentation grafting could be as simple as creating a small buccal pouch and inserting xenograft particles.[19,20]

Failing to place the implant centrally in the socket

Locating an IMI centrally in the molar socket in the mesiodistal plane is not quite as crucial as it is in the buccolingual/palatal plane, but it will compromise ideal crown design and size of implant-to-adjacent tooth proximal spaces remaining between the implant and adjacent teeth. The safest way to achieve optimal positioning is to utilize anatomically[10] or computer-guided osteotomy development. Figure 13-3 shows an example where an IMI was placed too far mesially as well as too far buccally.

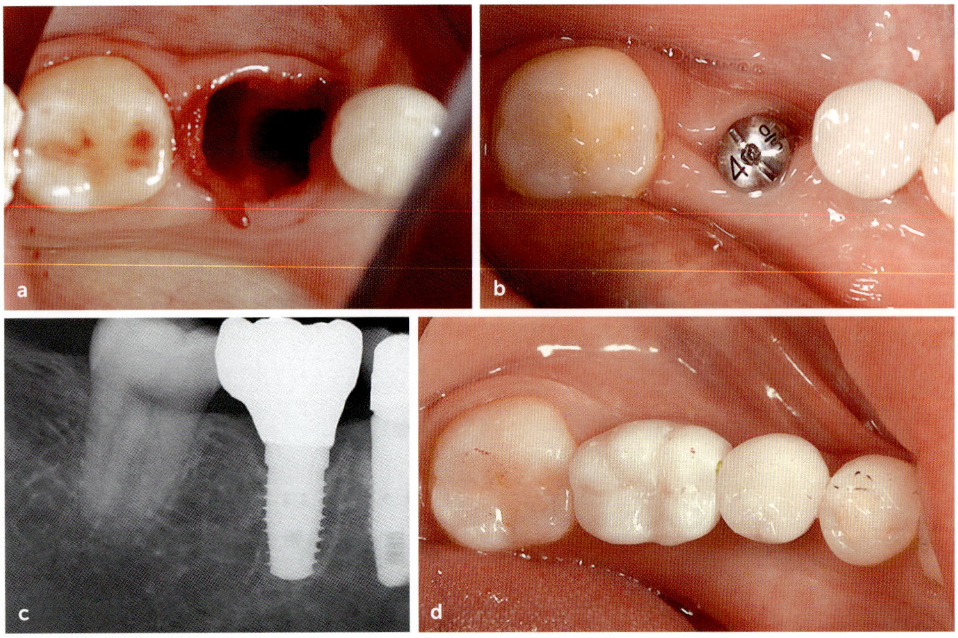

FIG 13-3 *(a)* After atraumatic tooth extraction, the IRS was confirmed to be type C, the most difficult IRS type to manage. *(b)* After osteotomy development, the implant can be seen to have been placed too far mesially and buccally. *(c)* The posttreatment radiograph shows unequal interproximal distances with adjacent teeth. *(d)* Buccal collapse of the hard and soft tissues occurred during site healing, leaving a food trap in the buccal vestibule.

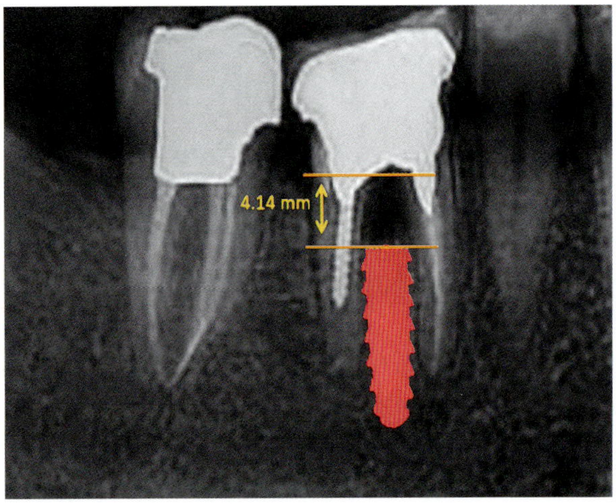

FIG 13-4 If an IMI were to be placed for this periodontally affected first molar, overseating would be the result.

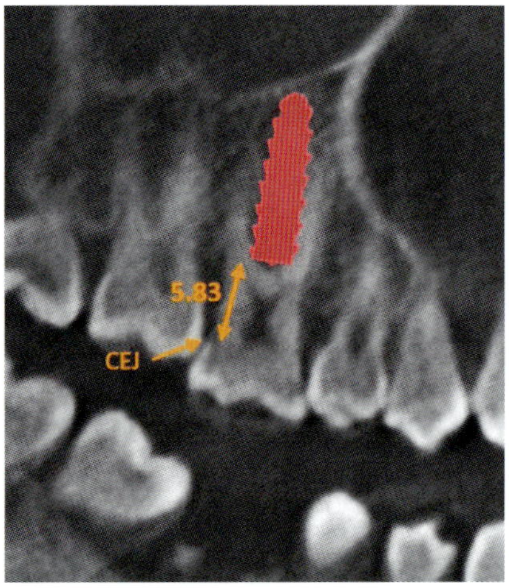

FIG 13-5 The first molar seen here has an excessively long root trunk. If it were to be replaced by an IMI, overseating of the implant could be the result.

Overseating or underseating the implant

Generally, the prosthetic platform of a threaded IMI should be at least 3 to 4 mm apical to the free gingival margin of adjacent teeth. This apicocoronal distance between the platform and the gingival margin is referred to as *running room*.[21] It can be helpful to overseat IMIs by 1 to 2 mm subcrestally in order to ensure sufficient running room to develop a favorable emergence profile for the final molar crown and compensate for any minor crestal bone loss during site

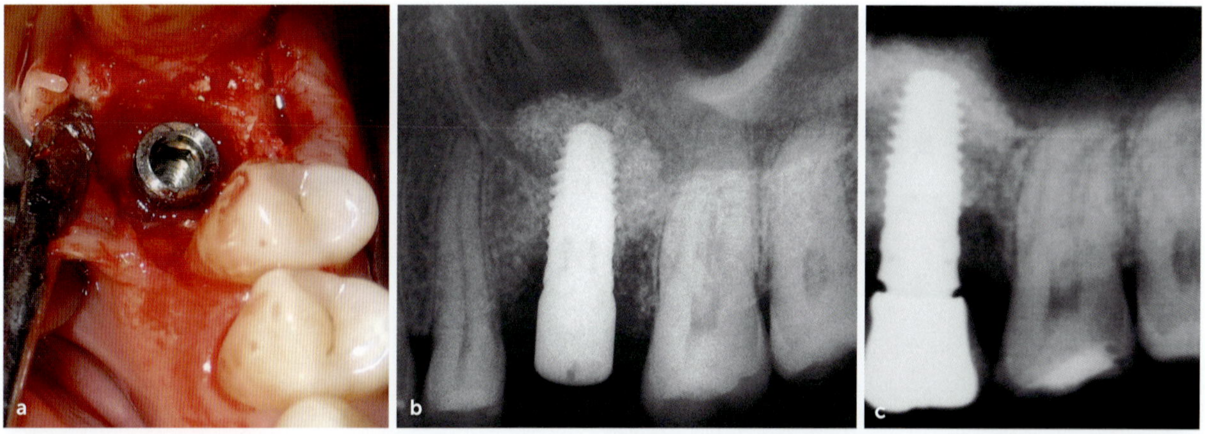

FIG 13-6 *(a)* This molar implant was not submerged 1 to 2 mm subcrestally as recommended. *(b)* The immediate postoperative radiograph. *(c)* After a short period of function, the implant can be seen to have lost significant bone height due to peri-implantitis.

FIG 13-7 A large space was left between this molar implant and its proximal tooth, the result being food retention and root caries.

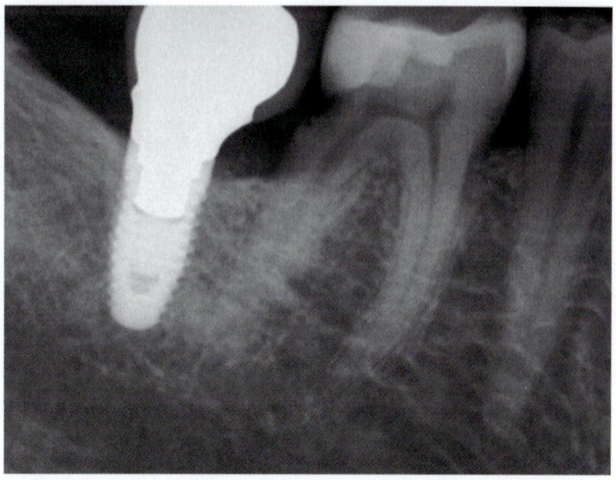

healing.[22] However, excessive overseating can occur if a molar presents with loss in height of the IRS due to periodontal disease (Fig 13-4) or if the tooth has a long root trunk (Fig 13-5). Molar implants placed too deeply can result in excessive running room for the final crowns, leading to inadequate access for daily hygiene and persistent soft tissue inflammation, possibly predisposing the area to mucositis and peri-implantitis. In such situations, rather than placing an IMI, it may be more appropriate to perform a ridge preservation procedure with delayed implant placement.

Too shallow placement of implants, ie, less than 3 mm below the free gingival margin, can lead to implant threads showing after the bone resorption phase of socket healing. A gray hue may show through the gingiva and give an unpleasant esthetic outcome. Underseating also may predispose the patient to peri-implantitis, with threads being exposed following normal crestal bone remodeling (Fig 13-6).

Leaving inappropriate spacing between an IMI and adjacent teeth

Achieving appropriate spacing between an IMI and its adjacent teeth or implants can be challenging. Leaving too little space can have a negative impact on the periodontium of the adjacent tooth. In addition, marginal bone loss around implants has been shown to be significantly greater for implants placed less than 3 mm from the adjacent tooth.[23] On the other hand, leaving too much space between an IMI and its adjacent teeth can predispose these teeth to root caries[24] and result in overhanging restorations in order to close the space (Fig 13-7; see chapter 11). Accidentally or intentionally placing an IMI into one of the tooth's root sockets also will result in inappropriate spacing. Figure 13-8 shows a situation where a failed endodontic treatment had resulted in chronic infection with major damage to the mesial root socket. While placing an IMI in the IRS could have been done

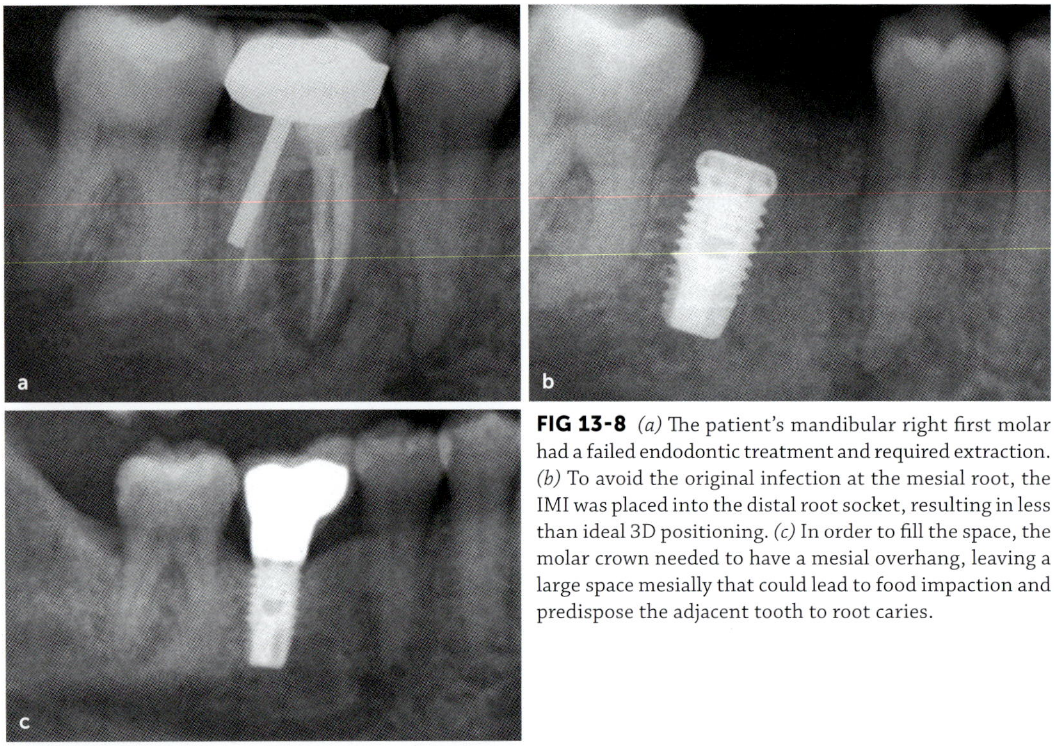

FIG 13-8 *(a)* The patient's mandibular right first molar had a failed endodontic treatment and required extraction. *(b)* To avoid the original infection at the mesial root, the IMI was placed into the distal root socket, resulting in less than ideal 3D positioning. *(c)* In order to fill the space, the molar crown needed to have a mesial overhang, leaving a large space mesially that could lead to food impaction and predispose the adjacent tooth to root caries.

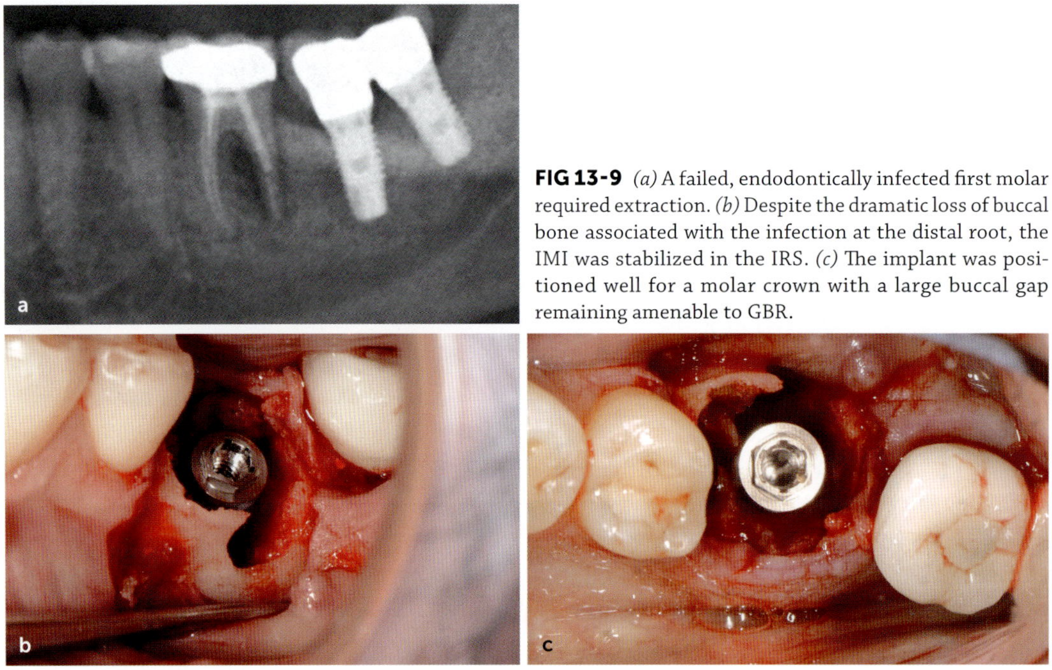

FIG 13-9 *(a)* A failed, endodontically infected first molar required extraction. *(b)* Despite the dramatic loss of buccal bone associated with the infection at the distal root, the IMI was stabilized in the IRS. *(c)* The implant was positioned well for a molar crown with a large buccal gap remaining amenable to GBR.

as long as the infection had been fully debrided, the clinician elected to use the distal root socket instead. As a result, the final crown ended up with a mesial overhang, creating a food trap.

For the most part, existing chronic periapical infection at a potential IMI site should not be an issue (see chapter 5). If a reasonable IRS remains and the infection can be thoroughly debrided, placing the implant in a prosthetically friendly location is preferred. An example is shown in Fig 13-9, where chronic infection had destroyed a major section of the buccal cortical plate of bone, but the implant was stable and GBR successfully undertaken.

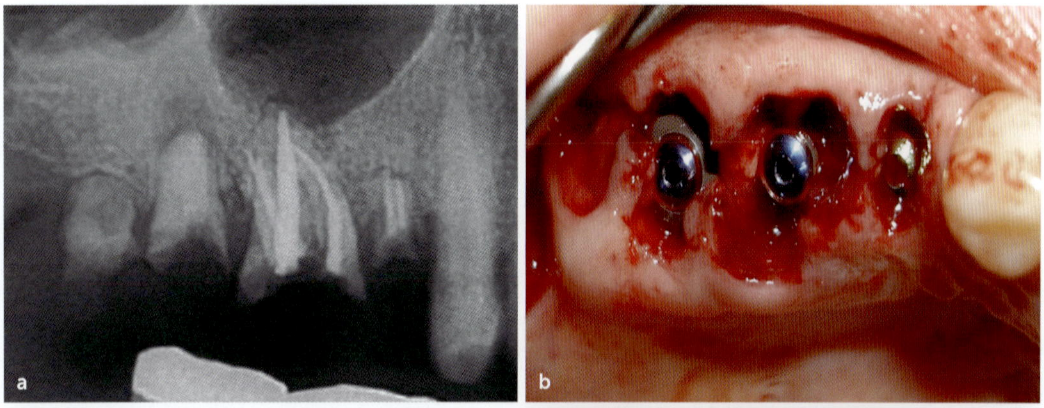

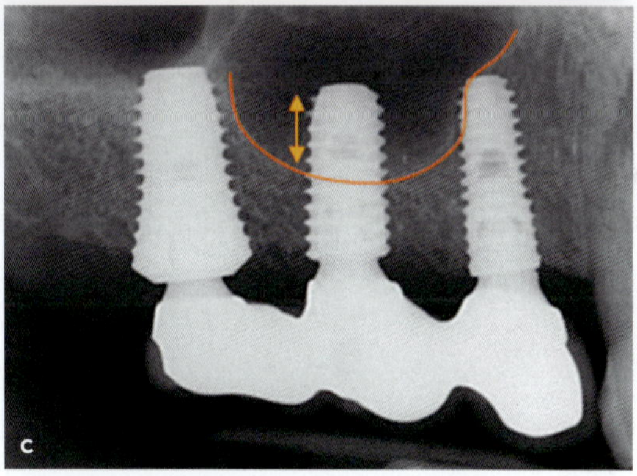

FIG 13-10 *(a)* The patient required extraction of the remaining maxillary posterior tooth fragments. *(b)* Immediate implants were placed in the remaining sockets of the second premolar and both molars. *(c)* The first molar implant, once seated, had half of its length protruding beyond the original sinus floor.

Anatomical Complications

Inadequate width and thickness of keratinized soft tissues

Gingival tissue biotype is moderately related to underlying bone thickness. For example, in the anterior maxilla, studies using CBCT linked thicker biotype with thick underlying bone and thin biotype with thin bone.[25] Moreover, a thick gingival biotype is associated with lower severity of peri-implantitis.[26] Therefore, the ideal site to receive an IMI is one with a thick gingival biotype as this will help in minimizing both hard and soft tissue recession buccally.[27,28] Thick and flat biotype (as opposed to thin or thick and scalloped) also presents with wider bands of keratinized tissue, and this remains a favorable factor in maintaining long-term peri-implant health, with studies showing increased plaque and bleeding scores at implant sites with less than 2 mm of keratinized tissue width.[29]

Sinus issues

In their CBCT radiographic study of maxillary first molars, Matsuda et al[30] estimated the mean distance from molar furcation to sinus floor (ie, IRS) as 6.51 ± 2.94 mm. Therefore, when placing a maxillary IMI into an IRS, it is more likely than not that the sinus floor will be breached. Nevertheless, investigators have confirmed that IMIs can be placed successfully in the IRS along with localized indirect, ie, transcrestal, sinus floor elevation. During the past two decades, we have learned that the sinus is far less of a risk than originally thought when placing maxillary implants. As long as the sinus membrane is minimally damaged and the IMI is adequately stable, breaching the sinus floor during implant insertion appears not to be an issue (Fig 13-10). Ragucci et al[31] undertook a systematic literature review reporting implant penetration into the sinus domain of *(1)* 4 mm or less or *(2)* more than 4 mm. Eight studies reporting 493 such implants

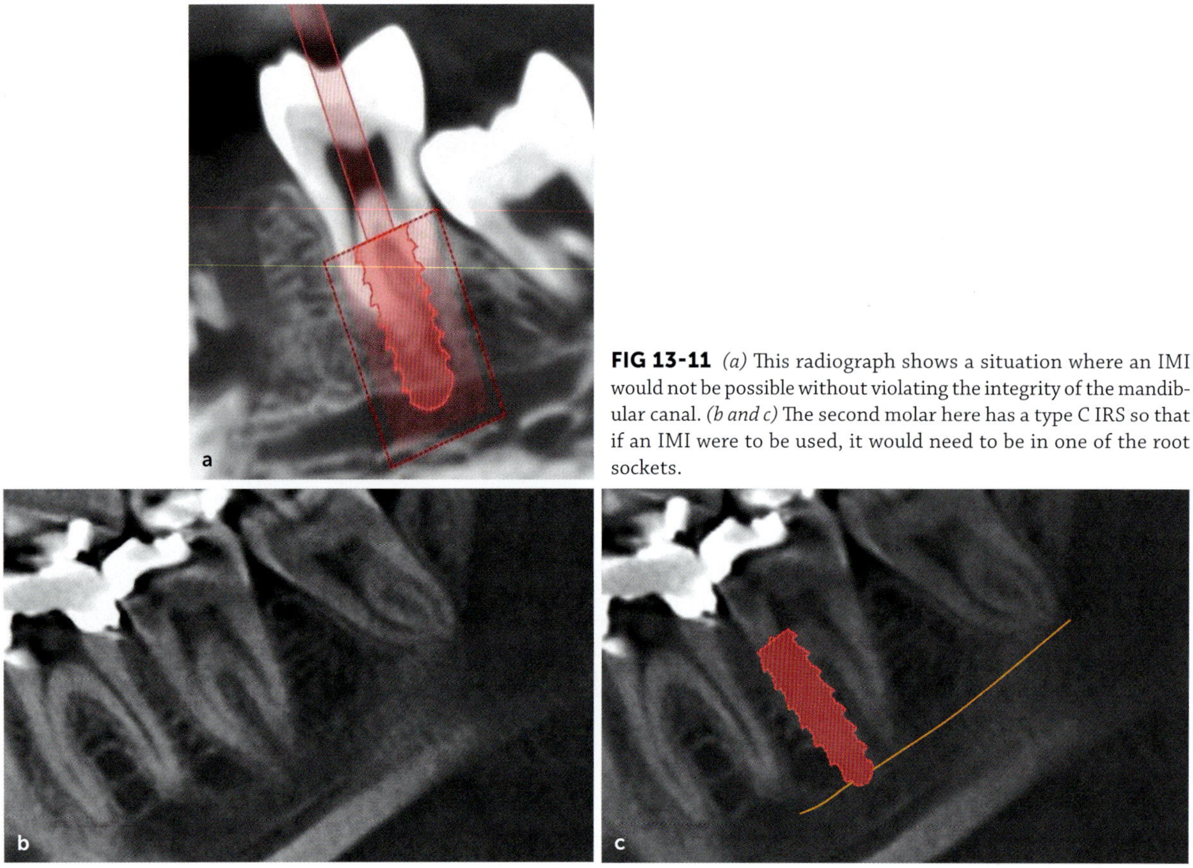

FIG 13-11 *(a)* This radiograph shows a situation where an IMI would not be possible without violating the integrity of the mandibular canal. *(b and c)* The second molar here has a type C IRS so that if an IMI were to be used, it would need to be in one of the root sockets.

provided information on survival rate, the weighted mean being 95.6% after 52.7 months of follow-up. The level of implant penetration (≤ 4 mm or > 4 mm) did not result in significant differences ($P = .403$). Seven studies provided information on the mean rate of clinical complications, which was 3.4%. The most frequent clinical complication was transitory postoperative epistaxis, while the most common radiographic complication was thickening of the sinus membrane, with a weighted mean of 5.29% for sinus penetration of 4 mm or less and 29.3% for penetration greater than 4 mm. Other complications include infection, inadequate primary stability, and (rarely) implant displacement into the sinus cavity.

Precautions that may be taken to avoid sinus complications include using hand osteotomes[32] or specialized burs run in counterclockwise motion[33] to develop the osteotomy and upfracture the sinus floor, together with inserting a bit of collagen sponge or an autologous platelet-rich fibrin clot immediately before inserting the implant.[34] These will serve as a cushion to prevent membrane tear during implant insertion. However, unintentional penetration through the sinus floor is not an infrequent occurrence and appears to have minimal to no untoward effect. Anatomical variations such as antral septa need to be taken into consideration in the planning stage, as close proximity to the developing osteotomy can contribute to higher and larger sinus membrane perforation rates.[35] Prescribing antihistamines and nasal decongestants will rarely be required.

Violating the mandibular canal

The complication of greatest concern is undoubtedly violation of the mandibular canal, but fortunately, this can be avoided by careful study of preoperative CBCT scans. Figure 13-11 shows an example where the risk could be high because of a long root trunk. To avoid the canal, there must be at least 2 mm of intact bone apical to the intended implant apex to avoid temporary or permanent paresthesia resulting from damage from the burs or implant seating.

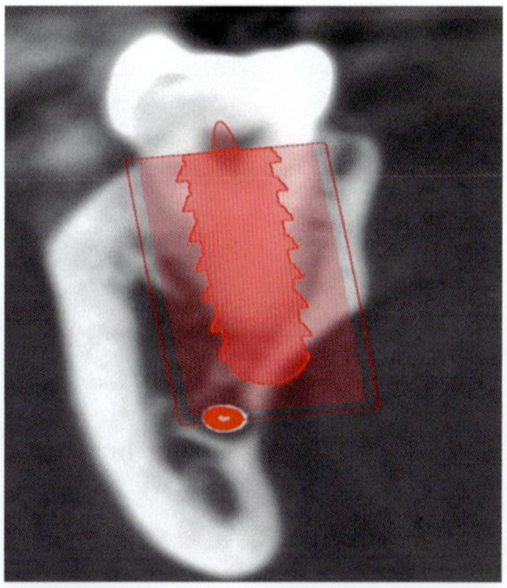

FIG 13-12 Lingual plate perforation in the posterior mandible presents a risk should severe undercuts in ridge shape exist.

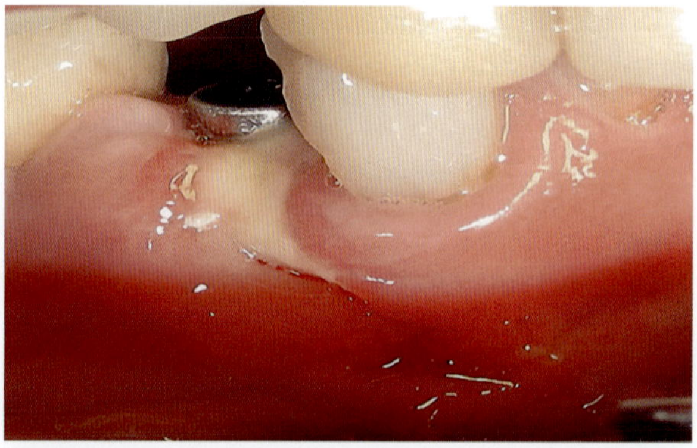

FIG 13-13 Infection after GBR due to membrane exposure.

Procedural Complications

Lingual plate perforation during osteotomy preparation

Avoiding perforation of the mandibular lingual plate of bone is largely preventable if CBCT scans have been obtained as part of treatment planning, as these will allow identification and assessment of lingual undercuts in the mandibular anatomy (Fig 13-12; see chapter 2). Lingual plate perforation can result in life-threatening hemorrhage due to close proximity to major blood vessels such as the lingual and submental arteries. Hemorrhage may result in swelling and airway obstruction. Therefore, in the event of lingual plate perforation resulting in severe bleeding, homeostasis should be attempted via local pressure, and the patient should be transferred to a hospital emergency room.[36] To help in avoiding lingual plate perforation, the surgeon should place a finger against the lingual plate during drilling to be able to sense vibrations related to the drill being too close to the plate. If a minimal plate perforation occurs without signs or symptoms, the implant may be left undisturbed. A computer simulation study using CT scans from 300 patients (1,279 teeth) found a higher frequency of lingual concavities in the mandibular second molar (62.7%) than the first molar (56.2%) or second premolar sites (25.6%).[37]

Complications following GBR at the time of IMI placement

The most predictable approach in using IMIs is to ensure that all four socket walls remain intact after tooth extraction, with most early investigators specifying this as a requirement. However, with experience, clinicians are now prepared to do simultaneous GBR as part of the implant procedure even without raising a mucoperiosteal flap. The original format for GBR was to use a particulate bone substitute material covered by a barrier of some sort, most commonly collagen membranes. However, infection and failure of the grafting were always a risk[38] (Fig 13-13). Most GBR complications come from membrane exposure. For example, 13.8% membrane exposure has been reported to be associated with the use of nonresorbable membranes. Other complications include membrane collapse, soft tissue dehiscence, infection, and bone loss. The complication rate could be as high as 23.6% of GBR cases.[39]

Conclusion

Placing IMIs is a difficult intervention and does come with the risk of complications without careful planning and execution. The most common errors include improper 3D positioning, inadequate initial stability, damage of vital anatomical structures, and early infection.

KEY POINTS

- The most common error or complication with the use of immediate molar implants is malpositioning of the implant too far buccally or not placing it centrally in the mesiodistal dimension. Delaying tooth root removal until after osteotomy creation will allow anatomically guided placement into the IRS.
- The optimal distance between an IMI and its adjacent tooth or teeth is 2 to 4 mm; otherwise, root caries risk can be a complication.
- Overseating IMIs is a risk for molars with long root trunks or furcal bone loss. Ideally, threaded implants should be placed subcrestally but only by 1 to 2 mm relative to the lowest bone crest buccally.
- Lingual plate perforation can occur with placement of mandibular IMIs, but this can be avoided by examining pretreatment CBCTs.
- Sinus violation is always a risk with reduced subantral bone height, intrusion of maxillary molar roots into the sinus, or where the distances for root apices to sinus floor are < 5 mm. Inadvertent sinus floor perforation is frequent but generally of no clinical significance.
- Soft and hard tissue collapse over time, particularly on the buccal aspect, can be minimized by correct 3D implant positioning and, if necessary, buccal onlay grafting of particulate xenograft and/or soft tissue grafting should the site have a thin buccal plate (≤ 1.5 mm) and/or thin gingival biotype.

References

1. Chen ST, Buser D. Clinical and esthetic outcomes of implants placed in postextraction sites. Int J Oral Maxillofac Implants 2009;24(suppl):186–217.
2. Adell R, Lekholm U, Rockler B, Brånemark PI. A 15-year study of osseointegrated implants in the treatment of the edentulous jaw. Int J Oral Surg 1981;10:387–416.
3. Albrektsson T, Dahl E, Enbom L, et al. Osseointegrated oral implants. A Swedish multicenter study of 8139 consecutively inserted Nobelpharma implants. J Periodontol 1988;59:287–296.
4. Schropp L, Wenzel A, Kostopoulos L, Karring T. Bone healing and soft tissue contour changes following single-tooth extraction: A clinical and radiographic 12-month prospective study. Int J Periodontics Restorative Dent 2003;23:313–323.
5. Zitzmann NU, Schärer P, Marinello CP. Factors influencing the success of GBR. Smoking, timing of implant placement, implant location, bone quality and provisional restoration. J Clin Periodontol 1999;26:673–682.
6. Lazzara RJ. Immediate implant placement into extraction sites: Surgical and restorative advantages. Int J Periodontics Restorative Dent 1989;9:332–343.
7. Schwartz-Arad D, Chaushu G. The ways and wherefores of immediate placement of implants into fresh extraction sites: A literature review. J Periodontol 1997;68:915–923.
8. Wagenberg B, Froum SJ. A retrospective study of 1925 consecutively placed immediate implants from 1988 to 2004. Int J Oral Maxillofac Implants 2006;21:71–80.
9. Froum S, Casanova L, Byrne S, et al. Risk assessment before extraction for immediate implant placement in the posterior mandible: A computerized tomographic scan study. J Periodontol 2011;82:395–402.
10. Rodriguez-Tizcareño MH, Bravo-Flores C. Anatomically guided implant site preparation technique at molar sites. Implant Dent 2009;18:393–401.

11. Scarano A. Traditional postextractive implant site preparation compared with pre-extractive interradicular implant bed preparation in the mandibular molar region, using an ultrasonic device: A randomized pilot study. Int J Oral Maxillofac Implants 2017;32:655–660.
12. Smith RB, Tarnow DP, Sarnachiaro G. Immediate placement of dental implants in molar extraction sockets: An 11-year retrospective analysis. Compend Contin Educ Dent 2019;40:166–170.
13. Deporter D, Khoshkhounejad AA, Khoshkhounejad N, Ketabi M. A new classification of peri implant gaps based on gap location (a case series of 210 immediate implants). Dent Res J (Isfahan) 2021;18:29.
14. Spray JR, Black CG, Morris HF, Ochi S. The influence of bone thickness on facial marginal bone response: Stage 1 placement through stage 2 uncovering. Ann Periodontol 2000;5:119–128.
15. Qahash M, Susin C, Polimeni G, Hall J, Wikesjö UM. Bone healing dynamics at buccal peri-implant sites. Clin Oral Implants Res 2008;19:166–172.
16. Monje A, Chappuis V, Monje F, et al. The critical peri-implant buccal bone wall thickness revisited: An experimental study in the beagle dog. Int J Oral Maxillofac Implants 2019;34:1328–1336.
17. Hu C, Gong T, Lin W, Yuan Q, Man Y. Immediate implant placement into posterior sockets with or without buccal bone dehiscence defects: A retrospective cohort study. J Dent 2017;65:95–100.
18. Alexopoulou M, Lambert F, Knafo B, Popelut A, Vandenberghe B, Finelle G. Immediate implant in the posterior region combined with alveolar ridge preservation and sealing socket abutment: A retrospective 3D radiographic analysis. Clin Implant Dent Relat Res 2021;23:61–72.
19. Brugnami F, Caiazzo A. Efficacy evaluation of a new buccal bone plate preservation technique: A pilot study. Int J Periodontics Restorative Dent 2011;31:67–73.
20. Birang E, Deporter D, Birang R, Mahabadi M, Atenafu E, Ketabi M. Effectiveness of buccal pouch grafting in minimizing loss of alveolar dimension: A canine investigation. Dent Res J (Isfahan) 2019;16:338–345.
21. Zamzok J. Nonsurgical soft tissue sculpting. Alpha Omegan 1997;90:65–69.
22. Smith RB, Tarnow DP. Classification of molar extraction sites for immediate dental implant placement: Technical note. Int J Oral Maxillofac Implants 2013;28:911–916.
23. Esposito M, Ekestubbe A, Gröndahl K. Radiological evaluation of marginal bone loss at tooth surfaces facing single Brånemark implants. Clin Oral Implants Res 1993;4:151–157.
24. Smith RB, Rawdin SB, Kagan V. Influence of implant-tooth proximity on incidence of caries in teeth adjacent to implants in molar sites: A retrospective radiographic analysis of 300 consecutive implants. Compend Contin Educ Dent 2020;41:e1–e5.
25. Fu JH, Yeh CY, Chan HL, Tatarakis N, Leong DJ, Wang HL. Tissue biotype and its relation to the underlying bone morphology. J Periodontol 2010;81:569–574.
26. Isler SC, Uraz A, Kaymaz O, Cetiner D. An evaluation of the relationship between peri-implant soft tissue biotype and the severity of peri-implantitis: A cross-sectional study. Int J Oral Maxillofac Implants 2019;34:187–196.
27. Linkevicius T, Apse P, Grybauskas S, Puisys A. The influence of soft tissue thickness on crestal bone changes around implants: A 1-year prospective controlled clinical trial. Int J Oral Maxillofac Implants 2009;24:712–719.
28. Schrott AR, Jimenez M, Hwang JW, Fiorellini J, Weber HP. Five-year evaluation of the influence of keratinized mucosa on peri-implant soft-tissue health and stability around implants supporting full-arch mandibular fixed prostheses. Clin Oral Implants Res 2009;20:1170–1177.
29. Wennström JL, Derks J. Is there a need for keratinized mucosa around implants to maintain health and tissue stability? Clin Oral Implants Res 2012;23(suppl 6):136–146.
30. Matsuda H, Borzabadi-Farahani A, Le BT. Three-dimensional alveolar bone anatomy of the maxillary first molars: A cone-beam computed tomography study with implications for immediate implant placement. Implant Dent 2016;25:367–372.
31. Ragucci GM, Elnayef B, Criado-Cámara E, Del Amo FS, Hernández-Alfaro F. Immediate implant placement in molar extraction sockets: A systematic review and meta analysis. Int J Implant Dent 2020;6:40.
32. Bruschi GB, Crespi R, Capparè P, Bravi F, Bruschi E, Gherlone E. Localized management of sinus floor technique for implant placement in fresh molar sockets. Clin Implant Dent Relat Res 2013;15:243–250.
33. Huwais S, Mazor Z, Ioannou AL, Gluckman H, Neiva R. A multicenter retrospective clinical study with up-to-5-year follow-up utilizing a method that enhances bone density and allows for transcrestal sinus augmentation through compaction grafting. Int J Oral Maxillofac Implants 2018;33:1305–1311.
34. Toffler M, Rosen P. Complications with transcrestal sinus floor elevation: Etiology, prevention, and treatment. In: Froum S (ed). Dental Implant Complications: Etiology, Prevention, and Treatment. Hoboken: John Wiley & Sons, 2016:428–455.
35. Reiser GM, Rabinovitz Z, Bruno J, Damoulis PD, Griffin TJ. Evaluation of maxillary sinus membrane response following elevation with the crestal osteotome technique in human cadavers. Int J Oral Maxillofac Implants 2001;16:833–840.
36. Mardinger O, Manor Y, Mijiritsky E, Hirshberg A. Lingual perimandibular vessels associated with life-threatening bleeding: An anatomic study. Int J Oral Maxillofac Implants 2007;22:127–131.
37. Huang RY, Cochran DL, Cheng WC, et al. Risk of lingual plate perforation for virtual immediate implant placement in the posterior mandible: A computer simulation study. J Am Dent Assoc 2015;146:735–742.
38. Urban T, Kostopoulos L, Wenzel A. Immediate implant placement in molar regions: A 12-month prospective, randomized follow-up study. Clin Oral Implants Res 2012;23:1389–1397.
39. Jensen SS, Terheyden H. Bone augmentation procedures in localized defects in the alveolar ridge: Clinical results with different bone grafts and bone-substitute materials. Int J Oral Maxillofac Implants 2009;24(suppl):218–236.

INDEX

Page references followed by "f" denote figures; "b" denote boxes; and "t" denote tables.

D

E

F

G

H

I

J

L

M

O

P

R

S

T

U

V

W

Z